D1715062

Hispanic Foodways, Nutrition, and Health

Diva Sanjur

Division of Nutritional Sciences

Cornell University

Allyn and Bacon

Boston London Toronto Sydney Tokyo Singapore

Printed in the United States of America
10 9 8 7 6 5 4 3 2 1   99 98 97 96 95 94

To Malden   . . . for his unfailing support and confidence in
me. . . .

and

A David y Robertito

. . . mis "Hispanos" favoritos, frutos del bicul-
turalismo, mi familia amorosa . . .

Contents

Foreword

The nutritional practices of populations and communities are important components of public health. Approaches to reducing mortality and morbidity from heart disease have identified factors that are associated with greater risk of these diseases in populations and individuals. A number of these risk factors are associated with dietary practices, and changes in food habits are often part of public health programs aimed at reducing disease risk.

Because dietary habits are determined by complex factors, often firmly rooted in cultural practices, an understanding of culturally related factors is essential for those designing and carrying out community nutrition programs. This text by Diva Sanjur provides such a background for work among the diverse populations of Hispanic origin found in the United States. It is based on research carried out in Hispanic communities over a lifetime by Dr. Sanjur. No other individual has done such extensive and varied community studies on food practices of various Hispanic populations, both in the United States and in those parts of the world from which most immigrants to the United States have come. The material in the chapters that follow provides background essential for community workers to understand the nature of the U.S. Hispanic community and the dietary practices, health problems, and intervention strategies of importance.

The food practices of the principal Hispanic groups are covered in considerable detail in this book. Of special interest and value are the dictionaries and glossaries that identify foods and their basic ingredients. This information is essential for assessment and evaluation of nutrient intake, and this book draws together a unique set of information not readily available elsewhere. Furthermore, the special health problems found in Hispanic communities are assessed in the book with the use of newly analyzed data from the Hispanic Health and Nutrition Examination Survey carried out in 1983–84. This information should also be of interest to those concerned with public health programs.

The book has practical information relative to nutrition counseling and nutrition education programs, particularly as applied to Hispanic populations. Collection and analysis of food consumption data are also considered.

Such information should be of particular interest to those involved in assessing food practices in communities.

I believe this is a book long overdue that can facilitate nutrition programs in Hispanic communities. I am pleased to commend it to you.

M. C. Nesheim
Professor, Nutritional Sciences
Cornell University

Preface

Nutritionists and other health professionals are often called on for advice for improving diets. More and more the advice is intended for people who come to the United States from other cultures. The effect of culture on diet is undeniably strong. Although the intent of any advice may be worthy, if it is not based on a firm cultural understanding, the information offered will be ineffective or ignored. While being sensitive to the cultural backgrounds of clients, nutritionists also need to be sure that the advice offered is not only practical but also culturally relevant by incorporating traditional foods and celebrating inherent diversity.

Although cultural diversity is a reality in the United States, there is disagreement on how best to meet the needs of multicultural clients. Some believe that existing counseling strategies are effective for all people and that trying to categorize the traits of different subcultural groups only perpetuates stereotypes. Others believe that existing couseling models, based on dominant middle-class cultural values, are ineffective with people from other cultures.

This book reviews sociodemographic data concerning Hispanics in the United States, their migration patterns, and their economic, health, and nutritional situations. Although the book uses the term *Hispanic* as a generic category, this author acknowledges that there are a great many differences among Hispanic subgroups. Nevertheless, the central intent of the book is to examine the many similarities and parallels among the various Hispanic/Latino groups relative to their food and nutrition situation, in order to provide a more meaningful context for program planners and practitioners to implement action.

Though many other books have examined the dynamic effects of racial, sociopolitical, and economic barriers on Hispanics in the United States, Hispanic foodways, nutrition, and health have generally been neglected. The subjects of diet, nutrition, and health were particularly chosen as the thrust of this book because this author feels they are a crucial piece of the present and future Hispanic health experience in the United States.

This book relies on a combination of national data, quasi-experimental field studies, and qualitative research throughout. Chapter 1 profiles the major Hispanic groups and their migration history, and Chapter 2 discusses the persistence of ethnic effects on food habits and the role of women in nutrition. Chapters 3, 4, and 5 detail dietary strengths and weaknesses among various Hispanic/Latino groups: Mexican-Americans, Puerto Ricans, Dominicans, Cubans, Central Americans.

In Chapters 6 and 7, diet-related diseases and obesity and overweight are identified as current problems among certain segments of the Hispanic population. A discussion of the U.S. Dietary Guidelines and their application to Hispanic diets is presented in Chapter 8. Chapter 9 details how to reach Hispanics through diet counseling and nutrition education. Finally, Chapter 10 provides useful techniques and approaches for assessing food intake among Hispanics. This chapter also makes a case for the critical need to create a National Nutrient Data Bank in order to analyze Hispanic diets. Unless this need is met, the author argues that there will continue to be serious questions about the validity of existing Hispanic nutrient intake data.

This book is directed toward teachers and students who have limited familiarity and understanding of Hispanic food traditions and their nutritional consequences in the United States. As a textbook or as supplementary reading, this book should be a valuable reference for health practitioners engaged in clinical nutrition, nutrition counseling, diet surveys, nutrition education, cultural foodways, or international nutrition.

This book may also be useful to nutrition planners and policymakers, as well as others working with or concerned with U.S. Hispanics and other urban Latino populations, because it describes and analyzes socioeconomic profiles, health behaviors, food ideologies, attitudes, and nutrition situations.

Finally, this book could be of interest to those who want to improve the quality of life in the United States, for in many ways, this book is as much about the United States as a multicultural society as it is about the foodways, nutrition, and health of Hispanic migrants in America.

ACKNOWLEDGMENTS

This book represents an extension of research work and field experience developed over a 20-year period at Cornell University. The contributions of many of my graduate students, friends, and colleagues are hereby acknowledged. Most importantly, I thank the contributing authors who wrote the guest chapters and those who assisted them.

Special thanks are extended to the many Hispanic women who inspired me and assisted me, serving as subjects in our studies. Their cooperation and friendliness still warm the memory.

It is impossible to name all those others who have contributed in some manner to this book. Those who prepared specific material are cited at appropriate points in the book. To all others—those who provided information, illustrations, or services and who critized or encouraged me when I needed it most—I am content to say a grateful "Thank you." May you feel rewarded by the gratitude of all those who find this book useful.

Diva Sanjur
Cornell University

1

Hispanic Migrants in a Nation of Immigrants

Hispanic Migrants: Strangers, Neighbors, Friends
The Pains of Acculturation: Old Issues, New Questions
America: A Multicultural Nation
Ethnocentric Labeling and Fear of Difference

Identifying the Hispanic Population
Who Is Hispanic?
Hispanics and U.S. Census Classification
Beyond the Census Classification: The Hispanic
Self-Perception
How Many Hispanics? Where?

The Process of Migration
The "Push and Pull" Theory
Motives for Migrating
Migration as a Stepwise Process
Women as a Significant Segment of the Migrant Population

Migration History of Hispanics
Mexican Immigration
Dominican Immigration
Cuban Immigration
Puerto Rican Immigration

Hispanic Migrant Agricultural Workers
Migrant Agricultural Labor in California
Migrant Agricultural Contract Workers from Puerto Rico
Migrant Agricultural Workers in the Midwest

Hispanic Demographic Trends in the 1990s

1

HISPANIC MIGRANTS: STRANGERS, NEIGHBORS, FRIENDS

The Pains of Acculturation: Old Issues, New Questions

Oscar Handlin, in his Pulitzer Prize winning book remarks:

> Once I thought I would write a history of the immigrants in America—then I discovered that the immigrants WERE American history. . . .[1]

Handlin's observations echo those made a decade later by Father Greely, who pointed out the pains and dilemmas faced by immigrant groups in America.[2] Father Greely's observations remain as timely today as they were in 1969, when he published Why Can't They Be Like Us?, in which he reminded us that peoples, as well as states, have been both the glory of the American republic and its torment—and that "from many, we became one. . . ."

Early in its history, the New World offered its bounty to the curious, the lucky, and the brave, whatever their social status or nationality. But the freedom and diversity that a nation of minorities and newcomers encourages can inflict hardship and torment on individuals and generate stress and tension for societal and public institutions.[3] The traditions of family and group do not reinforce, naturally or easily, the substance of government. Frequently, one set of traditions works against the other; for example, schools are charged with the task of "Americanization," while the family reinforces former loyalties and traditions.[4]

Americans today remain simultaneously *alike* and *different* in details of their behavioral patterns, lifestyles, and food habits. Even though the concept of the "melting pot" has lost its scholarly respectability, ethnic influences are still a latent but powerful force in American society. The melting pot notion is essentially a *political* one, designed to define citizenship, but citizenship alone does not resolve the conflicts endemic in a nation of ethnics. Sadly enough, the rich cultural influences and positive social and cultural contributions (family cohesiveness, group solidarity, family networks, and social supports) by past generations of immigrants of all ethnic backgrounds have been lost or grossly neglected in the analyses of America as a multicultural nation.

An increasing dependence on one another for many necessities of life, including food, poses the challenge to understand ethnic relations and meet basic human needs with enthusiasm and vigor.

This author, echoing Todhunter, feels that "history gives meaning to the present. . . ."[5] In order for students, scholars, and practitioners of nutrition and health to be effective, they must become familiar with the historical background of the groups they are working with. Hispanic nutrition and health cannot be fully understood unless viewed within the context of the Hispanic migration experience in America.

This chapter first examines issues concerning Hispanic migration, including the pains and dilemmas of acculturation in a nation of ethnics, as well as the difficulties faced by the U.S. Census in classifying "Hispanics." Perspectives on Hispanics' self-perception are provided by two Latino scholars, along with a historical account of Latin Americans' search for identity. The second part of the chapter describes patterns of settlement of specific Hispanic groups. Finally, U.S.-Hispanic demographic trends in the 1990s are discussed.

This chapter is intended to bridge the large gap in understanding the foodways, nutritional and health adaptations, coping strategies, and survival efforts of a significant segment of the urban American population. Continuity and change in migrants' dietary patterns are one of the many stresses that migrants face as they acculturate and adapt to new environments.

This migration perspective is meant to enhance understanding of the variations, as well as the similarities, among Hispanic migrants. It is hoped that this will contribute to the development of more effective nutritional and health intervention programs at various levels.

America: A Multicultural Nation

The formation of a nation on the North American continent made up of widely different nationalities may amaze social historians of the twenty-third or twenty-fourth century. They will find it hard to believe, notes Greely,[6] how it could have happened that in America, the English, Scots, Danes, Welsh, Irish, Germans, Africans, French, Italians, Finns, Spaniards, Swedes, Lebanese, Armenians, Greeks, Poles, Chinese, Japanese, Indians, Portuguese, Filipinos, and Puerto Ricans all came together to form a nation that not only survived but, all things considered, survived reasonably well.

Historians have documented European immigration and ethnic history for the earlier part of the twentieth century. However, much remains to be analyzed about the newer surge of immigrants and refugees who arrived in America, especially for those who came after 1960. Mohl notes that in many ways the immigration of the past few decades has reshaped some of the major metropolitan areas of the Unites States.[7] In 1983, for instance, the Los Angeles metropolitan area was home not only to more than 2 million Mexicans and Mexican-Americans but also to some 200,000 Iranians, 200,000 Salvadorans, 175,000 Japanese, 150,000 Chinese, 150,000 Koreans, 150,000 Filipinos, 130,000 Arabs, and to smaller concentrations of Israelis, Colombians, Hondurans, Guatemalans, Cubans, Vietnamese, East Indians, Pakistanis, and Samoans and other Pacific Islanders.

Similarly, Mohl reports that New York City has become a magnet for Asian, Caribbean, Hispanic, and other new immigrant and refugee groups. Large concentrations of Haitians, Dominicans, Colombians, and West Indians have created new ethnic neighborhoods in areas formerly populated by Italians, Jews, Germans, Scandinavians, and Irish. The *New York Times* observed on May 6, 1991, "Immigrants are coming to New York City from virtually every country, island and territory on the globe, creating a city more diverse in race, language and ethnicity than it was at the turn of the century when immigrants from Europe poured through Ellis Island. . . ." Ambition, hope, courage, and differential economic opportunities are some of the major motivations that cause people to move voluntarily from their native land to new and strange areas.

Ethnocentric Labeling and Fear of Difference

The Judeo-Christian tradition counsels people "to love thy neighbor as thyself." However, Senior notes that this is more likely to happen if the newcomer belongs to the same racial, ethnic, or nationality group, church, union, and/or socioeconomic class.[8] When individuals come from different ethnic, racial, nationality, religious, or class group, they may have habits, feelings, ideas, and ideals that do not coincide. Unless strangers can establish some common ideas and feelings to which they both owe allegiance, a neighborly, friendly life will be difficult.

In the strangeness of the new environment, immigrants seek people with whom they have something in common. "Their kind of people" can be trusted to offer help in the difficult adjustment to the new social setting. As Greely points out, in the Italian neighborhoods of New York's Lower East Side in the early 1920s, it was possible to trace, block by block, not only the region in Italy but also the very villages from which the inhabitants had come.[9] The ethnic group provided a "pool of preferred associates" for the more intimate dimensions of life. When it came to choosing a spouse, a doctor, a lawyer, or a construction contractor, a person was likely to feel much more at ease if she or he could choose "my kind of people."

To one degree or another, all newcomers to America have faced two universal social phenomena: ethnocentric labeling and fear of difference. "Sticks and stones may break my bones, but names will never hurt me" is a rhyme recited by children in self-defense. However, Senior argues that names *do* hurt, particularly when they injure the self-esteem of members of a minority group who are already struggling to make their way in the new world.[10]

The other social phenomenon, fear of difference, has sometimes emerged and focused on one ethnic or racial group. It is an irrational fear that afflicts communities as well as individuals, and it becomes more menacing as rapid transportation brings the peoples of the world closer together physically. Both ethnocentrism and fear of difference are *negative* behaviors that undermine democratic ideals. Ethnocentrism and fear of difference must be eliminated in order to establish friendly, neighborly relations in a nation of immigrants.

IDENTIFYING THE HISPANIC POPULATION

Who Is Hispanic?

Hispanic Americans, who may be of any race, generally are defined as those who share a Spanish-language heritage and trace their roots to the Spanish-speaking countries of Central and South America, Puerto Rico, the Dominican Republic, Cuba, and Mexico.[11] *Webster's New International Dictionary* (2nd ed., unabridged, 1971) defines Hispanic as "pertaining to or deriving from the people, speech, or culture of Spain or of Spain or Portugal; often specifically Latin America." Thus there are substantial variations in the racial composition of the individual Hispanic groups.

Hispanics can be correctly classified as white, black, American Indian, or Asian. In the 1980 census, 55.6% of self-identified Hispanics reported their race as white, 2.7% as black, 0.6% as American Indian, Eskimo, or Aleut, 1.1% as Asian or Pacific Islander, and 40% as "other."

With respect to the appropriate terminology, Hispanics have given a lot of thought to what they want to be called. Latino, Chicano, Mexican-American, Mexican, Boricua, Raza, Latin American, Spanish-American, Hispanic American, *Hispano,* and Hispanic have been some of the proposed choices. *Hispanic,* though not perfect, has widespread acceptance among both Hispanics and non-Hispanics and seems to be better understood than some other terms. In addition, the scientific literature as well as the news media accept the term. *Latino* is perhaps the second most preferred term, but some consider it a regionalism most often used in the state of California and thus not as widely accepted as Hispanic.

Hispanics and U.S. Census Classification

Historically, the U.S. Census has had difficulty with the racial classification of Hispanics, and there has been continuing debate over how to count Hispanics. According to Rodríguez, in 1930, "Hispanics/Latinos" were included in the census as a racial category.[12] In 1950 and 1960 they surfaced as "Persons of Spanish Mother Tongue." In 1970 they were "Persons of Spanish Surname and Spanish Mother Tongue." By 1980, Hispanics had lobbied for a new question to be included in the 100% count of the decennial census. In the 1970 census, a similar question had been asked, but only on the 5% sample form. This question asked specifically whether a person was "Hispanic" or of "Spanish origin or descent" and allowed individuals to specify whether they were Mexican, Puerto Rican, Cuban, or other Spanish/Hispanic.

McKenney et al. point out that the U.S. Census provides the most complete statistical picture of the diverse population groups in our society.[13] For the 1990 census, answers to each of the three questions on race, Spanish/Hispanic origin, and ancestry depended on self-identification, an individual's perception of his or her racial/ethnic identity. Figure 1.1 shows the 1990 census Hispanic question and the instructions to respondents. With respect to why the dual terminology of "Hispanic" or "Spanish" was used in the census, McKenney explains that pretesting showed that both terms were needed to get the most complete answer to any Hispanic question. For instance, some younger Hispanic people believe that "Spanish" refers only to persons from Spain, whereas other persons interpret "Hispanic" as having that meaning.

FIGURE 1.1   Spanish/Hispanic origin: Recommended 1990 question

7. Is this person of Spanish/Hispanic
   origin?   o No, (not Spanish/Hispanic)
   Fill ONE circle for person   o Yes, Mexican, Mexican-American, Chicano
                                              o Yes, Puerto Rican
                                              o Yes, Cuban
                                              o Yes, other Spanish/Hispanic (Print one
                                                 group, for example: Argentinian,
                                                 Colombian, Dominican, Nicaraguan,
                                                 Salvadoran, Spaniard, and so on.)

   If Yes, other Spanish/Hispanic,   _____
   print one group ————————>   _____

Instructions to Respondents—Hispanic Question

7. A person is of Spanish/Hispanic origin if the person's origin (ancestry) is Mexican,
   Mexican-American, Chicano, Puerto Rican, Cuban, Argentinian, Colombian, Costa
   Rican, Dominican, Ecuadoran, Guatemalan, Honduran, Nicaraguan, Peruvian,
   Salvadoran; from other Spanish-speaking countries of the Caribbean or Central or
   South America; or from Spain.

   If you fill the <u>Yes,</u> other Spanish/Hispanic circle, print one group.

   A person who is not of Spanish/Hispanic origin should answer this question by
   filling the <u>No</u> (not Spanish/Hispanic circle). Note that the term "Mexican-American"
   refers only to persons of Mexican origin or ancestry.

   All persons, regardless of citizenship status, should answer this question.

SOURCE: U.S. Bureau of the Census, Department of Commerce, Economics and Statistics
Administration, *Race Hispanic origin*, 1990 Census, no. 2, June 1991.

Beyond the Census Classification: The Hispanic Self-Perception

Two additional perspectives—one offered by Puerto Rican sociologist Clara
Rodríguez and the other by Chilean scholar Miguel Rojas Mix on Latin Americans' search for identity—help elucidate the ongoing debate over Hispanic
identity.

Rodríguez[14] sees contrasts between the way that North Americans perceive race (usually as the colors white or black, yellow, red, and brown) and
the way that Latin Americans perceive race (as cultural and social classifications as well as color-based). In Puerto Rico, specifically, racial categories are
based on color, class, facial features, and texture of hair. Rodríguez points out
a spectrum of racial classifications as used in Puerto Rico: *blancos,* equivalent
to whites in the United States; *indios,* similar to (Asian) Indians in the United
States, that is, dark-skinned and straight-haired; *morenos,* dark-skinned, with
a variety of Negroid or Caucasian features; and *negro,* equivalent to dark-
skinned African-Americans in the United States.

As an aside, she points out that the term *negro* (literally Spanish for
"black") is used as a term of endearment, at which time it bears no connotation

of color. And finally, there is the term *trigueño,* applied to people considered brunettes in the United States, or to blacks or *negros* who have high social status. Now, it may become clearer why Puerto Ricans are also known as the "Rainbow" people. In short, it is important to understand that for Hispanics racial classification is much more complex than it is for Americans.

Rojas Mix[15] offers his interesting perspective in his *Reinventing Identity,* where the Latin Americans' 500-year search for identity[16] is discussed from colonial times to the present:

> Unable to bear to think of ourselves as Indians—which in fact, we are not—we are far from being the Europeans that many have "claimed" us to be. . . . Identity is history, and in America, ours is an alien, imposed history. Without agreeing on who we are, we cannot agree on who are our allies, and who are our enemies. . . ."[17]

Rojas Mix notes that people seek identity at different levels—race, class, nation, continent. He seeks to explain how these different conceptual notions of identity over time have affected how Latinos view themselves and how this search for identity continues today.

Because Hispanics have classified themselves in so many different ways, it is not surprising that the U.S. Census has had so much difficulty in classifying Hispanics in the United States.

> During the colonial period, the word *"nation"* referred to the aboriginals. In woodcuts, the Mexican, Honduran, Chilean or Paraguayan was represented as an Indian, while the white person born in the New World was called a *"Spaniard of the Indies."* Thus, it was the indigenous element that first gave meaning to nationality. The nation became associated with the *la patria,* the homeland, and thus with the "patriots" who fought for independence. . . . Thus, in 1815, at the dawn of independence, Simón Bolívar, the Venezuelan *Libertador,* and first proponent of integration of the American republics, put it as this: "We are not Europeans, we are not Indians, but a hybrid species between the aborigines and the Spaniards. Americans by birth and Europeans by right. . . ."

> A Chilean writer, Francisco Bilbao, was the first proponent of the name Latin America in 1865, as a formula for unity against "Saxon America." Interventions by the industrialized countries in search of raw materials and U.S. interventions in Mexico (1845) and Nicaragua (1855); and the French in Mexico (1861); and the Spaniards in Peru (1964) stimulated feelings of Hispanic American solidarity against aggressors. . . .

> This union of Latin America, a confederation of the South, watered by the Amazon and the Plata and shaded by the Andes, is the picture of the American and Latin identity, which will perpetuate the race and permit the creation of the great American nation. . . . Only this union . . . can hold back the imperialism of the United States of the North, which believes in its empire as Rome believed in its own. . . .

> The notion of "Pan-Americanism" is a project of integration without identity— viewed as an imperialist concept. Thus, for Cuban revolutionary Jose Martí, Pan-Americanism meant the "union of the condor and the lamb . . ." and he instead proposed the concept of "Our America" (Nuestra América), united from "the Rio Grande to the Straits of Magellan."

Yet another term "Ibero-America" was launched in Spain in the wake of the Spanish defeat in the Spanish-American-Cuban War of 1895–1898. If Pan-Americanism was an attempt at integration without identity, Ibero-America represented identity without integration. It was meant to describe Spain's cooperation with its former colonies and to counter the term "Latin America."

More recently, Sandino in Nicaragua, and Che Guevara in Cuba, presented a revolutionary image of Latin America against capitalism and imperialism. Salvador Allende in Chile carried the idea further in his phrase *"Pueblo Continente"* or "Continental People" where the task of liberation from poverty could only be achieved through "socialist homeland."[18]

Rojas Mix concludes by reminding us that

The quest for identity, as Bolívar, Martí, Allende, and others understood it, was not an attempt to find ourselves in the past. Rather, it is a common project, defined by our common struggle. The history of our definitions of our identity, whether as "Creoles" and "Indians," "Hispanic Americans," "Indo-" or "African-Americans," "Pan-Americans," "Latin Americans" or "Continental People," is a record of a commitment to unity on particular bases. This quest for identity is not about the past but about the future we choose to construct. . . .[19]

How Many Hispanics? Where?

The population of the United States increased by 9.8% in the past decade, from 226.5 million in 1980 to 248.7 million in 1990. The number of people of Hispanic origin (regardless of race) increased by 53%, from 14.6 million to 22.4 million in 1990, a large portion of which was attributable to immigration. The number of persons of Hispanic origin as a percent of total population by county in the 1990 census is shown in Figure 1.2.

Hispanics of Mexican ancestry are by far the largest U.S. group covered under "Hispanic origin." Figure 1.3 shows the composition of the Hispanic origin population in millions for 1990. Among all Hispanics, Mexicans account for 62%; Central and South Americans 12%; Puerto Ricans 12%; Cubans 5%; and "Other Hispanics" 9%.[20]

Point of Entry   Interestingly, the point of entry for each Hispanic group has largely determined its current geographic distribution (Figure 1.2). According to Valdivieso and Davis, Mexican-Americans are concentrated in the Southwest, particularly in California and Texas.[21] In 1980, only about one-

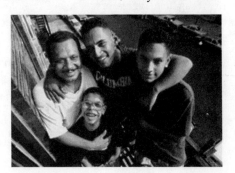

"The Rainbow People." Even within a single Hispanic group there may be much variation.

FIGURE 1.2 Persons of Hispanic origin as a percentage of total population, 1990

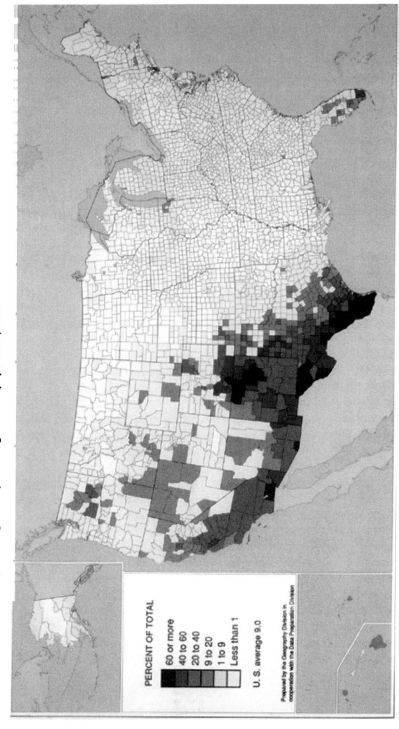

PERCENT OF TOTAL

60 or more
40 to 60
20 to 40
9 to 20
1 to 9
Less than 1

U. S. average 9.0

Prepared by the Geography Division in cooperation with the Data Preparation Division

SOURCE: U.S. Bureau of the Census, Department of Commerce, Economics and Statistics Administration, *Race Hispanic origin*, 1990 Census Profile, no. 2, June 1991.

Boundaries are as of January 1, 1990.

FIGURE 1.3   Composition of the Hispanic origin population, 1990 (in millions)

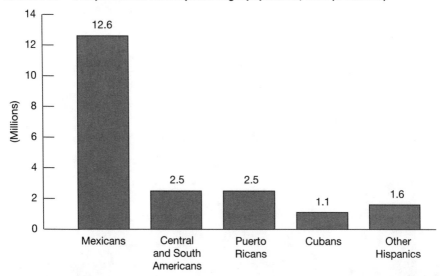

SOURCE: U.S. Bureau of the Census, Department of Commerce, Economics and Statistics Administration, *Race Hispanic origin*, 1990 Census Profile, no. 2, June 1991.

quarter of them were foreign-born, underscoring that they are among the oldest group of Hispanics residing in the United States.

Puerto Ricans, the second largest subgroup, are clustered heavily in the New York metropolitan area. Unlike other Hispanics, as natives of a U.S. commonwealth, Puerto Ricans may enter or leave the U.S. mainland at will. In 1980, about one-half of those residing on the U.S. mainland had been born on the island of Puerto Rico.

The Cubans have migrated primarily into Florida, the point of entry for refugees who fled the Fidel Castro regime in the 1950s and 1960s. Remarkably, Dade County, Florida, still contains about one-half of the 1 million Cuban-Americans. According to the 1980 census, three-fourths of the U.S. Cuban population was foreign-born, but Valdivieso and Davis feel that this number does not reflect the influx of 125,000 Cuban refugees during the 1980 Mariel boatlift.[22]

Central and South Americans are among the most recent of the major immigrant groups. The majority live in California, a favorite entry point, but sizable communities also exist in large eastern urban areas. New York contains sizable communities of Dominicans and Colombians, for example, and many Central Americans live in the Boston and Washington, D.C., metropolitan areas. In 1990, the U.S. Census Bureau counted 545,852 Hispanics living in Chicago, the third largest city in the United States. This number represents 19.6% of the total population in Chicago and 60% of the 904,446 Hispanics in Illinois.[23]

"Other Hispanics" are heavily concentrated in the Southwest, particularly in New Mexico and Arizona. The group includes some Americans who

FIGURE 1.4   Ten states with largest Hispanic origin population, 1990

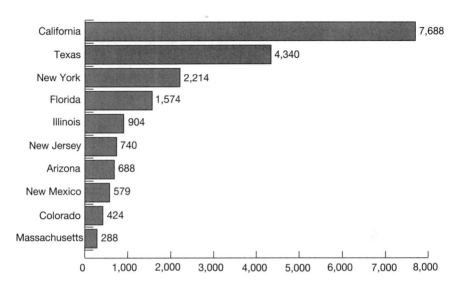

SOURCE: U.S. Bureau of the Census, U.S. Department of Commerce, Economics and Statistics Administration, *Race Hispanic origin*, 1990 Census Profile, no. 2, June 1991.

immigrated recently from Spain, as well as those who came centuries ago. Many of them are long-term residents who no longer identify themselves with Spain or a specific Latin America country, but still consider themselves to be "of Hispanic origin." The vast majority (80%) of them were born in the United States.[24]

Geographic Distribution   Figure 1.4 shows the 10 states that had the largest number of Hispanic residents according to the 1990 Census Profile. With the exception of Massachusetts, which replaced Michigan as the state with the tenth largest number of Hispanic residents, the 10 states with the largest Hispanic populations in 1990 were the same as in 1980. Arizona rose from eighth to seventh largest, changing place with New Mexico. California's Hispanic population increased by 69%, from 4,544,000 in 1980 to 7,688,000 in 1990. This exceeded the national Hispanic increase of 53%. Three other states had Hispanic populations of 1 million or more in 1990: Texas, New York and Florida.

The Hispanic population is geographically concentrated. A majority of all Hispanics lived in just two states (California and Texas) in 1990, and 87% of all Hispanics resided in 10 states. The largest increase in the number of Hispanics in the last decade occurred in California (3,144,000), followed by Texas and Florida (Figure 1.5). California alone accounted for 41% of Hispanic population growth in the United States during the decade, whereas the 10 states with the largest Hispanic growth together accounted for 89% of the increase.

FIGURE 1.5   Ten states with largest increases in Hispanic origin population, 1980–90 (in thousands)

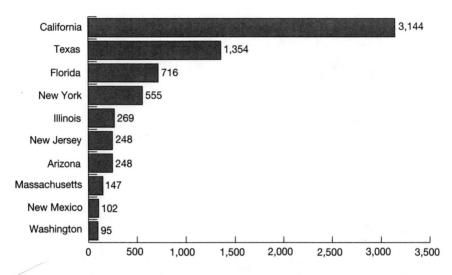

SOURCE: U.S. Bureau of the Census, Department of Commerce, Economics and Statistics Administration, *Race Hispanic origin*, 1990 Census Profile, no. 2, June 1991.

Among the 15 states with Hispanic origin populations of 100,000 or more in 1980, the highest percentage increases between 1980 and 1990 occurred in Massachusetts (104%), Florida (83%), and Washington (79%). Table 1.1 compares regional and state-by-state distribution of all persons in the United States and of Hispanics in 1980 and in 1990.

Five contiguous southwestern states (New Mexico, California, Texas, Colorado, and Arizona) had the highest numbers of Hispanics as a percentage of total population, ranging from 38.2% in New Mexico to 12.9% in Colorado (Figure 1.6). These five states also had the highest percentage of Hispanics in 1980, although California's rank rose from third to second, changing places with Texas. The percentage of Hispanics in Texas rose sharply from 21.0% to 25.5%; however, the percentage of Hispanics in California rose even more rapidly, from 19.2% to 25.8%.

Outside the five southwestern states, in 1990, four states had percentages of Hispanics above the national average of 9.0%: New York, Florida, Nevada, and New Jersey. There were 11 states in which Hispanics represented less than 1% of the total population in 1990 (see Table 1.1).[25]

THE PROCESS OF MIGRATION

Migration is defined by the U.S. Bureau of Census as "any change of residence across a county boundary. . . ." This kind of migration is also known as "in-

TABLE 1.1   A Comparison of All Persons in the United States and Those of Hispanic Origin (of Any Race), by States, 1980 and 1990 (in thousands)

Division and States	All Persons			Hispanic Origin		
	1990	*1980*	*% Change*	*1990*	*1980*	*% Change*
New England	13,207	12,348	7.0	568	299	90.0
Maine	1,228	1,125	9.2	7	5	36.4
New Hampshire	1,109	921	20.5	11	6	102.8
Vermont	563	511	10.0	4	3	10.8
Massachusetts	6,016	5,737	4.9	288	141	103.9
Rhode Island	1,003	947	5.9	46	20	132.2
Connecticut	3,287	3,108	5.8	213	124	71.2
Middle Atlantic	37,602	36,787	2.2	3,186	2,305	38.2
New York	17,990	17,558	2.5	2,214	1,659	33.4
New Jersey	7,730	7,365	5.0	740	492	50.4
Pennsylvania	11,864	11,864	0.1	232	154	50.9
East North Central	42,009	41,682	0.8	1,430	1,068	34.5
Ohio	10,847	10,798	0.5	140	120	16.5
Indiana	5,544	5,490	1.0	99	87	13.5
Illinois	11,431	11,427	——	904	636	42.3
Michigan	9,295	9,262	0.4	202	162	24.1
Wisconsin	4,892	4,706	4.0	93	63	48.0
West North Central	17,660	17,183	2.8	289	209	38.4
Minnesota	4,375	4,076	7.8	54	32	67.7
Iowa	2,777	2,914	−4.7	33	26	27.8
Missouri	5,117	4,917	4.1	62	52	19.5
North Dakota	639	653	−2.1	5	4	19.6
South Dakota	696	691	0.8	5	4	30.5
Nebraska	1,578	1,570	0.5	37	28	31.9
Kansas	2,478	2,364	4.8	94	83	47.9
South Atlantic	43,567	36,959	17.9	2,133	1,194	78.6
Delaware	666	594	12.1	16	10	63.8
Maryland	4,781	4,217	13.4	125	65	93.2
District of Columbia	607	638	−4.9	33	18	85.0
Virginia	6,187	5,347	15.7	160	80	100.7
West Virginia	1,793	1,950	−8.0	8	13	−33.2
North Carolina	6,629	5,882	12.7	77	57	35.4
South Carolina	3,122	3,122	11.7	31	33	−8.6
Georgia	6,478	5,463	18.6	109	61	77.8
Florida	12,938	9,746	32.7	1,574	858	83.4
East South Central	15,176	14,666	3.5	95	120	−20.3
Kentucky	3,685	3,661	0.7	22	27	−19.8
Tennessee	4,877	4,591	6.2	33	34	−3.9
Alabama	4,041	3,894	3.8	25	33	−26.0
Mississippi	2,573	2,521	2.1	16	25	−35.6
West South Central	26,703	23,747	12.4	4,539	3,160	43.6
Arkansas	2,351	2,286	2.8	20	17	11.0
Louisiana	4,220	4,206	0.3	93	99	−6.1
Oklahoma	3,146	3,025	4.0	86	57	50.1
Texas	16,987	14,229	19.4	4,340	2,986	45.4

TABLE 1.1   A Comparison of All Persons in the United States and Those of Hispanic Origin (of Any Race), by States, 1980 and 1990 (in thousands) (*continued*)

Division and States	All Persons			Hispanic Origin		
	1990	1980	% Change	1990	1980	% Change
Mountain	13,659	11,373	20.1	1,992	1,443	38.0
Montana	799	787	1.6	12	10	22.1
Idaho	1,007	944	6.7	53	37	44.6
Wyoming	454	470	−3.4	26	24	5.1
Colorado	3,294	2,890	14.0	424	340	24.9
New Mexico	1,515	1,303	16.3	579	477	21.4
Arizona	3,665	2,718	34.8	688	441	56.2
Utah	1,723	1,461	17.9	85	60	40.3
Nevada	1,202	800	59.1	124	54	130.9
Pacific	39,127	31,800	23.0	8,114	4,811	88.7
Washington	4,867	4,132	17.8	215	120	78.8
Oregon	2,842	2,633	7.9	113	66	71.2
California	29,760	23,668	25.7	7,688	4,544	69.2
Alaska	559	402	36.9	18	10	87.3
Hawaii	1,108	965	14.9	81	71	14.2

SOURCE: U.S. Bureau of the Census, U.S. Department of Commerce, Economics and Statistics Administration, *Race Hispanic origin*, 1990 Census Profile, no. 2, June 1991.

ternal" migration, as opposed to "external" migration, in which the change of residence takes place across national borders.

Migration can be either voluntary or involuntary. Voluntary migration occurs as people choose to move from rural to urban areas, usually in search of economic opportunities. Involuntary migration occurs when people are forced to move for reasons of war, political strife, drought, famine, disease, or natural disaster.

One of the most significant demographic phenomena in recent decades is the growth of urban populations in many countries. In low-income countries, recent migrants constitute a large percentage of the total urban population (at any particular time a significant fraction having arrived during the previous five years) and overurbanization is an overwhelming problem that is likely to continue for years to come. The United Nations Population Division predicts that by the year 2000, 50% of the population in developing countries (and 75% in Latin America) will live in urban areas. Currently, two-thirds of population growth in developing countries is in urban areas, with migration accounting for 50% of this.

The "Push and Pull" Theory

Much has been written about the movement from rural areas to cities, but its etiology seems best summarized by the *"push and pull" theory* of migration described by Herrick.[26]

Figure 1.6   Ten states with the highest percentage of Hispanics, 1990

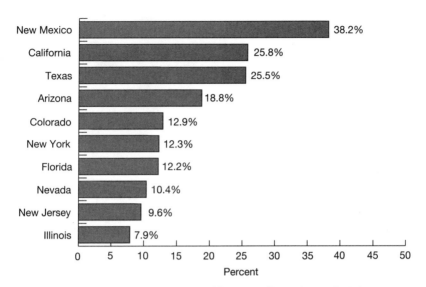

SOURCE: U.S. Bureau of the Census, U.S. Department of Commerce, Economics and Statistics Administration, *Race Hispanic origin*, 1990 Census Profile, no. 2, June 1991.

Migration is not a random process. It is self-selective in the sense that "push and pull" factors associated with origin, destination, and differential intervening obstacles play an important role. Intervening obstacles include such factors as travel costs, personal issues, destination distance, immigration policy, quotas, and control on movements. These "push and pull" factors have varying degrees of importance in the decision to migrate.

The "push" stems primarily from the pressure of rural poverty caused by increased population, decreased availability of land per capita, low agricultural production, and increased use of mechanization. The "pull" factors include higher wages, better quality and more available public services (e.g., health care, schools, water, electricity), and the belief that urban life is more dynamic, exciting, and modern.

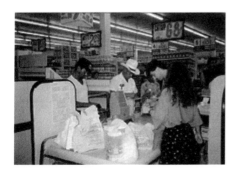

Hispanic migrants are clustered heavily in the southwest region of the United States.

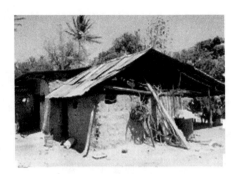

The pressures of rural poverty, including poor dwellings, "push" Hispanics to migrate.

Motives for Migrating

In developing economies, particularly those at very early stages of development, most of the country's labor force is engaged in subsistence agriculture because of the biological necessity for food and because of the low labor productivity in traditional agriculture. As industrialization begins, incomes rise and agricultural employment declines in relative importance. The shift from a rural to an urban economy begins.

In an intermediate stage of development, industrialization is given impetus by technological innovation, and the rate of productive investment rises. The manufacturing sector employs increasing amounts of labor. Lastly, as the country achieves its full economic development, there is a decline in the industrial labor force and a rise in employment in the service sector. Industrial production expands, but it is efficient enough so that more and more labor can be released from industry.

Parts of Latin America seem to be moving from the first to the third stage of development without creating a solid industrial sector. As a result, the employment surplus is concentrated in the service sector, income distributions are heavily skewed in favor of a small elite, and poverty is widespread.

Migration as a Stepwise Process

Given the motivations behind migration, persons most likely to respond to the push and pull are the landless or unemployed and those seeking future opportunities, often the young and better educated.

Further investigation reveals that migration may be a stepwise process. From rural areas, migrants often move first to a small local city or to the provincial capital. Only later do they or their children move again to a large city or to the nation's capital. Migration is usually of a relatively short distance, with people often moving to the capital city of the province in which they live. Migrants usually visit a city before moving there, and they often live with friends or relatives upon first moving.

Herrick described the stepwise process in Chile.[27] He found that Chilean migrants in the early 1960s came to Santiago mostly from cities and towns instead of from agricultural districts.

Women as a Significant Segment of the Migrant Population

Black and Sanjur, in their study of internal migration and maternal diets in Puerto Rico,[28] describe the "typical migrant" as someone from a smaller city or rural area, fairly young, who views the move as permanent, and who may not be educationally hampered in searching for jobs. Although their chances of finding jobs may be greater than those of their urban counterparts, these jobs will most likely be in low-paying service occupations.

Increasingly, however, women make up a significant part of the migrating population. After decades in which the flow was made up overwhelmingly of men traveling for seasonal work, the number of Mexican women crossing into the United States has risen sharply in recent years. Census and immigration data indicate that women now account for about half of the Mexican immigrants who settle in the United States.[29] Their shift from an impoverished rural environment to an urban environment may cause a considerable reduction in their cultural and social support networks. Women may lose the extended kin and personal support networks that helped them to survive in economically marginal situations. Potential conflicts (or benefits) between a mother's participation in market work and the nutritional status of her young children is reviewed in Chapter 2.

MIGRATION HISTORY OF HISPANICS

Mexican Immigration

The number of Mexicans immigrating to the United States increased steadily during the twentieth century and has accelerated rapidly since the 1940s. Furthermore, in the last two decades, the number and proportion of undocumented Mexican immigrants have increased sharply. Although migration has recently been on the increase, many Mexican-Americans are long-term residents.

The ancestors of Mexican-Americans came voluntarily to the United States, some as long as 360 years ago. The Spaniards arrived in California a century before the *Mayflower* reached Plymouth Rock in 1620, and their influence in the Southwest is evident even today. One needs only to look at the names of older towns in the Southwest to appreciate the extent of early Spanish settlement.[30]

Mexico, to which California belonged about 120 years ago, has contributed to the culture and traditions of that state. Early Mexican settlers contributed their rich cultural heritage and language. Mexicans were active in developing mining regions, opening new routes for travelers, and founding schools. In California, Mexicans are classified as *Chicano* (native to the area), *bracero* or green card holder (a Mexican national who entered the United States legally), or *wetback* (a derogatory term for illegal immigrants who may have swum the Rio Grande to cross the border).

Acosta and Aranda have described four groups of Mexicans in California in various states of acculturation (the process by which individuals learn the beliefs, attitudes, and behavioral patterns in a new society):[31]

Middle-class Mexican-Americans, descended from many generations born in California and exhibiting many characteristics of the dominant U.S. middle-class culture.

Second- and third-generation Mexican-Americans, at various stages of acculturation but still clinging to some of the customs, culture, and traditions of their parents and grandparents.

First-generation or Mexican nationals, who are well versed in all the traditions, cultures, and customs of Mexico, holding tenaciously to these beliefs and practices, while speaking nostalgically of returning home.

Migrant farm workers, who may be drawn from any of the other groups, but for reasons of constant travel, low income, and extremely low educational level are less likely than the other groups to acculturate to dominant middle-class customs.

A fundamental distinction between the immigration of Mexicans and that of others to the United States is that the Mexicans can and do freely travel back and forth across a shared border of more than 3,000 kilometers, renewing their culture, customs, traditions, and folklore.

Phases of Mexican Immigration[32]   According to Vernez and Ronfeldt there have been three phases of legal Mexican immigration to the United States during the twentieth century.[33] These are summarized in Table 1.2.

Phase I: 1901–1940. This phase was characterized by a steady increase of Mexican immigrants, at the same time as aggregate immigration from other countries was declining. Before 1900, Mexican legal immigration to the United States never exceeded 500 individuals per year, whereas by the 1920s, it represented 11% of the total legal immigration.

Phase II: 1941–1964. This period began after a temporary slowdown during the depression of the 1930s. As the U.S. economy recovered in the early 1940s, Vernez and Ronfeldt note that Mexican immigration increased. It was spurred by the Bracero Program, a 1942 U.S.-Mexican treaty that allowed importation of an unlimited number of temporary workers (*braceros*) to make up for war-induced labor shortages in the agricultural industry. By the end of the Bracero Program in 1964, more than 4.5 million Mexicans had come to work temporarily in the United States. These temporary immigrants exceeded the number of permanent legal immigrants by eightfold.

Phase III: 1965–1988. The last phase began with the cessation of the Bracero Program and the passage of the Immigration Reform Act of

TABLE 1.2   Average annual Mexican immigration activities to the United States, 1901–88

Decade	Immigrants Admitted[a]		Undocumented Immigration	
	Mexican-born	Percentage of Total Immigrants	Estimated Net Undocumented Immigrants	Aliens Apprehended[b]
		Phase 1		
1901–10	4,964	0.5		
1911–20	29,900	5.2		
1921–30	45,928	11.2	100,000	25,769
1931–40	2,231	4.2		14,745
		Phase 2		
1941–50	6,058	6.0[b]		137,721
1951–60	29,981	11.9[b]		359,894[c]
1961–64	46,748	15.9[b]		89,222
		Phase 3		
1967–70	45,393	12.3	25,000[d]	208,578
1971–80	64,029	14.2	110,000[d]	832,498
1981–86	66,936	11.4	135,000[d]	1,260,855[e]
1987–88	83,675[f]	13.4		1,099,165

[a] Gross yearly average unadjusted for subsequent departures and mortality.
[b] Were not recorded until 1925. The number of alien apprehensions exceeds the number of undocumented individuals crossing into the United States because the same person may be apprehended more than once.
[c] Peaked in 1954 at 1,089,583.
[d] Total undocumented Mexican-born immigrants legalized under the Immigration and Reform Act (IRCA) distributed according to reported date of first entry into the United States.
[e] Peaked in 1986 at 1,767,400.
[f] Includes yearly average of about 15,000 previously undocumented immigrants admitted under the IRCA Registry provision which legalized undocumented immigrants who have continuously resided in the United States since 1972.
SOURCE: Adapted from G. Vernez and R. Ronfeldt, The current situation in Mexican immigration. *Science, 251* (March 1991), 4498.

1965. Although the latter placed the first ceiling on immigration from the Western Hemisphere, including Mexico, permanent Mexican legal immigration continued to increase steadily, and more rapidly than total legal immigration, until the late 1970s.

Undocumented Mexican Immigration   As shown in Table 1.2, Vernez and Ronfeldt suggest that legal immigration (temporary and permanent) has been accompanied by continuous undocumented immigration. The number of illegal immigrants is estimated to range from about 100,000 yearly in 1920 to 135,000 yearly in the mid-1980s.

Factors associated with the most recent wave of illegal immigration include a widening gap between wages in Mexico and the United States, decreased employment opportunities in Mexico, and migrant networks that are established between places of origin in Mexico and destinations in the United States. These networks lower the cost of migration because friends and relatives provide newcomers with housing and other kinds of social and economic support.

From the 1940s to the 1980s, the stream of Mexican immigrants continued, although in some years it was considerably diminished. Based on this pattern, it appears that current immigration law will not markedly affect the immigration of Mexicans.

Dominican Immigration

Dominicans have been immigrating to the United States, legally and illegally, for many years. However, their influx increased dramatically in the early 1960s, probably in response to political factors, especially Trujillo's death and the Juan Bosch revolution. Many of the early immigrants were from the middle class; however, since then, many more from the lower economic status have also come, lured by the promise of economic gains.[34] Family reasons and education, particularly for the higher economic class, are also high priorities, but political reasons do not seem to play a major role at the present time.

Since 1968, the U.S. immigration policy has tried to reunite families, but families are defined only as parents, spouses, and legitimate children. Although common-law marriages are usual in the Dominican Republic, the "spouses" and "illegitimate" children resulting from such unions are not eligible for visas.[35] One strategy to cope with this problem is marriage "as a favor." A legal resident of the United States marries a Dominican to facilitate his or her entry into the country, but neither party considers it a lasting commitment. Marriage "for business" is also common, costing between $500 and $1,000.[36] Other tactics used to enter the United States include "purchasing" a passport (actually renting one) for as much as $1,200. Also, Dominicans may "pass" as Puerto Ricans, who are U.S. citizens. But probably the most common mechanism is the semilegal one of entering on a tourist visa and staying on after its expiration.[37]

Reasons for Dominican Immigration The Dominican Republic occupies the eastern two-thirds of the Caribbean island of Hispaniola, which it shares with Haiti. The country's 48,100 square kilometers (19,000 square miles) are bounded to the north by the Atlantic Ocean and to the south by the Caribbean Sea. Two-thirds of the country is mountainous highlands, which makes internal transportation difficult. Many rivers that originate in the mountains supply the rest of the country with water.[38] Rainy seasons are in the spring and fall. Its subtropical climate, which makes it possible to grow coffee almost down to sea level, ranges from extreme aridity in the valleys and coastal areas of the southwestern part to the very humid slopes and lowlands of the northeast. The Dominican Republic has some of the most extensive pine forests in the Caribbean area. Its principal cities include Santo Domingo, the capital and the oldest city in the Western Hemisphere, Santiago de los Caballeros, San Pedro de Macoris, Barahona, La Vega, San Francisco de Macoris, La Romana, San Juan de la Maguana, and Puerto Plata.

Like most low-income countries, the Dominican Republic suffers from high unemployment and a growing population.[39] In 1991, the population of the Dominican Republic was estimated at 7.3 million.[40] With a high birth rate of 29 per 1,000 and a declining death rate of 6 per 1000, the population continues to increase rapidly.

In 1990, more than 60% of the population was unemployed or underemployed.[41] Unemployment is expected to increase further because almost half of the population is under 14 years old and will soon be expected to enter the already oversaturated labor force. Nearly half the working population is engaged in agriculture, and about three-quarters of the industrial labor force works in sugar mills. Tourism also provides a number of jobs.

The distribution of income in the country is highly skewed, with the top 10% of the population earning more than one-third of the nation's income and the bottom 50% earning only one-fifth.[42] Per capita income in 1991 was reported as $820.[43]

Legal and Illegal Immigrants   There are conflicting reports as to the real size of the Dominican population in the United States. Although Ugalde et al. reported some time ago that Dominicans were the third largest Hispanic immigrant group (after Mexicans and Cubans),[44] they are not listed by the U.S. Census as a major Hispanic group. The conflicting reports may be due to the number of undocumented Dominicans.

Tiffany notes that estimates of the number of illegal immigrants vary widely, according to the interests of the group gathering the data.[45] She contends that the best estimates are those of the Roman Catholic Church, which is the only institution that the immigrants trust. In the early 1980s, the church estimated that at least 40,000 Dominicans, many illegal, were living in New York City. This is more than three times greater than estimates by the U.S. government and is equivalent to about 7.3% of the entire Dominican population. One source contributing to this figure is the number of "nonimmigrants" (people who arrive in the United States with a visa to visit, study, or work as diplomat) or visitors with expired visas. The number of legal immigrants increases each year. However, Tiffany feels that there may be a recent decline in net migration, because many immigrants return to the Dominican Republic.

The Dominican Migrant in New York City   Ninety percent of all Dominican immigrants to the United States settle in New York City. In fact, for many Dominicans New York and the United States are synonymous.[46] Tiffany provides an in-depth perspective of the pains and dilemmas, alienation and joys experienced by Dominican immigrants in New York City. She argues that maintaining contact with their homeland is essential because the hope of returning home is often more than a dream. The Asociación Nacional de Dominicanos Ausentes (ANDA), the National Association of Absent Dominicans, was formed to get the right to vote in elections in the Dominican Republic, an example of the continuous contact that Dominicans want with their homeland. In fact, recreational and social organizations such as ANDA often augment linkages with the Dominican Republic rather than aid in cultural assimilation.

However, the nostalgic notion of returning home is jeopardized by economic realities. It is expensive to return home, and many relatives there are supported by money sent to them by workers in New York. Illegal residents cannot return home because they fear being caught and deported. Economic stress coupled with the knowledge that their stay is tenuous may accentuate Dominican immigrants' feelings of loneliness and distrust.

Tiffany concludes her analysis by noting that although they encounter many difficulties, Dominican immigrants are generally satisfied. Even though they may have had to settle for less than they expected, most of them are grateful for any small opportunity to better themselves economically and educationally. They have some mixed feelings, however. As one woman explains: "New York is the best place to get ahead, to improve your life, to live better, but the Dominican Republic is the best place to be when you are down and out or have problems. . . ."[47]

Cuban Immigration

There are many historical bonds between Cuba and the United States, and the presence of Cubans in southern Florida dates back more than one hundred years. It was in Key West and Tampa where José Martí found support to create his Revolutionary Party to free Cuba from Spain.[48] According to Sandoval, during the first half of the twentieth century, after Cuba became a republic, Florida remained the destination for many Cubans who experienced political persecution or dissatisfaction during Machado's dictatorship in the 1930s and Batista's in the 1940s and 1950s.

Four Stages of the Cuban Exodus   Portes and Mozo have classified four major turns in Cuban migration to the United States:[49]

> **1.** *January 1959–October 1962.* Approximately 215,000 Cubans beyond immigration quotas were admitted during this period. This exodus included Cuban upper classes, supporters of the fallen Batista regime, joined by many professionals and smaller merchants. After the 1962 missile crisis, direct transportation between Cuba and the United States was halted.
>
> **2.** *November 1962–November 1965.* Because it was possible to leave Cuba only through clandestine means or restricted flights to third countries, mostly Mexico, the number of refugees dwindled during the next three years. However, about 74,000 Cubans entered the United States during this period, mostly because in September 1965, a family reunification

program was established. The Cuban government permitted the departure of individuals to join relatives in the United States.

3. *December 1965–April 1973.* The governments of Cuba and the United States signed a memorandum of understanding that launched an airlift from Varadero Beach in Cuba to Miami. The two daily flights that operated during this period brought in more than 340,000 new refugees, mostly of lower-middle and urban working classes.

4. *May 1973–September 1980.* In April 1973, the Cuban government unilaterally terminated the airlift. Clandestine escapes and travel to third countries, mainly Spain (but also Mexico, Jamaica, Puerto Rico, Venezuela, and Panama) became the only means of leaving Cuba. Emigration again decreased and by 1979 amounted to fewer than 3,000. In April 1980, however, the occupation of the Peruvian embassy in Havana triggered the largest Cuban emigration in a single year. In five months, May to September of 1980, 124,769 new Cubans arrived, more than the combined total for the preceding eight years. In the month of May alone, more refugees arrived than during all of 1962, previously the record year of Cuban emigration.

The flow of Cubans to the United States is expected to continue in the years ahead, because the Migration Agreement of 1984 allows up to 20,000 Cubans to enter the United States annually under the U.S. preference system.[50] (According to Bach,[51] the agreement collapsed when the United States allowed Radio Martí to begin broadcasting in Cuba. In retaliation for the broadcasts, the Cuban government suspended the Migration Agreement, but it was reinstated in November 1987.)

Reasons for Cuban Immigration   Two important features of the Cuban exodus to the United States are its socioeconomic composition and its motivations.[52] The waves of Cuban immigration, as described by Portes and Mozo, brought to the United States a population that increasingly resembled the socioeconomic characteristics of the Cuban population on the island, with the early wave bringing mostly upper middle class and the later period including a more significant proportion of the working class. In terms of the motivational impetus for immigration, the Cuban exodus was prompted by political reasons rather than by economic hardship. Sandoval argues that Cubans have chosen to immigrate to Florida because it is geographically close and familiar. Also, the United States has welcomed Cuban exiles and given them help in resettling.

In short, between 1959 and 1980, more than 800,000 Cubans left their homeland for the United States. Unlike the Mexican and Puerto Rican immigrants, the Cubans who came to the United States during the early 1960s were often well schooled, with occupational skills, and many of them spoke English. These early immigrants were a select segment of the total population living in Cuba.

Settlement Patterns   Despite federal government efforts to relocate Cuban exiles throughout the United States, most of them eventually settled in the Miami area. By the early 1970s, Miami had become the world's second largest "Cuban" city, smaller only than Havana. Clark notes that throughout the years the number of Cubans in Florida has increased through natural growth, arrivals from abroad, and also from a steady flow of "returnees" who, after having been resettled elsewhere by the former Cuban Refugee Program, have come back to a climate and culture more akin to those of Cuba.[53]

But not all of Miami's Hispanics are Cuban; perhaps as many as 150,000 have originated from Colombia, Venezuela, Panama, Ecuador, Peru, and Argentina, as well as from Mexico, Puerto Rico, and the Dominican Republic. In addition, Mohl reports that revolutions in Nicaragua and El Salvador have created large new communities of exiles in Miami in the past years.[54] Thus the Hispanic population of Miami, although mostly Cuban, is actually quite diverse.

Environmental Adjustment or Cultural Assimilation?   Questions raised by scholars about Cuban immigration patterns pertain to the issue of adjustment versus assimilation. To what extent have Cuban immigrants become assimilated into American culture? To what extent do second- or third-generation Cuban-Americans retain Cuban identity? What factors account for Cubans' rapid and relatively successful adjustments, such as high levels of citizenship, voting participation, education, occupational success, and socioeconomic mobility? Is this adjustment due to economic prosperity, support by the U.S. government, a feeling of "being at home" in the United States, or a combination of these and other factors?

Mohl, citing sociologist Milton Gordon's classic study, *Assimilation in American Life,*[55] contends that a distinction must be drawn between *behavioral assimilation* and *structural assimilation.* Behavioral assimilation occurs when an individual learns the language, acquires survival skills, gets a job, and becomes a citizen. Structural assimilation requires further integration into mainstream society.

Another indicator used by sociologists to measure cultural assimilation is the rate of marriage to people outside the ethnic group. Among second-generation Cuban-Americans the rate of marriage to non-Hispanics is quite high. Mohl argues that this is directly related to the geographic concentration of ethnic groups. In New York City, where Cubans are geographically dispersed, marriage to outsiders is more prevalent than in Miami, where Cubans are clustered in Little Havana and Hialeah.

Cuban Achievements   As one reviews the historical accounts of the socioeconomic impact and cultural contributions brought to America by Cubans and developed in America by Cuban-Americans, one is impressed by both the breadth and depth of such accomplishments, as well as by the short time frame in which they have taken place. On this topic, Chávez finds much to applaud in the Cuban community.[56] She cites the extraordinary success of Cuban-Americans today, who within two generations, "through diligence and hard work," have achieved success in such fields as banking and real estate development.

Using recent work from some historians and other scholars studying the Cuban experience in America, this author reviews a few selected factors that have contributed to the Cuban success in the United States. These issues warrant further attention and will provide the reader with a better appreciation of certain aspects of the Cuban migration. Efforts to keep traditions and culture alive and at the same time achieve rapid assimilation in their new homeland appear to have been more successful among Cuban immigrants than any other Hispanic immigrant group.

Naturalization Patterns　Cubans, probably more than any other Hispanic group, hold more political power because they vote in elections. They are able to vote because they become citizens. The Cuban naturalization rate consistently exceeds the rates for all countries and those for individual countries and regions except Asia.[57] As more Cuban refugees become citizens, their involvement in local, state, and national elections will influence the political picture of Florida and of other states as well. Sandoval points out that already ten Cuban-Americans serve in the Florida legislature and a Cuban-American congresswoman serves at the federal level.[58] The socioeconomic and political impact of the naturalization process for an immigrant group cannot be overemphasized.

Economic Contributions　Cuban exiles have found enormous success in business and finance. The early upper-class immigrants demonstrated, after a brief period of adjustment, their economic abilities and influence. According to Mohl, by the 1980s, Cubans in Miami had established some 20,000 businesses, from retail stores to fishing fleets. Jorge and Salazar-Carrillo highlight several important factors or conditions that help explain the relative economic success of Cubans in southern Florida:[59]

1. The singular most important factor was the entrepreneurial ability of the Cubans.

2. The structural nature of South Florida's economy was not too dissimilar from that of the economy in Cuba. Thus, Cubans were able to undertake a wide variety of economic activities with a familiar level of technology and organization.

3. The high level of educational attainment of Cubans prior to their immigration approached that of the white population in Miami. This allowed Cubans to compete efficiently in the American markets.

4. A *host* of interrelated factors, ranging from personal to closely knit residential patterns of immigrants, constituted the basis from which the Hispanic market would grow.

5. Government programs, capital markets, and financial facilities and institutions played a critical role in propelling the Cuban economic per-

formance. The relative abundance of capital accessible to Cubans, almost from the start, was very important.

Language Maintenance, Bilingualism, and Spanish Media   Cubans have long been aware of the importance of bilingualism. They have insisted that their children learn both English and Spanish. Speaking Spanish helps preserve their traditions and cultural heritage and also enhances their economic opportunities. According to Mohl, the Cubans are perhaps the only immigrant group in American history to perceive an economic value (as opposed to a cultural imperative) in maintaining their language.[60]

In 1973, Dade County, Florida, passed an ordinance that officially made the county bilingual. The intention was to reduce the language barrier that kept many citizens from obtaining government services or employment opportunities, as well as to promote commerce and tourism with Latin America.[61] However, by 1980, following a divisive and emotional campaign, Dade County passed an ordinance stipulating that public funds were not to be used to teach languages other than English or to "promote a culture other than the American culture." It also limited the county's power to use Spanish for official business.[62]

In spite of the antibilingual ordinance, Spanish continues as an important language in southern Florida. Sandoval believes that this intersection of Spanish and English is extremely important because they are the two most important languages in the Western Hemisphere.[63] Thus southern Florida has the potential to become an economic and cultural broker of the Americas.

The continued use of Spanish in Miami has been enhanced by Spanish-language radio and television stations and daily and weekly newspapers and magazines. Sandoval notes that bilingual journalism has increased sales of several daily newspapers, and that there are more than 25 Spanish-language tabloids in southern Florida. Similarly, Editorial America publishes 13 Spanish-language magazines with a monthly circulation of almost 300,000 in the United States and Latin America.

Puerto Rican Immigration

Clara Rodríguez, in the introductory remarks to her book *Puerto Ricans—Born in the U.S.A.*, states:

> Since 1898, all Puerto Ricans have been born in the U.S.A., for that was the year the United States invaded Puerto Rico as part of its war with Spain and proceeded to make Puerto Rico an unincorporated territory of the United States. All Puerto Ricans born in Puerto Rico since that time have been born on U.S. soil. . . .[64]

Puerto Ricans have been migrating to the United States mainland for more than a hundred years, but only since the end of World War II has this migration taken on social and economic significance. Rodríguez, citing

Stevens-Arroyo and Díaz Stevens[65] and Maldonado,[66] classifies the migration of Puerto Ricans after the U.S. takeover into three major periods. During the first period, 1900–45, the pioneers arrived. The majority of them settled in New York City, especially in what is known as El Barrio in East Harlem, Brooklyn, the Lower East Side, and sections of the South Bronx. During this first period, contracted industrial and agricultural laborers also arrived. Longtime residents relate that, in the late 1940s and early 1950s, at the beginning of the postwar boom, U.S. agricultural growers began to recruit farm labor from Puerto Rico to offset a manpower shortage. At first, the men came by themselves and returned to the island each fall. Gradually, as opportunities to support their families increased, they began to settle, with their wives and children, in areas outside New York and in Hawaii, California, Arizona, and other southwestern states.

The second period, 1946–64, is known as the "great migration" because of the large numbers of Puerto Ricans who arrived. In the aftermath of World War II, the availability of inexpensive air transportation and increased job opportunities in the United States, especially in the New York area, motivated large numbers of Puerto Ricans to migrate northward. During this phase, Rodríguez points out that the already established Puerto Rican communities of East Harlem, the South Bronx, and the Lower East Side increased their numbers and expanded their borders. Thus, at the same time as Puerto Ricans began to settle in new areas of the country, the majority of them continued to live in New York City. By about the mid-1950s, migration slowed down and was exceeded in some years by reverse migration. Many Puerto Ricans who came to the United States during the 1950s were from rural areas, were in economic need, had agrarian, nontransferable skills, and had a low level of schooling.

The third and last period, from 1965 to the present, called the "revolving-door migration," involves fluctuating patterns of net migration, as well as greater dispersion of Puerto Ricans to other parts of the United States. By 1980, Rodríguez notes, the majority of Puerto Ricans in the United States were living outside New York State.

Puerto Ricans: Colonial Immigrants but also U.S. Citizens   Rodríguez argues that the fact that Puerto Rico and the United States were joined through an act of conquest has often been understated. Although various scholars have viewed Puerto Ricans as "the last in the continuum of immigrant groups to the United States, . . ."[67] Rodríguez points out their differences. Although Puerto Ricans were, and to a large extent still are, like earlier immigrants, with their foreign culture, language, and experience, they differ from European immigrants in a number of ways. Unlike European immigrants, Puerto Ricans enter the United States as citizens, serve in the U.S. armed forces, have accessible transportation to their country of origin, come from a strategic base of the United States, and have a Caribbean rather than a European cultural and racial background.[68]

HISPANIC MIGRANT AGRICULTURAL WORKERS

John Steinbeck, in *The Grapes of Wrath,* points out:

> Migratory farm laborers move restlessly over the face of the land . . . but they neither belong to the land, nor does the land belong to them. . . . They pass through community after community, but they neither claim the community as home, nor does the community claim them. . . . The migratory workers engage in a common occupation . . . but their cohesion is scarcely greater than that of pebbles on a seashore. . . .[69]

A migrant agricultural worker is an individual whose primary employment is in agriculture on a seasonal or other temporary basis, and whose permanent residence is out of the country or state where he is working. In contrast, a nonimmigrant domestic agricultural worker is an individual employed at least 110 consecutive days under one employer.[70] In 1970, the U.S. Senate Subcommittee on Migratory Labor said of migrant laborers: "No other segment of our population is so poorly paid, yet contributes so much to our nation's wealth and welfare. Despite their vital role in modern agriculture, particularly in filling the crucial need at harvest time, these people have been grossly neglected by our society. . . ."[71]

Although the number of migrant farm workers has steadily decreased in the last 20 years, there are still enough interstate rural seasonal workers to merit consideration. Vernez and Ronfeldt[72] note that during the last two decades Mexican immigrant participation in the agricultural industry has been halved to 15% of all native-born Mexicans in the labor force, whereas their role in the manufacturing industry has increased nearly twofold. Similarly, the Puerto Rican migrant agricultural labor population has declined steadily, from 12,986 in 1960 to 4,191 in 1977.[73] Although not all migrant agricultural laborers are of Hispanic origin, many of them are, and the following section provides a historical perspective of Mexican and Puerto Rican migrant laborers, as well as their working conditions and other health issues.

Since the 1970 White House Conference on Food, Nutrition and Health, Subpanel on Migrant and Seasonal Farm Workers, various local, state, and federal agencies have tried to improve the socioeconomic conditions and well-being of migrant workers. However, many negative conditions still persist, and renewed concern and efforts are needed to improve the lot of the seasonal rural agricultural worker. Some of these negative conditions include:

1. *Pesticide exposure:* Health statistics indicate that agricultural workers experience the highest occupational disease rate of all occupation groups. Rashes, nausea, vomiting, diarrhea, chest pains, eye trouble, and other serious health problems are common among agricultural workers and their children as a result of pesticide exposure.

2. *Extreme poverty:* Large families, payment by piece rates, and low wages all contribute to conditions of extreme poverty for a vast majority of seasonal rural workers. Limited access to such governmental programs as nutritional subsidies plus humiliating procedures to determine eligibility for programs have undermined participation in government programs.

3. *Lack of educational opportunities:* As communities, schools, and teachers face changes from one year to the next, the task of educating migrant children has been difficult, as for many of them, it must begin anew each season. Schooling has generally been inadequate and school lunches often have not been available for children of poor farm workers.

4. *Lack of political power:* Seasonal workers are among the most difficult to organize, and when these workers come from more than a thousand miles away and are scattered over hundreds of farms, the problems multiply. Similarly, the political power of eligible migrant workers is reduced if elections occur when migrants are out of the state. However, as more Hispanic migrant farm workers reach voting age, and more acquire citizenship, their voting strength and political power may increase accordingly. Yet the areas where migrants live often lack sewers, pavements, fire protection, and other basic municipal services.

Migrant Agricultural Labor in California

To understand the problems faced by migrant workers in California today, it is necessary to be aware of California's agricultural history. Burma notes that after World War I, when European immigration was limited and many southerners—African-Americans and whites—began to move to northern industrial centers, many Mexican immigrants began to arrive, settling mostly in the Southwest. Early in the 1940s, during World War II, many Mexican residents left California to join the armed forces, thereby creating a labor shortage. Consequently, in 1942, the United States and Mexico began the Bracero Program, the importation of Mexicans as seasonal laborers on a contract basis. By August 1944, 36,000 Mexican nationals were working in California. In 1964, the program ended, and the agricultural labor force dropped from 64,000 in 1964 to less than 6,000 Mexicans in the peak month of 1967.

Migrant Agricultural Contract Workers from Puerto Rico

According to Seidl et al.,[74] Puerto Ricans are second only to Mexicans as a source of cheap imported labor for U.S. growers; on the East Coast, they are unrivaled. However, unlike Mexicans, Puerto Ricans need not worry about quotas or deportations. Because Puerto Ricans are citizens of the United States, the Department of Labor and the Immigration and Naturalization Service consider them "domestic workers"—often referred to as "interstate migrants," not "illegals." Rodríguez notes that Puerto Rican contract labor migration began soon after 1898 and has continued throughout the twentieth century.[75] The very first Puerto Ricans to migrate to the United States after 1898 was a group of contract laborers who went to Hawaii. A "Report of the Commissioner of Labor on Hawaii," published in 1903 and cited by Seidl, tells about that migration, describing the working conditions and the racism that was prevalent among North Americans of that era.

According to Maldonado, for many Puerto Ricans the farm labor system was a stepping stone to residence in the United States, usually in urban areas.[76] These migrants formed the nucleus of subsequent Puerto Rican communities in less urban areas of Hawaii, California, Arizona, and other southwestern states.[77] Communities in Gary, Indiana, in Lorain, Cleveland, and Youngstown, Ohio, began this way. Similarly, between 1960 and 1970, the Puerto Rican population of the Hartford, Connecticut, area more than tripled. In 1975, when 4,100 "local" workers were hired to replace Puerto Rican contract workers, half of them were Puerto Rican residents of the Connecticut Valley.[78] As of the late 1970s, estimates of the number of Puerto Ricans who migrated to work in U.S. agriculture each year varied, from 60,000 to 200,000. Some came independently in search of work, and others were recruited on the island by private agencies, crew leaders, or growers.

In the late 1940s, a "contract program" was instituted by the commonwealth government to regulate the recruitment and employment of workers in mainland agriculture. Seidl et al. report that over the past 27 years more than 350,000 Puerto Rican contract workers have been employed in the harvests of 22 states, harvesting peaches in South Carolina, apples in Vermont, beets and cabbage in western New York, shade tobacco in Connecticut, and vegetables in New Jersey.[79]

Migrant Agricultural Workers in the Midwest

Torres contends that the migrant worker represents a segment of the Hispanic population that has always had the lowest health status, earnings, job security, educational attainment, and political power.[80] Mobility makes it especially difficult for migrants to have regular or continuous health care. Torres cites the serious health problems found by Slesinger et al. in migrant workers in Wisconsin.[81] Ninety percent of these workers were Mexican-Americans, who reported a higher than expected prevalence of acute and chronic conditions.

In assessing reports of chronic health conditions, Slesinger found that mothers who spoke English were more likely to report that a child had a chronic condition.[82] He postulates that women who do not speak English may not label various childhood conditions as chronic illnesses. Because a large proportion of women spoke only Spanish, they may have substantially underreported the chronic conditions of their children.[83]

De la Rosa also reports that migrant workers in Ohio have a variety of health problems, including respiratory ailments, diseases of the digestive system, skin problems, and disorders of the nervous system.[84] In Michigan, migrants experience higher rates of tuberculosis, diarrhea, hepatitis, and gastrointestinal disorders. In addition, migrant workers have an average life expectancy at birth of under 50 years.[85]

The health picture that emerges is quite alarming, especially with respect to child mortality. This is particularly disconcerting because babies born to Mexican and Central and South American mothers are no more likely to be of low birth weight than babies born to white, non-Hispanic women. Given that the incidence of low birth weight is quite favorable for most Hispanic groups,[86] especially for Mexican-Americans (5.6%), Cubans (5.9%), and Puerto Ricans (9.4%), other factors must account for higher child mortality among migrant children in the Midwest. One could speculate that poor living conditions may be a cause. Further discussion of the health status of Hispanic children is presented in Chapter 6.

HISPANIC DEMOGRAPHIC TRENDS IN THE 1990S

As we approach the beginning of a new century, population scholars foresee significant demographic trends in the 1990s relative to U.S. Hispanics. Valdivieso and Davis have outlined several broad trends:[87]

1. The Hispanic population will continue to grow more rapidly than the U.S. population. This growth will be fueled by a young age structure, high fertility rates, and immigration.

2. Projections show a Hispanic population of nearly 29 million by the year 2000.

3. The growth of the Hispanic population will not be spread evenly, with numbers of Cubans likely to decline (due to a low fertility rate and a low rate of immigration) and numbers of Central Americans likely to increase.

4. Better educated, upper-class Hispanics may immigrate to the United States if political and economic problems worsen. Recently introduced immigration legislation suggests that the United States may be more receptive to wealthier immigrants in the 1990s. Several social, demographic, and economic trends within the United States may also encourage the immigration of more Hispanics. The proposed Simpson-Kennedy immigration bill would expand the percentage of immigrants who enter the country for work-related reasons and limit those entering under family reunification provisions. This legislation may reflect the thinking about immigration policy that will dominate the 1990s.

5. Hispanics will become a more potent force in politics and business, particularly in California, Texas, Florida, and New York.

Valdivieso and Davis acknowledge that as long as much of the growth in the Hispanic population is due to immigration of refugees and unskilled workers, the overall socioeconomic status of Hispanics will remain low. But this may mask the significant upward mobility of many earlier Hispanic immigrants who have already entered mainstream American society. Chávez also argues that data on Hispanics are often misleading because they do not distinguish between long-term residents and new arrivals.[88] The newly arrived Hispanics, generally poor, unskilled, and uneducated, create a statistical bottom that diminishes awareness of the advances by other Hispanic citizens and long-term residents.

In view of the increasing numbers of Hispanics, Valdivieso and Davis suggest that policymakers should seek ways to

Ease Hispanics' transition into mainstream society

Increase their productivity through improved education and training

Encourage their participation in the decision-making and political processes.

Valdivieso and Davis help us conclude this chapter with their statement that "perhaps the recognition that improving the position of Hispanics is in the best interest of all Americans offers policy makers the best incentive to focus more attention on Hispanic concerns. . . ."[89]

SUMMARY

This chapter has provided an overview of the Hispanic migrant experience in a nation of immigrants. Issues of ethnocentrism and fear of difference, as well as the historically important role played, and being currently played, by America as a nation of immigrants and thus as a multicultural nation, were also briefly presented.

The thrust of the chapter centered on the migration history of individual Hispanic groups, for understanding the migration history of the different groups is the basis for understanding the overall Hispanic experience in America. The level of presentation was descriptive rather than analytical, as the idea was to provide "flavor" and to highlight the major stages of the Hispanic migration.

The second and most important goal of this chapter was to provide a demographic picture of the diversity of the Hispanic population and to recognize common bonds and similarities among Hispanics. The definition of who is Hispanic according to the U.S. Census, as opposed to how Hispanics define themselves, may contribute to the achievement of these goals. The summary of U.S.-Hispanic demographic trends in the 1990s reveals the necessity of continuing efforts to improve the quality of life for Hispanics in America.

NOTES

1. Handlin, O., *Newcomers* (Boston: Harvard University Press, 1959).
2. A. M. Greely, *Why can't they be like us?* (New York: Institute of Human Relations Press, American Jewish Committee, 1969).
3. Ibid.
4. R. C. Wood, Foreword, in A. M. Greely, ibid.
5. E. N. Todhunter, in M. E. Lowenberg, et al., *Food and people,* 3rd ed. (New York: Wiley, 1979).
6. Greely, *Why can't they be like us?*
7. R. A. Mohl, An ethnic boiling pot: Cubans and Haitians in Miami. *Journal of Ethnic Studies, 13* (1985), 51–74.
8. Clarence Senior, *The Puerto Ricans— Strangers—Then neighbors* (Chicago, Quadrangle Books, 1965).
9. Greely, *Why can't they be like us?*
10. Senior, *Puerto Ricans.*
11. Jobs and poverty increase for Hispanic Americans. *New York Times,* November 8, 1991.
12. Clara E. Rodríguez, *Puerto Ricans—Born in the U.S.A.* (Boulder, CO: Westview Press, 1991).
13. N. R. McKenney, A. R. Cresce, and P. A. Johnson, Development of the race and ethnic items for the 1990 census, paper presented at the 1988 annual meeting of the Population Association of America, New Orleans, April 1988.
14. Rodríguez, *Puerto Ricans.*
15. Miguel Rojas Mix, *Reinventing identity,* NACLA Report on the Americas, Columbian Quincentenary, 24, February 5, 1991.
16. "Identity" as defined by Webster is the "fact of being a specific person or thing." Rojas Mix defines identity as "who we are and what culture we belong to . . ."
17. Rojas Mix, *Reinventing identity.*
18. Ibid.
19. Ibid.
20. U.S. Bureau of the Census, U.S. Department of Commerce. Economics and Statistics Administration, *Race Hispanic origin,* 1990 Census Profile, no. 2, June 1991; also F. L. Schick and R. Schick, *Statistical handbook on U.S. Hispanics* (Phoenix, AZ: Oryx Press, 1991).
21. R. Valdivieso and C. Davis, *U.S. Hispanics: Challenging issues for the 1990s.* Population Trends and Public Policy, Population Reference Bureau, no. 17, December 1988.
22. Ibid.
23. Midwest Consortium for Latino Research, Illinois makes top ten lists for Latino population growth. *Michigan State University Quarterly Newsletter, 1*(3) (Fall 1991).
24. Valdivieso and Davis, *U.S. Hispanics.*
25. Most of the 1980 and 1990 census data included in this section were published in Bureau of the Census press release CB-91-100, March 11, 1991, and 1990 Census Profile, no. 2, June 1991.
26. B. Herrick, *Urban migration and economic development in Chile* (Cambridge, MA: MIT Press, 1965).
27. Ibid.
28. S. Black and D. Sanjur, Nutrition in Río Piedras: A study of internal migration and maternal diets. *Ecology of Food and Nutrition, 10*(25), (1980).
29. More Mexican women, casting off traditional warp, join flow to U.S. *New York Times,* June 7, 1992.
30. John Burma, ed., *Mexican-Americans in the United States* (Cambridge, MA: Schenkman, 1970).
31. P. B. Acosta and R. Aranda, Cultural determinants of food habits in children of Mexican descent in California. In *Practices of low-income families in feeding infants and small children.* HEW Pub. [HSA] 75-5605 (Washington, DC: U.S. Government Printing Office, issued 1972, reprinted 1975).
32. This section draws heavily from Vernez and Ronfeldt. For additional information on this topic, see E. Galarza, *Merchants of labor: The Mexican bracero history* (Charlotte, VA: NcNally and Loftin, 1964); L. A. Cardoso, *Mexican immigration to the United States* (Tucson: University of Arizona Press, 1980); and U.S. Department of Justice, *Statistical yearbook of the Immigration and Naturalization Service, 1943 to 1988* (Washington, DC: U.S. Government Printing Office, 1989).
33. G. Vernez and R. Ronfeldt, The current situation in Mexican immigration. *Science, 251* (March 1991), 4498.

34. S. Sassen-Koob, Formal and informal associations: Dominicans and Colombians in New York. *International Migration Review*, 13(2) (1979), 314–332.

35. Throughout Latin America, including the Caribbean, a fairly common occurrence is to rear other people's children as one's own. These children are known as *hijos de crianza* and they usually are taken as part of one's family, particularly by a godparent, or if they become orphans, by a close relative of their parents. *Hijos de crianza* are also not legally eligible to immigrate.

36. V. Garrison and C. T. Weiss, Dominican family networks and U.S. immigration policy: A case study. *International Migration Review*, 13(2) (1979), 264–283.

37. Jean Tiffany, Dietary patterns and nutritional status of immigrant women from the Dominican Republic living in New York City, masters thesis, Cornell University, May 1984.

38. G. T. Kurian, *Encyclopedia of the third world*, Vol. I (New York: Facts on File, 1987).

39. Margaret M. Mort, Effects of women's characteristics, household characteristics, and food acquisition practices on the dietary practices and nutritional status of rural Dominican women, masters thesis, Cornell University, January 1990.

40. UNICEF, *The state of the world's children, 1987* (New York: Oxford University Press, 1993).

41. *Unemployment* refers to the process of actively seeking work and being unable to find it; *underemployment* refers to working at a level below one's capacity or technical skills. For example, a physician working as a lab technician or a certified teacher working as a teacher's aide could be considered underemployed.

42. Mort, Effects of women's characteristics.

43. UNICEF, *State of the world's children*.

44. A. Ugalde, F. D. Bean, and G. Cárdenas, International migration from the Dominican Republic: Findings from a national survey. *International Migration Review*, 13(2) (1979), 235–254.

45. Tiffany, Dietary patterns.

46. Ugaldi, Bean, and Cárdenas, International migration.

47. Tiffany, Dietary patterns.

48. M. C. Sandoval, Cultural contributions of the Cuban migrations into south Florida. In A. Jorge et al. (eds.), *Cuban exiles in Florida: Their presence and contributions* (Miami: University of Miami, 1991), pp. 14–37.

49. A. Portes and R. Mozo, The political adaptation process of Cubans and other ethnic minorities in the United States: A preliminary analysis. *International Migration Review*, 1(35) (1985), 35–63.

50. R. L. Bach, *Migration as an issue in U.S.-Cuban relations*, Occasional Paper no. 29, School of Advanced International Studies, John Hopkins University, March 1988.

51. Ibid.

52. Juan M. Clark, The social impact of Cuban immigration in Florida. In A. Jorge et al. (eds.), *Cuban exiles in Florida: Their presence and contributions* (Miami: University of Miami, 1991), pp. 39–61.

53. Juan M. Clark, Los cubanos de Miami: Cuántos son y de donde provienen. *Ideal* (Miami), July 1973.

54. Mohl, An ethnic boiling pot.

55. Milton M. Gordon, *Assimilation in American life* (Cambridge: Oxford University Press, 1964), pp. 60–83.

56. Linda Chávez. *Out of the barrio: Toward a new politics of Hispanic assimilation* (New York: Basic Books, 1991).

57. Portes and Mozo, Political adaptation process.

58. Sandoval, Cultural contribution.

59. A. Jorge and J. Salazar-Carrillo, The contribution of Cuban exiles to the Florida economy. In A. Jorge et al. (eds.), *Cuban exiles in Florida: Their presence and contributions* (Miami: University of Miami, 1991).

60. Mohl, An ethnic boiling pot.

61. Adolfo L. De Varona, The political impact of Cuban-Americans in south Florida. In A. Jorge et al. (eds.), *Cuban exiles in Florida: Their presence and contributions* (Miami: University of Miami, 1991).

62. Ibid.

63. Sandoval, Cultural contributions.

64. Rodríguez, *Puerto Ricans*.

65. A. Stevens-Arroyo and A. M. Dìaz Stevens, Puerto Ricans in the States: A struggle for identity. In A. G. Dworkin and R. J. Dworkin (eds.), *The minority report: An introduction to racial, ethnic, and gender relations*, 2nd ed. (New York: CBS College Publishing/Holt, Rinehart & Winston, 1982).

66. Edwin Maldonado, Contract labor and the origin of Puerto Rican communities in

the United States. *International Migration Review, 13* (1979), 103–121.

67. Rodríguez, *Puerto Ricans.*

68. José L. Vázquez Calzada, *La población de Puerto Rico y su trayectoria histórica,* Universidad de Puerto Rico, Recinto de Ciencias Médicas, May 1988.

69. John Steinbeck, *The Grapes of Wrath* (New York: Viking Penguin, 1989).

70. Stevens-Arroyo and Díaz Stevens, *Puerto Ricans.*

71. *White House Conference on Food, Nutrition and Health* (Washington, DC: Section on Migratory Labor, 1970).

72. Vernez and Ronfeldt, The current situation.

73. T. Seidl, J. Shenk, and A. DeWind, The San Juan shuttle: Puerto Ricans on contract. In Adalberto López (ed.), *The Puerto Ricans: Their history, culture and society* (Cambridge, MA: Schenkman, 1980).

74. Ibid.

75. Rodríguez, *Puerto Ricans.*

76. Maldonado, Contract labor.

77. Rodríguez, *Puerto Ricans.*

78. Seidl et al., San Juan shuttle.

79. Ibid.

80. Roberto E. Torres, *Health status assessment of Latinos in the Midwest,* Working Paper no. 5, Julian Samora Research Institute, Michigan State University, July 1990.

81. D. P. Slesinger, *Health needs of migrant workers in Wisconsin* (Madison: Department of Rural Sociology, University of

Wisconsin Extension Center, 1979); D. P. Slesinger and E. Cautley, Medical utilization patterns of Hispanic migrant farmworkers in Wisconsin. *Public Health Reports,* 96 (1981), 255–263; D. P. Slesinger, Health status of Wisconsin's migrant agricultural workers. *As You Sow, 19* (1988).

82. Slesinger, *Health needs.*

83. D. P. Slesinger, B. A. Christenson, and E. Cautley, Health and mortality of migrant farm children. *Social Science and Medicine, 23* (1986), 65–74.

84. M. De la Rosa, Health care needs of Hispanic Americans and the responsiveness of the health care system. *Health and Social Work, 14* (1989), 104–113.

85. R. I. Rochin, A. M. Santiago, and K. S. Dickey, *Migrant and seasonal workers in Michigan's agriculture: A study of their contributions, characteristics, needs, and services,* Research Report no. 1, Julian Samora Research Institute, Michigan State University, 1989.

86. S. J. Ventura, *The health and development of Puerto Rican mothers and children in the mainland,* presentation at conference, Brown University, Providence, RI, November 1990.

87. Valdivieso and Davis, *U.S. Hispanics.*

88. Chávez, *Out of the barrio.*

89. Valdivieso and Davis, *U.S. Hispanics.*

2

Hispanic Food Habits: Women, Nutrition, and Health Concerns

Persistence of Cultural Effects on Food Habits

Understanding Food Habits and Ethnicity
What Is Meant by Food Habits?
What Is Meant by Ethnicity?
The Multiple Meanings of Food
What Characterizes Staple Foods or Traditional Diets?
The Cultural Acceptance of Foods: Implications for Change
Changing Food Habits, or Food Influencing Change?

Food Ideology Systems
Etiology of Hispanic Food and Folk Medicine Beliefs
How Is Health and Nutrition Valued by Hispanics?
Reasoning Underlying Some Food Ideologies
Food Ideologies during Pregnancy and Lactation
Traditional Methods of Weaning
Breast-feeding "Principles"
Subcultural Variations
Implications for Health Practitioners

Women and Nutrition:
Linkages between Education and Work
The Concept of Women's Empowerment
Women and Nutrition
Women and Education
Women and Work
Women's Workload and Time Use
Female-headed Households
Women and Health

PERSISTENCE OF CULTURAL EFFECTS ON FOOD HABITS

All humans require the same basic nutrients, yet the foods that supply these nutrients are as different as the environments in which people exist and the cultures through which people have adapted to their environments. The consequences of food intake are biological; individual biological functioning is affected by food intake over the course of a lifetime. But the nature of food intake—what people eat, how, when, where, and how much—is heavily influenced by socioeconomic and cultural processes.

The reciprocity between humans and their environment involves the intersection of biological needs with physical, social, and cultural environments. And thus there is little doubt that the environmental changes occurring in many societies today have profound biological as well as social consequences, with particular reference to maintaining traditional food habits. Take, for example, the so-called urbanization or industrialization effect, which had its beginnings in the spread of urban values and attitudes, especially among migrating populations. The transfer of underdevelopment and poverty from a rural to an urban setting can be stressful and unhealthy among newcomers to an urban setting.

The early part of this chapter reviews and elaborates on general concepts regarding food habits and ethnicity and interactions between the concepts. The persistence of cultural effects on food habits is addressed, along with some symbolic meanings of food and food ideology systems.

Latino communities in the United States have identified the *ineffectiveness of monocultural models* used by health care professionals as a major problem of health care delivery systems in the United States (see Chapter 6, Table 6.1). Therefore this chapter reviews some basic information about ethnicity and food habits in order to assist health practitioners to deliver more culturally sensitive and relevant health and nutrition messages. The other major problem identified by Latino communities, *lack of access to medical services and health promotion efforts*, is also discussed in Chapter 6. Other contemporary issues, such as the role of women in the nutrition of families, the effect of maternal education and employment, and the effect of female-headed households are also briefly discussed.

What, why, and how often human populations eat depend on many factors, but most important is where people live. In a large portion of the developing world, food is mostly consumed where it is produced. Household purchasing power is also a major influence on dietary patterns. But beyond these physical and economic determinants, food habits are fundamentally cultural. An individual's cultural background and orientation, in conjunction with personal characteristics, ultimately determine his or her dietary pattern.

Given the cultural determinants of food habits, it is useful to review briefly certain attributes of culture and to consider their nutritional implications, especially in regard to modifying dietary patterns:

One important attribute of culture is that *culture is learned rather than biologically determined.* Cultural behavior is the product of interaction among generations of men and women, and it always changes over time. The notion that culture is learned also implies that it can be unlearned.

Change is another attribute of culture, and cultural processes change at different rates. Food habits are an example of a dynamic cultural process, always changing. All cultures resist change by self-generated mechanisms that perpetuate cultural traits and maintain boundaries. (*Boundary maintenance* is the reaffirmation of ethnicity by engaging in cultural activities—use of traditional foods and customs, celebration of holidays, etc.—in order to help distinguish and clarify boundaries between cultural groups.) Food habits, like all cultural habits, although far from fixed, are also resistant to change.

UNDERSTANDING FOOD HABITS AND ETHNICITY

What Is Meant by Food Habits?

A conventional definition of food habits is the "way in which individuals or groups of individuals in response to both physical and sociocultural situations, select, consume and utilize portions of the available food supply. . . ."[1] Another way of defining food habits in more operational terms is by viewing their development as being conditioned by what the environment produces and by what cultural traditions dictate as edible. Thus food habits, which include consumption, preference, and ideology of any population group, are basically the product of two major forces:

1. *Physical availability of food:* People eat what they can get from the environment.
2. *Cultural availability of food:* Given a choice, people eat what their ancestors ate.

Although indigenous food habits of any population group are deeply rooted in local environment as well as local culture, food habits constantly change and are influenced by many factors. Thus traditional foodways are a dual process: rigid and resisting change but also dynamic and always changing. These dual characteristics make the modification of food habits a challenging and complex process.

Ethnicity is an important factor in patterning and modifying dietary intake. In the following sections conceptual definitions of ethnicity, symbolic meanings of foods as a reaffirmation of ethnic identity, and the dual impact of culture and ethnicity on food intake are discussed to gain further appreciation of the underlying sociocultural bases of ethnicity and food habits.

The importance for health practitioners to understand the overlap between culture and ethnicity was highlighted in the national report, *Healthy People 2000,* which contends that improving the health of all Americans depends on improving the health of certain groups that are at high risk.[2] The report encourages health practitioners to understand the needs of these special groups in order to target health programs to meet their needs. The report also states that general characteristics used to define populations can be dangerous because exceptions are many. The challenge is to refine knowledge and understanding of different cultural groups so that health policies can be translated into effective community-based prevention programs and clinical preventive services.

What Is Meant by Ethnicity?

Weber defines an ethnic group as a "human collectivity based on an assumption of common origin—real or imaginary."[3] Others refer to ethnic groups as a group of people who share a similar cultural and regional origin, hold common norms and beliefs, and form part of a larger population, interacting with people from other segments of society.[4] Barth categorizes ethnic groups as those sharing the following criteria:[5]

Members share fundamental cultural values and norms that differ from other groups making up the larger population or nation.

Members communicate and interact together, reaffirming their ethnic identity.

Members and others recognize the group as distinguishable from other groups.

Most definitions of ethnic groups stress the "distinct sense of culture which is fostered by an individuals' participation in or identification with a specified group."[6] *The sense of sharing is the ethnic identity.* The concept of ethnic groups represents ties deeply rooted with a sense of "blood and land." Being a member of an ethnic group has different implications, depending on whether a person is first-, second-, third-, or fourth-generation. A first-generation Mexican-American, for example, was born in Mexico; second-, third-, or fourth-generation Mexican-Americans were born in and grew up in the United States.

Often many members of an ethnic group settle in the same section of a community (for example, Puerto Ricans in the South Bronx, New York, or Cubans in Little Havana, Florida), making the group highly visible. Ethnic members living in those areas are likely to share many common cultural characteristics, ensuring that cultural ways become even more pervasive and deeply rooted. Conversely, members of ethnic groups who live outside such enclaves are more likely to adopt the cultural ways of the dominant society and may eventually lose their cultural boundaries. In other words, as individuals become more assimilated, they eventually lose their cultural traits and ethnic distinctiveness. Ethnic food habits, like other aspects of culture, change as a result of this contact.[7]

Migrant ethnic groups can play positive and negative roles. Among the positive roles, ethnic groups help to

1. Keep cultural traditions alive

2. Provide preferred associates

3. Contribute to primary, secondary, and tertiary sectors of the economy

4. Offer other recent immigrants opportunity for mobility and success

5. Enable men and women to identify themselves in the face of threatening chaos of a large impersonal urban society

Conversely, ethnic groups can also

1. Create exclusiveness and isolation

2. Reinforce suspicion, distrust, and resentment, which serve as foci for conflict

3. Adhere firmly to traditional ways, thus preventing members from seeking new alternatives

The overlap between food habits and ethnicity is so pervasive that food habits are viewed by many as cultural markers of ethnicity. Brown and Mussell note that foodways in subcultural groups "bind individuals together, define the limits of identity, and celebrate cultural cohesion."[8]

One common pitfall among nutrition researchers insufficiently trained in cultural anthropological methods is to categorize any change in dietary patterns of an immigrant group as an early indication that ethnic food patterns are disappearing. Dietary changes have often been measured by examining the use or nonuse of ethnic dishes or specific food items by different generations of immigrants. In this respect, Brown and Mussell caution that foodways research relative to issues of persistence and change may be addressed more fruitfully if a broader, multifaceted measure of acculturation is employed. Rather than using single measures of food items or traditional dishes to measure dietary change among members of an ethnic group, researchers should also examine meal cycles, use of traditional foods during holidays, or other related variables.

The Multiple Meanings of Food

Another significant point has to do with the cultural meanings that underlie culture-specific behavior relative to foods and traditions. Ethnic pride—translated into an internal perspective of being the only members of a particular ethnic group who know authentically how to prepare the food—becomes a strong element of cohesiveness and identity among immigrant groups.[9]

What Characterizes Staple Foods or Traditional Diets?

Central to issues related to dietary change and continuity among migrant groups are characteristics of staple foods and traditional diets. Flores characterizes food patterns as static and dynamic with respect to the ease with which they are modified.[10] More static food patterns are associated with consumption of staple foods. For example, static patterns are commonly associated with farming systems that are strongly traditional. Consumption of staple foods is difficult to change because their use is deeply embedded in the cultural values of a society.

Flores notes that in the rural areas of Central America, for instance, maize has persisted as a staple food for many centuries, and it has always been the major crop. For the cultivation of maize, people still use the same implements and follow the same methods as their ancestors. Furthermore, the process of converting maize into food has not changed since the time of the ancient Mayan civilization. Similarly, in various Central American countries, yams and cassava, supplemented with rice, corn, and bananas, have remained the staple items; people still use the same implements and methods of cultivation as in times past. No changes in the preparation of these foods have been observed for many centuries; prolonged boiling and roasting of tubers and bananas continue undisturbed.

The Cultural Acceptance of Foods: Implications for Change

Culture has a pervasive influence on human diets. In the modern American culture, insects, horses, frogs, and reptiles are not defined as edible, but they are highly esteemed foods in other cultures. Indeed, iguanas are consumed frequently, and turtles and armadillos to a lesser extent, in many rural communities of Panama. Not only does culture influence what is defined as food, but it also influences how food should be prepared. For example, people in different cultures prepare meat and fish in different ways. Some Americans prefer beef rare or almost raw; most Hispanics prefer it well done. Peruvians and Panamanians enjoy fish raw in a dish known as *ceviche* (raw, marinated seafood, with generous amounts of onions and hot pepper). Hispanics like dried meat, as the Mexican *machaca* (dry, salted meat, shredded by pounding) or the Panamanian *tasajo* (sliced dried beef).

The "cultural availability" of a given food also carries significance relative to sources of the food, ways of eating it, methods of preparation, and cooking techniques. Cultural acceptability is also related to eating schedule, order of dishes served, and even age- and gender-specific foods. According to Bourges, in Latin America, in general, it is not acceptable to have soup for breakfast (except in Colombia, where soups and broths are enjoyed for breakfast) or to serve dessert as the first dish, or to serve bony fish to a child.[11]

In short, food habits are conditioned by both the physical availability of food (kinds and quantity, for people cannot eat what is not there) and cultural availability of the food (what a society deems "edible, harmful, or unacceptable").

What a particular cultural group considers "edible" food, regardless of its scientific or nutritional characteristics, carries tremendous importance for that group. Passim and Bennett proposed a classical food categorization scheme several years ago, distinguishing frequency of consumption and importance of foods, that is still useful:[12]

> **1.** *Core foods* are universal, regular, staple, important, and consistently used.
>
> **2.** *Secondary foods* are widespread but not universally consumed. They are more variable in use and form, less important emotionally, and include recently introduced store-bought foods.
>
> **3.** *Peripheral foods* are the least common foods, infrequent in occurrence. Their use is characteristic of individuals rather than groups; they are often very recent additions to the diet, and their use may be stimulated by specific economic conditions.

From a practical point of view, these distinctions help predict that the greatest emotional resistance to dietary change will be encountered in the core foods. Core foods have a special emotional meaning for individuals and the community; sometimes they are invested with religious or magical connotations. People do not tire easily of core foods, and they are difficult to substitute for in the diet. In most cultures, cereals and grains are considered core foods. Cereals and grains provide the most abundant and cheapest energy source (even though many people may not consciously prefer them for these reasons).

Because secondary foods carry less emotional meaning than core items, they may be easier to replace in the diet. Peripheral foods have very limited emotional significance, and because people are less attached to them, they can be substituted for with minimum effort.

Changing Food Habits, or Foods Influencing Change?

A number of sociotechnological, political, and economic changes also impact and dramatically change certain food habits. Take, for example, developments in food technology and processing. The phenomenal growth of the fast-food industry and the large number of fast-food establishments attest to these changes. Similarly, vending machines are increasing in number and appearing in office buildings, stores, hospitals, institutions, airports—wherever people eat.

Also, note that the increased use of convenience foods reflects modern lifestyles that place high value on newness, saving time, and variety. Similarly, other changes in lifestyles, including women working outside the home, may mean that other family members become more responsible for their own diets. The extended family has been gradually replaced by a highly mobile nuclear family, with nonrelated members, in which eating can be and is an individual, nonscheduled event.

Lastly, increased food advertising has also contributed to exposure to and acceptance of new foods. Television, radio, newspapers, and magazines, all common in homes today, have encouraged people to buy new and different foods.

How these societal forces have affected the nutrition and health behavior of the Hispanic migrant population, and even more important, how they have affected the continuity of traditional diets vis-à-vis the adoption of new foods and dishes, are addressed in subsequent chapters.

FOOD IDEOLOGY SYSTEMS

A *food ideology system* is a set of ideas, attitudes, and beliefs that affects diet and nutrition. Whereas attitudes have been classified as *affective* (one may feel for or against something), beliefs serve as *cognitive* elements of attitudes. Therefore a person may "believe in" or have a "belief about" the existence of a thing or event or have a "belief about" the way in which it exists. Thus, if a person gets information so that the probability of an event's existence is increased, she or he then develops a belief in this event. A food belief is something thought to be true by those adhering to it. It can be *restrictive,* as when Panamanian children "avoid eating too many mangoes because they cause diarrhea," or it can be *prescriptive,* as when Mexican lactating women drink boiled milk to produce more breast milk.

This section summarizes selected issues relative to food ideology systems not just to give a "flavor" of this issue; its main purpose is to help health and nutrition practitioners become aware of the importance of food ideology on food choices and to take it into consideration when designing health and nutrition education programs, particularly those for dietary change. Health practitioners should explore food belief systems by asking: (1) how strong or weak are mothers' specific adherence or commitment to these belief systems? and (2) what are the health and nutrition consequences, from a biomedical point of view, of the beliefs that mothers follow?

Etiology of Hispanic Food and Folk Medicine Beliefs

Food and folk medicine beliefs and practices are often inextricably combined in an extensive, complex web of cultural beliefs and attitudes. The etiology of folk medicine in Latin America has emerged from classical Spanish medicine theory as well as from American Indian and *mestizo* cultures. (*Mestizo* refers to the mixture of European white and American Indian cultures.)

The most important single set of ideas governing food-related behavior in some rural societies of Latin America is a folk manifestation known as the "hot-cold dichotomy." In brief, foods, herbs, illnesses, and bodily states are characterized by degree of "hot" or "cold." However, this hot-cold concept is not related to the food's actual temperature but, rather, to innate, symbolic qualities of each food that are unclear to outsiders. Usually, the female members of the community learn from their elders and peer group the classification of each food. Because foods are believed to be intimately involved in the general conception of health and disease, almost any degree of illness leads to the withdrawal of certain foods from a child's diet.

Although Mexican and Puerto Rican dietaries differ, Cassidy notes that many people in both cultures rely on the hot-cold theory of health to select food. She illustrates the hot-cold dichotomy by noting that "a good meal provides a balance, and a person can get sick by eating foods whose temperatures are wrong for him or her. A pregnant women is 'hot'—hence she must avoid both very 'hot' (chili peppers, salty, fatty, sweet) foods and very 'cold' (acidic, sour, fresh lemons, tomatoes, or watermelon) foods."[13]

How Is Health and Nutrition Valued by Hispanics?

There are contradictory reports about how Latin Americans value food, nutrition, and health. Some investigators contend that in Central and South America food is valued as conducive to good health and strength. People have a real desire to eat well, if funds permit, and to spend any extra money on food rather than on other goods, such as clothes, jewelry, livestock, or land.

Other researchers report that some traditional systems of medicine recognize a personal responsibility to avoid ill health. Similarly, some have noted that, at least in some parts of Central America, there seems to be a useful empiricism in a mother's attitude as to what her child can and cannot eat. Each child in the family is treated individually, and food is not withheld from one child because it seemed to disagree with another. Furthermore, it has also been observed that in Central America pregnant women are encouraged to eat well and to drink strengthening gruels and *caldos* (beef or chicken broths) during lactation. In very remote traditional rural areas, lactating mothers are encouraged to consume these *caldos* for 40 consecutive days postpartum.

Some investigators note that although Latin American villagers know that food is related to health and illness, they tend to see this relationship in a negative rather than positive fashion. They argue that Latin peasants have little idea that a balanced diet promotes good health; rather, people who enjoy good health are believed able to eat what they want and can afford. Conversely, during illness, foods that are thought to cause conflict with the equilibrium of the body and to cause the illness are withheld. A description of the pattern of feeding practices in a Guatemalan village seems to agree with these observations. It is reported that people in this village fed their children well, "not to make them healthy, but because they are healthy . . ."[14] A good appetite is associated with health; however, children are not forced to eat foods that they resist because their preferences are respected.

Reasoning Underlying Some Food Ideologies

Health values underlie certain food and feeding habits among Latin American families. Cravioto has reported that cow's milk sometimes is not given to small Mexican children because a mother or grandmother observed that it caused diarrhea.[15] Although observation of diarrhea following milk consumption was valid in this Mexican community, the mother did not know that the bacterial contamination of the milk was the agent and not the milk per se.

Cravioto notes that these Mexican families used empirical reasoning, in the absence of knowledge on the microbial theory of disease, to establish their own cause-and-effect relationship between certain foods and diseases. An unfortunate consequence of this is that foods of high protein value are the ones said to be harmful to small children and thus are omitted from the diet. This "fear of food" is the result of careful observations over several generations. A list of harmful foods is passed on from mother to daughter as part of the knowledge and practice of "nutrition education."

Food restrictions may also be related to nonmodern scientific concepts of body physiology. In Peruvian villages, the belief that the child's stomach is not fully formed during the first year, and thus cannot handle certain foods, has been reported. The appropriateness of various foods and the time at which they are first offered to the child vary greatly among individual families.

Food Ideologies during Pregnancy and Lactation

In Latin America, desires for particular foods or foods prepared in a certain way are called *antojos*. There is a widespread belief that unfulfilled desires of pregnant women may result in birthmarks. In general, although few restrictions are imposed on pregnant women, they are legion after birth.[16]

Whether or not a woman believes she can become pregnant while lactating sometimes has a bearing, one way or another, on the length of time she will breast-feed her child. A number of years ago Sanjur et al. reported that rural Mexican mothers were almost equally divided in their opinion as to the effect of lactation on possible impregnation.[17] Almost half the women stated unequivocally that they could not get pregnant while breast-feeding, and a little over half believed, or "knew through experience," that they could conceive while lactating. A few others remarked, "*Lo que Dios quiera* (it depends on God's will); there is not a set rule for this; some women get pregnant while others do not. . . ."[18] That prolonged breast feeding has a contraceptive function is a widely held belief in many parts of the world that affects length of lactation.

Traditional Methods of Weaning

The reasons for stopping breast feeding in many parts of the world vary, but traditionally cessation is dictated by the onset of another pregnancy. It is widely believed that if pregnancy occurs, breast milk will become "harmful" or "poisonous" to the suckling child. Separating the child from the breast is sometimes accomplished by applying bitter or unpleasant substances to the breast. In one Mexican village, use of *sábila*, a plant with bitter leaves, was the most frequently reported method.[19] Use of charcoal ashes, hot pepper, tomato, lemon, corn dough, and garlic was also mentioned. Usually these practices were accompanied by an explanation from the mother telling the child that the nipple was "dirty" or "hot." The mothers reported that in most cases one to three applications of these substances was sufficient.

Another traditional method of weaning was preventing the child from finding the breast. To do this, mothers sleep with their clothes on, tie a towel around their breasts, or simply avoid sleeping with the child.

The pervasiveness of these traditional attitudes and practices cannot be overemphasized. There are similarities in the principles of breast feeding and weaning with those reported by Millard and Graham, almost two decades later.

Breast-feeding "Principles"

Millard and Graham characterized Mexican women's explanations of their lactational behaviors and decisions as "principles" rather than beliefs because they were based on how these women regarded lactation and child development.[20] The researchers studied two small farming communities in the Valley of Mexico, 15 kilometers apart. One community was inhabited by Spanish-speaking mestizos whose main income was derived from wages earned in urban areas. The other village was inhabited by Nahuatl-speaking Indians, descendants of the Aztecs, who derived their income mainly from agriculture. Yet, despite these differences, women of both villages shared a number of principles that guided weaning practices. Incidentally, weaning was seen as "a process requiring maternal effort and discipline, and its objective was to maintain each child's health . . ."[21]

These weaning principles are summarized as follows:

1. Colostrum is unhealthy for babies, and breast feeding should start at the appearance of true, "healthful" milk.

2. Babies with teeth should no longer breast-feed because they are mature enough to eat weaning foods.

3. Prolonged breast feeding produces an ill-mannered child.

4. Combining mother's milk and other food makes a child sick, so weaning should not be done gradually.

5. Lactation should cease when the mother again becomes pregnant; continued nursing damages the fetus.

6. Lactating or pregnant women should avoid emotional stress, because it can lower the quantity or quality of her breast milk and endanger the infant's health.

7. Animal milk is unhealthy for babies and should not be given to them.

Subcultural Variations

Because certain beliefs about food and folk medicine are more pervasive in some Hispanic subcultural groups than in others, nutritionists and other health practitioners need to be careful not to assume that all Hispanic mothers strongly adhere to the same beliefs. For instance, though many grandmothers and older mothers may still classify foods as "hot," "neutral," or "cold," younger, more urbanized mothers may view this classification as old-fashioned. These women would be offended if a health worker assumed that they followed such "traditional, backward" ways. The following examples illustrate this point.

A number of years ago, Harwood, in a stimulating and much cited study among Puerto Ricans in New York City, contended that medications, too, have inherent temperatures, and that a woman may refuse to take "hot" medicines, such as iron supplements, during her pregnancy.[22] Conversely, Lieberman, in a study of New England Puerto Rican mothers, reported that they sought prenatal care and were quite compliant with medical instructions.[23] Furthermore, Kay found that her sample of pregnant southwestern Mexican-Americans regularly saw a doctor and took prescribed vitamins and minerals faithfully.[24] No traditional folk beliefs were reported among the last two groups.

Implications for Health Practitioners

A recent report on breast feeding and weaning in Mexico and the United States calls for health professionals to consider that "folk wisdom" and reasons for terminating breast feeding may conflict with established health doctrines.[25] Prescientific notions of food, health, and folk medicine held by a large number of rural women in Latin American countries may strongly influence the way in which they feed their families.[26] In sum, four important points about food ideology systems among Hispanic families should be considered: (1) to adherents of the "hot-cold" belief system, foods are medicines; (2) different Hispanic subcultural groups vary in their practice of food ideologies; (3) traditionally held beliefs may be a function of age or rural/urban origin; and (4) health practitioners must understand and integrate biomedical beliefs with traditional Latin American belief systems in order to improve health and dietary compliance.

WOMEN AND NUTRITION: LINKAGES BETWEEN EDUCATION AND WORK

The Concept of Women's Empowerment

Throughout most of the world women have the major responsibility for their families' nutrition. Therefore any efforts to prevent malnutrition and enhance health depend substantially on women's activities, indeed, on their *empower-*

ment. We use "empowerment" here as referring to the need for women to achieve equality of status in society and in the family and an equal role in making decisions. Such empowerment often involves major changes in attitudes, institutions, and possibly laws.[27]

Kent argues that "malnutrition (both under and over-nutrition) is due to poverty, but even more fundamentally to powerlessness. . . ."[28] People who are malnourished almost always suffer the effects of decisions made by others, with more power and conflicting priorities. Women and children are relatively powerless within the household. Thus, if malnutrition has roots in powerlessness, then remedies must lie in empowerment. In Kent's view, "to be empowered is to increase your capacity to define, analyze, and act on your own problems."[29] To illustrate the relationship of powerlessness to malnutrition, Kent cites data from the U.S. National Center for Health Statistics:

1. Women, regardless of age, are more likely to be obese than men.

2. Obesity, particularly among females, is more prevalent in lower socioeconomic groups.

3. Rural populations tend to be more overweight than urban populations.

4. Blacks (and Hispanics) as a group are more likely to be obese than whites.

Evidently, Kent concludes, politically weaker groups are more likely to suffer obesity. This newer concept relating empowerment of migrant ethnic groups, women, and children to their nutritional status is an interesting and different perspective to keep in mind when reading subsequent chapters that examine intervention strategies for dietary change.

Women and Nutrition

The successful integration of women's productive and reproductive lives is the basis for child survival. As Tiffany so forcefully states:

> We learn about ourselves by understanding the forces that have shaped the experience of people in different times and in different places. We cannot afford, in this period of global interdependency, to ignore the knowledge and experiences of people in other societies, who, like ourselves, are part of the mosaic comprising the human condition. Knowledge is power, and in this book we discover the ways in which women in different societies utilize their roles as workers and childbearers to control their lives and influence the worlds in which they live . . .[30]

Because it is women who influence family food choices, they generally hold the key to improved nutritional status and health for the family, particularly for infants and children. An understanding of household dynamics and how women influence decision making, particularly as it pertains to family food choices, requires detailed investigation, especially at the household level.

A case in point is illustrated in a study conducted by Bryant among Cuban, Puerto Rican, and Anglo families in Dade County, Florida.[31] Results showed that even though males were identified as dominant family members among the Latino families, women made most of the infant feeding decisions without consulting their husbands. Moreover, Bryant points out that the maternal grandmother had a major role in deciding what to feed infants. Many new mothers consult with grandmothers about what to feed the baby, and grandmothers often help care for and feed the baby, in addition to giving advice.

In contrast, Anglo families in the study relied mostly on advice from health professionals, husbands, and friends, and the maternal grandmother had relatively little influence over infant feeding patterns. Many women explained their reluctance to seek advice from their mothers by pointing out that feeding practices have changed in the last decades and that their mothers are "too old or outdated" to provide reliable information.

The study of the role of women in nutrition demands a multidimensional approach that accounts for women's biological nutritional needs, as well as environmental and sociocultural factors that, in turn, influence nutritional status and health. These factors also affect the nutrition of women's families because women play a major role in household food production, food acquisition, food purchase, food preparation, and intrahousehold distribution. Within communities and households, forces that give an individual leverage are socially and culturally specific.[32]

Among the myriad factors affecting the role of women in nutrition, two particularly enhance women's empowerment and thus the nutritional status and health of the family: level of female education and level of maternal employment. Conversely, the increasing trend for low-income families to be female-headed has some serious implications for nutrition.

Women and Education

Increased years of schooling for females is critical to enhance women's rights and to sustain social welfare objectives, including adequate nutritional status for all. Educational level attained, if taken as a proxy for income, appears to substantially minimize urban poverty. Some argue that education provides women with important tools with which to reason and take initiative, thus providing a sense of power and control over their own lives. In short, the ties between the level of health and nutrition and educational opportunities for women are extremely important.

Mounting evidence reveals that maternal education is one of the most important predictors of child nutritional status. The educational level of women has been found to be positively correlated with the nutritional status of children in Mexico,[33] in Puerto Rico,[34] and in the Dominican Republic.[35] Children of more educated mothers have better dietary intakes in Panama.[36]

More educated women have greater occupational choices and higher productivity in the marketplace. For example, in Panama, Tucker and Sanjur found that more educated women were more likely to be employed, and that women who participated in the market economy usually had better diets for themselves and their children.[37] One caveat, however: A certain spread of educational level may be needed in order to detect the *differential effect* of maternal education on dietary status. There is a question about the point at which women's educational attainment begins to make a difference on the nutritional status of her family. For example, in Peru, maternal education did not correlate with the dietary and nutritional status of children.[38] In this study of Peruvian families who were recent internal migrants living in the low-income peripheral settlements of Lima, known as *pueblos jóvenes*, the educational level of the mothers was very low; most women had not gone beyond primary school. Possibly, at these low levels of schooling, education does not affect child nutritional status.

To understand these relationships better, and to control somewhat for confounding effects, Piwoz and Viteri suggest the need to desegregate and disentangle the effects of education from those of other social and economic conditions (i.e., parental income, women's income, and maternal health) that may influence the decision-making process in the household.[39]

It is also important to explore the underlying mechanisms through which maternal education affects the nutrition of the family. Is it through a broader exposure to diverse communication channels, as a woman attains more schooling? Is it through a greater awareness of the health needs of her family? Is it by engaging in more productive activities that improve family income and thus nutrition? Or is it through other processes? As sociomedical research relative to these issues continues, future investigations may unravel some of these important yet unresolved issues.

While awaiting answers to these significant questions, for now it appears that formal and informal education provides women with greater confidence in making decisions that improve the quality of rural and urban life in many ways. For instance, instructing mothers about the benefits of prolonged breast feeding or about low-cost, nutritious weaning foods is beneficial, if mothers have enough educational background to analyze the information effectively and decide to put it into practice. In other words, education "empowers" women to be more selective and to make more rational decisions when bombarded with sound/unsound mass media messages or when urged to comply with health and nutritional messages.

Knowledge about health and nutrition, analytical skills to make informed nutritional decisions, and changed attitudes and behaviors toward food are all part of a package that can make women better informed contributors to a modern, complex society, where survival may ultimately depend on informed choices.

Lastly, and more importantly, education as a form of investment in human capital will have its greatest impact on income. Improving the economic lot of rural and urban women will enhance their ability to become politically active, to be more assertive as consumer advocates, to engage in self-gratifying activities, to become more aware of the relation among diet, health, and chronic diseases, and to be able to purchase more nutritious and healthful foods for the family.

Women and Work

Equally important to education is increased women's access to productive resources, particularly increased income and, more significant, control over it. As women's educational and economical empowerment increases, the overall condition of the household, including the nutritional situation, usually improves. However, the effect of maternal employment on the nutritional status of children is as yet unclear and conflicting. Although maternal employment increases household income available for food expenditures, it also decreases the time available for child feeding and care.

Engle and Pedersen reviewed maternal work for earnings and children's nutritional status in urban Guatemala, distinguishing among formal, informal, and domestic work.[40] They found that the infants of domestic workers weighed less than those of nonworkers and of formal and informal workers. Although breast feeding was of shorter duration among the working mothers compared with domestic workers and nonworkers, such short duration was not associated with lower nutritional status.

Breast-feeding practices of urban domestic workers may be particularly important to study because domestic service is one major source of employment for some low-income Hispanic women and is also one work context where one might expect that the integration of productive and reproductive activities would be possible. However, in reality, constraints are often put on domestics that make it difficult, if not impossible, to breast feed while employed. As with subsistence agriculture, the assumption that these work contexts are always compatible with breast feeding must be carefully examined.[41]

Research on women's work and child nutrition   Leslie has suggested that there is a fundamental difference in the way that the "women-in-development community" and the "nutrition community" look at women's work and child nutrition.[42] Whereas the first group has focused on women rather than on mothers, the second group has focused on the mother's reproductive and child care roles.

The women-in-development community has been interested in such topics as women's role in food systems, women's need for independent income, and women's control over their earnings, and the nutritional implications of all these. The nutrition community, on the other hand, has been more interested in finding out whether working mothers spend less time caring for their children, and whether being entrusted to caretakers affects the nutritional status of children. Figure 2.1 focuses on the linkages between mothers' work outside the domestic sphere and the nutrition of their children. Ac-

FIGURE 2.1   Linkages between women's education and work and the nutrition of their children

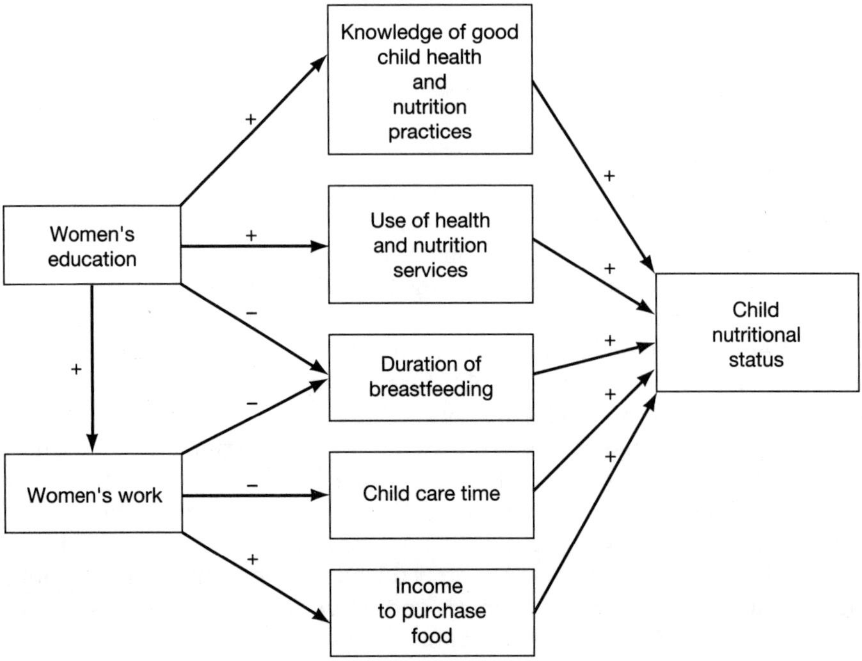

SOURCE: From Joanne Leslie, *Women's work and child nutrition in the third world* (Washington, DC: International Center for Research on Women, 1985).

cording to Leslie, the overall effect of mothers' employment on child care and feeding is influenced by both a positive effect on income and a negative effect on time for child care and feeding.

Figure 2.2 focuses on women as "nutrition intermediaries," showing factors that may affect mothers' effectiveness in the nutritional care of their children. These investigators also take into account the possibilities for help in child care. Such help often depends on the presence of older siblings or other adult women in the household. Child work, particularly caretaking of small children, is very common in developing countries, including some Latin American countries. The immediate effect of caretakers on nutrition will depend on the extent to which they take on the responsibilities of absent mothers in food preparation and feeding.[43] Van Esterik argues that women who make use of reciprocal child care among informal groups of relatives or neighbors can only work part time or sporadically because they must reciprocate by caring for other children.[44] Women need dependable, long-term child care with no reciprocal obligations if they are to take regular formal employment or travel long distances.

FIGURE 2.2 Women as nutrition intermediaries

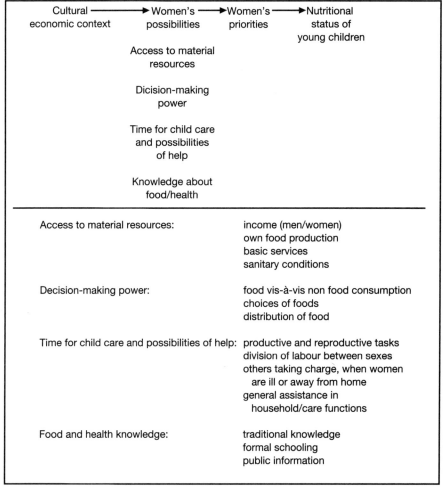

SOURCE: From M. Wandel and G. Holmboe-Ottesen, Women as nutrition mediators: A case study from Sri Lanka. *Ecology of Food and Nutrition*, 21 (1988), 117–130.

There are other "confounders" or mediating variables that tend to obscure the relationship between maternal income and nutrition. Such variables include household and community sanitation, monetary and nutritional value of home-produced foods, family size and composition, maternal health and nutrition knowledge, and locus of control of the additional female income, among others.

When women have more control over additional household income, then nutritional benefits may be realized. This was the case in a study conducted by Tucker in Panama, where maternal income was positively associated with preschooler dietary intake.[45] Sources of income in the professional occupations included teacher, nurse, and bank teller; unskilled occupations included maid, laundress, waitress, cook, and factory worker. A third category of self-employment included women who supplemented their incomes by initiating home income activities, the most common being the preparation and sale of foods from the home. Tucker reports that often older Panamanian children sold home-prepared fried foods in the early morning, door to door, or from a central location such as a school yard. From homes with refrigerators, women commonly sold ice and *"duros"* (popsicle-type frozen bars made either with powdered flavoring or, more frequently, with available tropical fruits).

Another investigation among rural households found that children of working mothers had a lower weight-for-age than children of mothers who did not work.[46] But within the poorest families this relationship was reversed. Increases in income achieved by men, however, were used to purchase "prestige" goods rather than additional food.

It has also been noted that women placed greater priority on the needs of their children than on those of their husbands, because women spend a greater percentage of their own income on food.[47]

Interesting and consistent findings are reported for both urban and rural Dominican women. Tiffany found that immigrant women from the Dominican Republic living in upper Manhattan, in New York City, showed a strong positive relationship between per capita income and intake of selected nutrients.[48] Similarly, Mort, studying rural Dominican women from the Cibao Sierra (highland area), noted that total household income had a positive association on women's dietary and nutritional status.[49] When components of income were considered, female income produced the greatest effect on women's dietary status.

Kaiser and Dewey did not observe, in rural Mexican households, a relationship between mothers' cash contribution to household income and nutritional status of preschoolers.[50] However, the authors note that given the fact that only 17% of the women reported any personal income at all, the lack of a relationship between maternal income and child nutrition is not surprising. The possibility of having underestimated the women's income is also acknowledged by these investigators. Maternal income in this particular study came from a variety of sources, such as making tortillas, ironing, sewing, weaving, and selling food.

Another interesting finding reported by Kaiser and Dewey relates to source of income. The researchers specifically report finding a negative relationship between the proportion of income received from migrant (foreign) remittances and the weight-for-age of preschoolers. These investigators reason that for many of these Mexican households remittances arrive sporadically, often once a month or less often. Thus, "malnutrition in households relying on migrant income may result from the tendency of these households to allocate less of their income to food, to allot relatively more for processed foods and less for traditional foods, as compared to other types of households. . . ."[51]

The deleterious nutritional implications of processed foods, in particular, high-sugar foods such as soft drinks, have been documented in other studies conducted in Mexico.[52] Interestingly, a subsequent study by DeWalt et al. found the incidence of child malnutrition to be higher in villages with more migration than in communities with low rates of out-migration.[53]

It appears that the relationship between maternal employment and nutrition should be examined in light of trade-offs between increased maternal income and reduced time for child care. Because economic need often drives women to work, negative associations between maternal income and child nutritional status may be an artifact of overall economic need rather than of the work situation per se.

Women's Workload and Time Use

In trying to illustrate different factors affecting the linkages among women, nutrition, and health, it is tempting to select almost everything. However, an important dimension that focuses on the woman herself, rather than on her role as mother, is the variable of workload and its corollary, time use. There has been concern that women, in both developed and developing countries, have very limited time for self-realization activities, leisure, personal needs, learning new skills, or improving formal education or vocational level. Ironically, empirical observations have suggested that when women have extra time, they use it for additional income-generating activities to help with household expenses.

A second important issue deals with women's workload. Women play a critical part in procuring, preparing, and even in processing foods. In de-

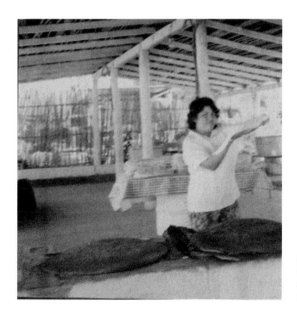

Selling home-made tortillas is an important income-generating activity for many Hispanic women.

veloping countries, women dry and smoke such foods as fish, vegetables, fruit, and grains. These preparations, necessary for food storage, minimize the "feast or famine" situation that can be caused by seasonal fluctuations. In industrialized societies, women also have social, political, and economic roles that leave little time for personal needs.

Women's workload has been a recognized but neglected topic by the nutrition community. However, it has important implications for health. For example, in rural areas, women's energy output for heavy work frequently does not correspond to increased food consumption, thus jeopardizing health and well-being. The incredibly long hours that women work is illustrated in the profile from *A Day in the Life of a Guatemalan Plantation Woman*, as summarized by Colle and Fernández-Colle:

> Francisca Gómez makes the meals for six men workers, but does not wash their clothes because it takes too much time. She wouldn't be able to take proper care of her own family. She has had four children and three are alive. They are 6 years, 4 years and 4 months old. Elfido would be 2 years old, but died at 11 months from fever. Yesterday Francisca got up at 4 in the morning. "I dusted the *poyo* [adobe wood stove], started the fire, washed myself and combed my hair, washed the coffee jug and put breakfast on the fire, made *atol* [cereal gruel], washed the corn and took it to the mill. I made tortillas, and at six, those that work had breakfast. At 6:30 I had breakfast with the children. I washed the dishes, swept, made beds and went to wash clothes at the *pila* [cement washtub] at 8 a.m., and came back at 9 a.m. Every other day we go and bathe in the river. On those days we come back home at ten. That is when we have *atol*. I warmed up the lunch for those coming from work; they have lunch at 11:00. At 11:30 the children and I had lunch. I put the children to bed for a nap from 12:00 to 2:00. I washed dishes, toasted coffee and ground it, played with the children and went to get water. At four we had coffee and bread and I made tamalitos and supper. The children had supper at five and the rest of us had supper at 5:30. I washed the dishes, prepared the corn for the next day and, at seven, put the children to bed. We got to bed at eight."[54]

Female-headed Households

The family is the primary context in which nutrition and health activities occur and thus is potentially the most immediate source of health-related support and education for the individual. It is in the context of the family that attitudes and behaviors regarding diet, food preferences, and health beliefs are learned and maintained. Given this situation, it follows, then, that the family also offers the primary opportunity for teaching children how to change or modify unhealthy dietary habits and other types of behaviors. It is also recognized that within the complexity of urban living, families should not be expected to assume these responsibilities in isolation. Families need and deserve the support of their communities in order to achieve and maintain good health and quality of life.

When women experience stress, such as desertion, widowhood, divorce, or separation, that may result in unhealthy outcomes for them or their children, the community's responsibility becomes increasingly urgent. Single parenthood and poverty are two factors that threaten the family's viability. Widowed and divorced women not only are threatened economically but also lose former family support systems.

Concern over female-headed households has emerged particularly because fewer economic resources have been available to such households. For example, the U.S. national statistics on the distribution of family income reveal that larger percentages of comparably sized female-headed households than male-headed households have been classified as living below the poverty thresholds. The growing number of households headed by women has been an evident trend in urban America and in many cities in developing countries. Mayer, examining nutritional problems in the United States, notes that many poor children today live in one-parent families headed by a single woman, victims of the "feminization of poverty."[55]

The increased percentage of Puerto Rican households headed by women (about 33% in New York City in 1980) is often cited as an important reason for the consistently low-income levels of Puerto Ricans. But even more significant is that the majority of these Puerto Rican female-headed households (57%) rely solely on public assistance to cope with their difficult economic situation; comparable figures for whites and African-American women who head their own families are 9% and 28%, respectively.[56]

A report by Buvinic notes not only the feminization of poverty through the rise in poor women-headed households in Latin America but also the increasing number of children living in poverty in female-headed households.[57] Rural to urban migration, search for employment in semiurban or urban cities, and an increase in overall impoverishment may account for the increase in woman-headed households. Specifically, when men move to urban centers to seek work, their families are often left behind.

Women in these households experience multiple difficulties with increased workloads and decreased access to resources. First, women alone cannot usually cultivate large enough plots of land to provide adequate food. Second, even if they are able to do so, they are likely to have problems with access to credit, agricultural technology, and extension service information when households lack male adults. Last, remittances from absent males are often inadequate and too irregular to provide their families with enough food and other necessities. A case that illustrates this issue is the large number of female-headed households that this author has observed in the rural highlands of the Dominican Republic. Women in these households perform multiple roles, economic and domestic, and must work strenuously to survive because their husbands left to find work in New York City, "in search of a better life."

According to McGuire and Popkin, data for five Latin American cities show that in all, except Bogotá, Colombia, households headed by women are much more prevalent among lower than higher income groups (Figure 2.3).[58] In lower-income groups, the percentage of female-headed households ranges

FIGURE 2.3   Percentage of female-headed households of all households in selected cities, by income

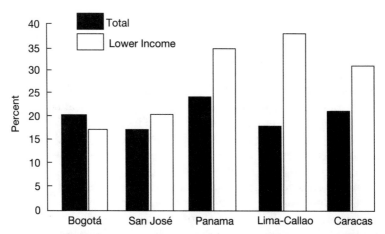

SOURCE: From J. McGuire and M.B. Popkin, Beating the zero sum game: Women and nutrition in the third world, presented at ACC/SCN Symposium on Women and Nutrition, United Nations, October 1990.

from 22% in San José, Costa Rica, to 38% in Lima and Callao, Peru. The lower incomes of female-headed households are readily apparent in Figure 2.3, and their nutritional implications cannot be ignored.

This author has been careful to present female-headed households as a significant proxy variable reflecting the income level or poverty level of the family. Health practitioners should not equate this variable with family dysfunction or associate or equate it with childhood neglect or deprivation. While no one can deny the constraints and difficulties experienced by men and women when raising children alone, there are also many instances when poor Hispanic single mothers in the United States have raised their children successfully, in spite of their dire economic circumstances. An illustration is found in a nutrition study conducted by Sanjur and Haines among 576 New York State low-income households.[59] Nearly one-third of the sampled families were headed by a female. Interesting and significant findings emerged with respect to the dietary assessment. When diets were evaluated using the Recommended Dietary Allowances (1980) for six nutrients (calories, protein, vitamin A, vitamin C, iron, and calcium), the authors concluded that, in general, urban female-headed households, of all races, purchased more nutritionally adequate diets than did male-headed households.

Another important finding, although of a nonnutritional nature, was reported by Pelto et al. in their study of 153 Puerto Rican households in New Hartford, Connecticut.[60] These investigators found that single-parent households were no more or less effective than dual-parent households in coping with the stresses of urban life. This study underlines that female-headed households are not necessarily destined for negative outcomes.

Women and Health

As stated in Chapter 1, it has long been recognized that Hispanics have been a disadvantaged minority in the United States, mostly because of ethnic discrimination, low levels of education, high unemployment rates and poverty levels, and consequently, limited health care utilization. An examination of recent U.S. Bureau of Census reports on population trends among U.S. Hispanics and other cross-sectional demographic studies on Hispanics attest to this. However, these disadvantages are not uniformly experienced by the different Hispanic groups, and thus we briefly note additional data, in light of the profound social and health implications of such disadvantages. One segment that appears to be clearly disadvantaged is women.

Three major health issues of concern among Hispanic women, as summarized by Ventura, using 1988 National Center for Health statistics, are the following:[61]

1. *Childbearing by Hispanic Unmarried Mothers:* A high percentage of Hispanic births are to unmarried women. One-third of all Hispanic births, as compared to one-quarter of all non-Hispanic births, were to unmarried women. The proportions for individual Hispanic groups differed considerably: Puerto Rican, 53%; Central and South American, 36%; Mexican, 31%; and Cuban, 16%. For comparative purposes, the births to unmarried women were 15% for white non-Hispanics and 64% for black non-Hispanics.

2. *Childbearing and Educational Attainment:* Except for Cuban women, Hispanic mothers are much less likely than non-Hispanic mothers to have completed high school. In 1988, 58% of all Hispanic women who gave birth were high school graduates compared with 83% of white non-Hispanic and 69% of black non-Hispanic mothers. Educational attainment, as with many other social indicators, varies considerably among the individual Hispanic groups. In 1988, 82% of Cuban mothers, 48% of Central and South American mothers, 55% of Puerto Rican mothers, and 43% of Mexican mothers were high school graduates.

3. *Births to Hispanic Teenage Mothers:* Another issue of substantial importance to health and nutrition policy relates to births to teenage mothers (Figure 2.4). According to Ventura, in 1988, about 1 in 6 of all Hispanic origin births were to teenage mothers, compared with 1 in 10 of all white non-Hispanic births and nearly 1 in 4 of all black non-Hispanic births. However, there are wide variations in the incidence of teenage child-

FIGURE 2.4   Percentage of births to teenage mothers

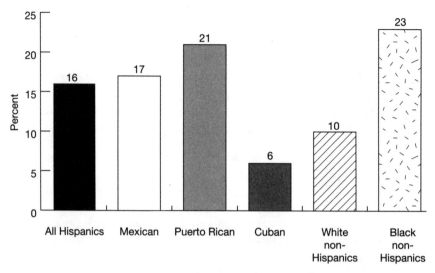

SOURCE: S. J. Ventura, The health and development of Puerto Rican mothers and children in the mainland, paper presented at NCHS conference, Brown University, Providence, RI, November 1990.

bearing among the various Hispanic groups. Seventeen percent of births to Mexicans and 21% of births to Puerto Ricans, compared with 6% of births to Cubans and 8% of births to Central and South Americans, were to teenage mothers (not shown in Figure 2.4).

SUMMARY

This chapter has addressed the relationship between food habits and ethnicity, particularly their overlap, and the nutritional and health implications for practitioners who work with and counsel members of ethnic groups. Emphasis has been placed on recognizing the important role played by culture and ethnicity in patterning food behavior. However, lack of economic resources or institutional neglect may also sometimes explain different health behaviors and outcomes among various ethnic groups.

Prescientific notions of food, health, and folk medicine held by Hispanic families were discussed, along with subcultural variations in adherence to and practice of these beliefs. Similarly, implications for the health practitioner and the need to integrate biomedical beliefs with traditional Latin American belief systems were addressed.

The linkages between women and nutrition have been discussed relative to maternal education, employment, workload, and time use. Additional health concerns relative to female-headed households and women's health were discussed as they affect the nutrition of children.

NOTES

1. H. Passim and J. W. Bennett, *Social process and dietary change*. National Research Council Bulletin 108 (Washington, DC, 1943).

2. USHSS/Public Health Service, *Healthy people 2000*, Publication no. [PHS] 01-50213 (Washington, DC, 1991).

3. Max Weber, The ethnic group. In Talcott Parsons et al. (eds.), *Theories of society*, Vol. 1 (Glencoe, IL: Free Press, 1961), p. 305.

4. C. A. Bryant, A. Courtney, B. A. Markesbery, and K. M. DeWalt, *The cultural feast* (St. Paul, MN: West, 1985).

5. Frederick Barth, *Ethnic groups and boundaries: The social organization of cultural difference* (Boston: Little, Brown, 1969).

6. Ibid.

7. Bryant et al., *Cultural feast.*

8. L. K. Brown and K. Mussell, eds. Ethnic and regional foodways in the United States (Knoxville: University of Tennessee Press, 1984).

9. Ibid.

10. Marina Flores, *Disponibilidad y utilización de alimentos de uso convencional como fuentes de proteínas y calorías*, paper presented at the International Conference of Nutrition, San José, Costa Rica, August 1976.

11. Héctor R. Bourges, Costumbres, prácticas y hábitos alimentarios. *Cuadernos de Nutrición* (Mexico, D.F.), 13(2), (March–April 1990).

12. Passim and Bennett, *Social process.*

13. Claire M. Cassidy, Subcultural prenatal diets of Americans. In *Alternative dietary practices and nutritional abuses in pregnancy* (Washington, DC: National Academy Press, 1982).

14. Diva Sanjur, Parámetros ambientales y socioculturales que afectan la alimentación en los países del tercer mundo. *Archivos Latinoamericanos de Nutricion*, 30(4), (December 1980).

15. Joaquín Cravioto, La alimentación del niño en el medio rural mexicano, en Seminario sobre la alimentación normal. In *Ediciones Médicas* (Hospital Infantil de México, 1961).

16. Diva Sanjur, J. Cravioto, L. Rosales, and A. Van Veen, Infant feeding and weaning practices in a rural preindustrial setting. *Acta Pediatrica Scandinavica* (Supplement 200), 2 (1970), 56.

17. Ibid.

18. Ibid.

19. Ibid.

20. A. V. Millard and M. A. Graham, Principles that guide weaning in rural Mexico. *Ecology of Food and Nutrition, 12* (1985), 195–202.

21. Ibid.

22. Alan Harwood, The hot-cold theory of disease: Implications for treatment of Puerto Rican patients. *JAMA, 216* (1971), 1153–1158.

23. L. S. Lieberman, Medico-nutritional practices among Puerto Ricans in a small urban northeastern community in the United States. *Social Science and Medicine, 13B* (1979), 191–198.

24. M. A. Kay, Health and illness in a Mexican-American barrio. In E. H. Spicer (ed.), *Ethnic medicine in the Southwest* (Tucson: University of Arizona Press, 1977).

25. Breastfeeding and weaning in Mexico and the United States, *Nutrition Reviews, 44* (1986), 104–106.

26. Kay, Health and illness.

27. ACN/SCN symposium report, *Women and Nutrition*, UN Nutrition Policy Discussion paper no. 6, October 1990.

28. George Kent, Nutrition education as an instrument of empowerment. *Journal of Nutrition Education, 20*(4), (1988).

29. Ibid.

30. S. Tiffany, *Women's Work and motherhood: The power of female sexuality in the workplace* (Englewood Cliffs, NJ: Prentice Hall, 1982).

31. Carol A. Bryant, The impact of kin, friend and neighbor networks on infant feeding practices: Cuban, Puerto Rican and Anglo families in Florida. *Social Science and Medicine, 16* (1988), 193–195.

32. D. Sanjur, J. Cravioto, and A. G. Van Veen, Infant nutrition and sociocultural influences in a village in central Mexico. *Tropical and Geographical Medicine, 22* (1970), 443–451.

33. L. Kaiser and K. Dewey, Migration, cash cropping, and subsistence agriculture: Relationships to household food expenditures in rural Mexico. *Social Science and Medicine, 33*(10) (1991), 1113–1126.

34. K. DiGiacomo, The effects of maternal employment on family income, food habits and health practices in Puerto Rico, M.S. thesis, Cornell University, 1976; Mirta Colón Archilla, Efecto de la producción agrícola casera y el ingreso familiar en la ingestión de nutrientes y la antropometría nutricional de madres y pre-escolares en Naranjito, Puerto Rico, Recinto de Ciencias Médicas, University of Puerto Rico, M.S. thesis, June 1981; Laura Bentz Rivera, Patrones de consumo de alimentos e ingestión de nutrientes en Río Grande, Puerto Rico: Un enfoque sociocultural, Recinto de Ciencias Médicas, University of Puerto Rico, M.S. Thesis, June 1981.

35. M. Smith, B. Santos, and M. Fernández, Nutrition and public health in the Dominican Republic. *Archivos Latinoamericanos de Nutrición, 32*(4) (1982), 867–881.

36. Alicia García, Socioeconomic and maternal determinants of nutritional status and ascaris infection among school children in Coclé, Panama, Ph.D. dissertation, Cornell University, May 1989.

37. K. Tucker and D. Sanjur, Maternal employment and child nutrition in Panama. *Social Science and Medicine, 26*(6) (1988), 605.

38. P. Herold and D. Sanjur, Home for the migrants: The pueblos jóvenes of Lima: A study of socioeconomic determinants of child malnutrition. *Archivos Latinoamericanos de Nutrición, 36*(4) (1986), 559–624.

39. E. G. Piwoz and F. E. Viteri, Studying health and nutrition behavior by examining household decision-making, intra-household resources distribution, and the role of women in these processes. *Food and Nutrition Bulletin, 7*(4) (1985).

40. P. Engle and M. Pedersen, Maternal work for earnings and children's nutritional status in urban Guatemala. *Ecology of Food and Nutrition, 22*(3) (1989), 211–223.

41. P. Van Esterik, *Women, work, and breastfeeding.* Cornell University Program in International Nutrition, Monograph Series no. 23, 1992.

42. Joanne Leslie. *Women's work and child nutrition in the third world* (Washington, DC: International Center for Research on Women, 1985).

43. M. Wandel and G. Holmboe-Ottesen, Women as nutrition mediators: A case study from Sri Lanka. *Ecology of Food and Nutrition, 21* (1988), 117–130.

44. Van Esterik, *Women, work, and breastfeeding.*

45. K. L. Tucker, Maternal time use, differentiation and child nutrition, Ph.D. dissertation, Cornell University, June 1986.

46. S. K. Kumar, Composition of economic constraints in child nutrition: Impact of maternal incomes and employment in low-income households, Ph.D. dissertation, Cornell University, 1977.

47. D. Dwyer and J. Bruce, eds., *A home divided: Women and income in the third world* (Stanford, CA: Stanford University Press, 1987).

48. Jean Tiffany, Dietary patterns and nutritional status of immigrant women from the Dominican Republic living in New York City, Master's thesis, Cornell University, May 1984.

49. Margaret M. Mort, Effects of women's characteristics, household characteristics, and food acquisition practices on the dietary practices and nutritional status of rural Dominican women, Master's thesis, Cornell University, January 1991.

50. Kaiser and Dewey, Migration, cash cropping.

51. Ibid.

52. K. M. DeWalt, P. B. Kelley, and G. H. Pelto, Nutritional correlates of economic microdifferentiation in a highland Mexican community. In N. W. Jerome, R. F. Kandel, and G. H. Pelto (eds.), *Nutritional anthropology: Contemporary approaches to diet and culture* (Pleasantville, NY: Redgrave, 1980); K. G. Dewey, Nutritional consequences of the transformation from Sub-

sistence to commercial agriculture in Tabasco, Mexico. *Human Ecology, 9* (1981), 151–187.

53. K. M. DeWalt et al., Agrarian reform and small farmer welfare: Evidence from four Mexican communities. *Food and Nutrition Bulletin, 9*(3) (1987), 46–52.

54. R. D. Colle and S. Fernández-Colle, *The Communication Factor in Health and Nutrition Programs,* Department of Communication Arts Monograph, New York State College of Agriculture and Life Sciences, Cornell University, 1981.

55. Jean Mayer, Nutritional problems in the United States: Then and now two decades later. *Nutrition Today* (January/February 1990), 17.

56. Clara E. Rodríguez, *Puerto Ricans—Born in the U.S.A.* (Boulder, CO: Westview Press, 1991).

57. Mayra Buvinic, *Women and poverty in Latin America and the Caribbean: A primer for policy makers,* prepared for the Interamerican Development Bank, ICRW, 1990.

58. J. McGuire and M. B. Popkin, Beating the zero sum game: Women and nutrition in the third world. In ACC/SCN Symposium on Women and Nutrition, United Nations, October 1990.

59. Diva Sanjur and Pam Haines, Nutrient availability and food expenditures among selected low-income households. *Federation Proceedings, 38*(3) (March 1979).

60. P. Pelto, M. Roman, and N. Liriano, Family structures in an urban Puerto Rican community. *Urban Anthropology, 11*(1) (1982), 39–57.

61. S. J. Ventura, Presentation at Conference, The Health and Development of Puerto Rican mothers and children in the mainland, paper presented at NCHS conference, Brown University, Providence, RI, November 1990.

3

Mexican-American Diets
and Nutrient Intake

A General Profile of Mexican Diets
Nutritional Strengths and Weaknesses of Mexican Diets

Diets and Meals in Central and Southern Mexico
Meal Patterns
Food Preparation and Preservation
Food Consumption of Adults and Children
Infant Feeding Practices

Diets and Meals in Northern Mexico
Changing Food Patterns
The "Food Consumption Basket" for Rural Sonora
Food Consumption of Adults and Children
Infant Feeding Practices
Food Preparation and Preservation

Overview of Mexican Diets
Differential Patterns in Northern/Southern Diets
Differential Patterns in Rural and Urban Diets

**Dietary Trends and Nutritional Status of Mexican-Americans
in the United States**
Breast-Feeding Trends
Food Group Contributions to Total Nutrients
Dietary Intakes of Essential Nutrients
Children's Diets
Elderly Mexican-Americans
Dietary Changes among Mexican-American Families

A GENERAL PROFILE OF MEXICAN DIETS

Mexican-Americans, who live primarily in the states of California, Texas, Arizona, Colorado, and New Mexico, constitute the largest segment (approximately 62%) of the U.S. Hispanic population. The traditional dietary habits of Mexican families reflect the richness and variety of their Mexican cultural heritage. Despite this diversity, Mexican-Americans have some common dietary practices that cut across age, gender, and socioeconomic categories.

Attempting to describe dietary patterns of such a diverse group is a complex task. For example, as any health-related or community worker already knows, dietary practices of rural Mexican-Americans living in Texas differ widely from those of Mexican-Americans living in urbanized East Los Angeles. Similarly, eating patterns in Tlaltizapán, in southwest Mexico, are likely to vary from those in Hermosillo, in northern Mexico.

This chapter focuses mainly on common dietary patterns of Mexican and Mexican-Americans, even as it recognizes differences among groups. The chapter attempts to provide a general profile of diet in Mexico and in the United States. The discussion of diets in Mexico comes mainly from information collected in central/southern and northern Mexico. This is appropriate because the largest number of Mexican immigrants and other *indocumentados* (undocumented immigrants) to the United States come mainly from these two regions. Seventy percent of the undocumented immigrants to the United States come basically from eight Mexican states: Michoacán, Guanajuato, Jalisco, Zacatecas, Durango, San Luis Potosí, Baja California, and Chihuahua.[1] In general, there is little information about the diets of Mexican-Americans living in the United States. A number of cross-sectional studies highlight specific dietary and nutritional trends that are especially informative and culturally relevant for nutrition counseling and nutrition education.

Nutritional Strengths and Weaknesses of Mexican Diets

There are three generally recognized nutritional strengths of traditional Mexican diets:

1. *The diets are high in complex carbohydrates and semivegetarian.* The traditional Mexican diet is primarily vegetarian, based on maize, beans, and *calabacitas* (squash). A wide variety of other foods—such as cactus parts, especially *nopales* (tender cactus leaves), *agave*, and several other

The substantial contribution of Professors M. C. María Isabel Ortega and Pedro Alejandro Castañeda to the section on food consumption in northern Mexico is gratefully acknowledged. Similarly, the contributions by Alma Campa Mada and Ana Lourdes Frisby on the nutrient composition of Mexican foods and the reviews and comments on this chapter by Emma Paulina Pérez L. and Dr. Mauro Valencia J. are also gratefully recognized.

wild leafy plants, such as *pápalos, verdolaga,* and *quelite*—are used in varying degrees to supplement the basic staples. In addition, other indigenous vegetables used, such as *chiles,* and *tomato verde,* are also high in vitamins A and C. Expensive, commercially processed foods are not usually eaten every day.

2. *The bioavailability of calcium and niacin is enhanced by traditional methods of maize preparation.* The traditional method of using lime to prepare maize in central Mexico (in other areas, ashes may be used) greatly increases the calcium content of maize. (Untreated ground corn contains about 25 milligrams of calcium per 100 grams; an equal amount of tortillas has about 140 milligrams of calcium.) Thus corn tortillas are an important source of calcium in the diet. In addition, the debilitating disease of pellagra, caused by niacin deficiency, is rare in Mexico. By heating the maize and soaking it in the lime solution for several hours, the bound niacin becomes biologically available to humans.

3. *Corn and beans eaten together are a good source of protein.* The significant nutritional contribution of the corn and beans diet resides in its protein content. In maize, the principal protein, zein, is very low in the amino acids lysine and isoleucine. Conversely, sulfur-containing amino acids, methionine and cystine, are low in beans. When eaten together, the lysine deficiency of corn is made up by the lysine of beans. Conversely, corn contributes methionine and cystine, which compensate for the limitation in beans. In short, corn and beans, two staples of the traditional Mexican diet, provide "complementary proteins" that increase the total amount of protein consumed and improve its quality. (*Complementary proteins* refers to the process of having a limited amino acid in one food "complemented" by the abundant amino acid in the other food. For example, corn and beans in the Mexican-American diet and rice and beans in the Puerto Rican diet illustrate well how the nutritional value of these diets is enhanced by eating these foods combined.) Thus it is important to preserve these strengths of the traditional Mexican diet.

In contrast to the nutritional strengths, traditional Mexican diets have three general weaknesses.

1. *Food preparation methods add liberal amounts of fat.* The liberal use of added fat in cooking and food preparation, as well as the generous toppings of Mexican cream on traditional dishes (such as *enchiladas*) and as spreads in Mexican sandwiches (*tortas*), is a major concern. However, this practice cannot be understood outside of the traditional ways in which many Hispanic families prepare food. In order to modify dietary fat intake successfully, the habit needs to be addressed within its cultural context.

Historically, the practice of frying foods and the preference for fried foods among Mexican families in particular and Hispanic families in general is intimately linked to traditional ways of cooking on stovetops or in a *fogón* (made of stones on the floor or raised above ground, with wood as fuel). When poor rural families in traditional societies lack the cooking appliances and facilities of a gas or electric stove or an oven, or even more importantly, are unfamiliar with other methods of food preparation such as baking and broiling, it is difficult to get them to change their ways overnight. Change is painful! Thus it is understandable that stewing or frying with fat or oil, which can be done easily on top of a stove, are their preferred methods of cooking. Thus, in Mexican cooking, as well as in many areas of Mesoamerica, meat, *menudo* or *mondongo* (tripe) and other organ meats, beans, tortillas, rice, green and ripe plantains, potatoes, and many other foods are liked best when fried.

2. *There is a preference for high-fat meats.* The second drawback of the traditional Mexican diet is the preference for high-fat meats, including *chorizos* or *longanizas* (sausages), *chicharrón* (fried pork skin), *cabeza de puerco* (pig's head), *patitas de puerco* (pig's feet), and several other high-fat organ meats. Poor Mexican families living along the U.S. border in the state of Arizona have been observed to purchase large quantities of organ meats. Two reasons may help explain the preference for high-fat meats among these families. One is satiety, because foods high in fat are filling, and another is cost, as these foods are relatively inexpensive. Haffner et al. have documented high fat and high cholesterol intakes among Mexican-Americans, especially men, living in Texas.[2]

3. *Food ideology limits use of some nutritious foods.* An indirect but associated drawback of traditional Hispanic diets, including Mexican diets, relates to food ideology and folk medicine practiced in varying degrees by some families. When pregnant and lactating mothers and children firmly adhere to these food beliefs, their nutrition and health may be compromised. (For more on food ideology, see Chapter 2.)

Subsequent sections in this chapter examine dietary and nutritional profiles in Mexico and in the United States. Breast-feeding trends and issues related to dietary change are also discussed. A glossary at the end of the chapter provides a comprehensive list of Mexican-American foods, dishes, and terms.

DIETS AND MEALS IN CENTRAL AND SOUTHERN MEXICO

Tortillas (flat corn cakes) and *frijoles* (beans) are the staples of the diet. The corn tortilla commonly consumed in this region contains only traces of fat, as opposed to the flour tortilla more typically consumed in the north. Flour tortillas each contain from one to two teaspoons of lard. Bread is mostly consumed as rolls, including sweet rolls, made in the local bakeries. Soups are usually consumed during the *comida* (early afternoon meal) and come in two varieties: *sopa aguada* (literally "watery soup") made from broth or bouillon powder, tomatoes, onions, garlic, and a thin noodle; and *sopa seca* (dry soup) made of spaghetti or rice cooked in a tomato and onion sauce. Slices of hard-boiled eggs usually accompany the *sopa seca* when it is made of rice. *Jitomate* (tomato), *tomate* (green tree tomato), onions, and *chili* (hot pepper) are consumed in great amounts as components of *salsa* (hot sauce), almost as essential to meals as are tortillas and beans. Mexican red or green *salsa*, made from diced tomatoes, garlic, chilis, and onion, is consumed raw and can be a good source of vitamins C and A. *Salsa* may be spread on the tortillas or used to prepare other dishes.

The most commonly eaten animal protein foods are eggs, pork, beef, and chicken. Eggs are well liked and inexpensive, and are often used in such dishes as *chiles rellenos* (green peppers filled with cheese or ground meat), *burritos* (wheat tortillas filled with cheddar cheese and refried beans), and scrambled eggs (prepared with potatoes, cactus, or sausage). Meat is usually eaten in *mole* or *guiso* (stew). Locally produced cheese is also eaten in *quesadillas* (folded tortillas with melted cheese and squash blossoms).

Milk, when consumed, is usually heated and flavored with sugar and coffee, chocolate, or cinnamon. Milk may also be used in *atole* (gruel), which is usually consumed, especially by children or lactating women, during the evening meal. When *atoles* are made from legumes such as *ajonjolí* (sesame seeds), they are thought to have great value as a *galactogue* (a promoter of increased production of breast milk).

In many rural villages, an abundance of tropical fruits is available in the marketplace. Families that can afford them choose from among such seasonally available items as bananas, oranges, guavas, papayas, mangoes, pineapples, apples, and the many indigenous Mexican fruits, such as *tunas, capulines, nanchis*, and *mamey*. Among the fruits, *plátano* (banana) seems to be the most popular. (Note that Spanish names for food items vary widely among various Hispanic subcultural groups. Mexicans call bananas *plátanos;* Central Americans call them *guineos*. To Puerto Ricans and Dominicans, *plátanos* are not fruits but starchy vegetables used to prepare *tostones,* slightly squashed, fried green plantains). A majority of the families in this region consume limes in home-made refreshments (*limonadas*) and in soups and salads. Most families have at least one lime tree growing behind their houses. Children like limes and eat them several times a day between meals.

Many fresh vegetables are available in the marketplace. Some of the most common are carrots, tomatoes, pumpkins, squashes, green peas, lettuces, cabbages, and a number of indigenous Mexican greens, such as *pápalos, pipizca, verdolaga*, and *quelite*. Vegetables are well liked, and their consumption seems to be limited only by income.

Interestingly, some women classify vegetables as *verduras de campo* (field vegetables, or greens that grow wild in open fields and are free) and *verduras de pueblo* (town vegetables, or vegetables that must be bought in the plaza market). Such indigenous classifications of vegetables must be considered when conducting dietary surveys among rural women in central and southern Mexico. During other dietary studies, it was noticed that women did not always report consuming field vegetables. When asked about this, they explained that they did not report eating *vegetables de campo* because they did not pay for them.

Meal Patterns

Three main meals are eaten during the day—*desayuno* and *almuerzo, comida,* and *cena*—taking place in the morning, early afternoon, and evening, respectively. The main meal of the day, the *comida* (eaten between 1:00 and 3:00 p.m.), is the most variable. If meat, eggs, *longaniza* (sausages), *chicharrón* (fried pork skin), or any other protein food is eaten during the day, it is most likely to be at this meal.

Some families have changed their morning meal patterns, especially those households where the mother gets up very early to prepare lunch for her early-rising husband. In this case, they may have a *desayuno* (eaten between 5:30 and 7:00 a.m.) of bread and sweetened coffee, herbal tea, or occasionally hot chocolate. Then an hour or two later, they may have an *almuerzo* (eaten between 8:00 and 9:30 a.m.) consisting of tortillas, boiled or fried beans, and coffee or tea. In some families, even fried eggs, meat, potatoes with *chiles* and tomatoes, bread, hot milk, or avocado are consumed during this meal. Avocado is very popular throughout Mexico, so much so that even small children will initiate the preparation of their own sandwiches with tortilla and avocado.

The *cena,* or evening meal (eaten between 6:00 and 8:00 p.m.), may be just bread or *pan dulce* (sweet bread), tea or coffee, and *tortillas* and beans. Some families consume at the *cena lo que sobre de la comida* (leftovers from noon) or *lo mismo* (the same as they had at noontime). Usually enough tortillas are prepared at noon to serve again in the evening with the beans. Consuming leftovers during the evening meal is also common among rural families in Central America and Panama, where tortillas or rice are prepared in sufficient

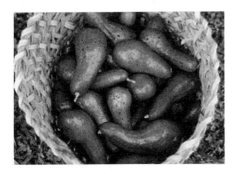

Avocados are popular among Hispanic families.

amounts to make sure there is enough for the latter meal. This practice saves fuel and time, two scarce resources in rural households.

Water, the usual beverage, is nearly always obtained from numerous local hydrants or home pipes. Bottled water may also be available for those who can afford it. Black coffee is the most common breakfast beverage, and tea the most common at evening. Traditional herb teas are often consumed by adults and children, including infants, in these Mexican villages. Black coffee is often served to children. *Té de hojitas* is a local tea made by steeping fresh citrus or spearmint leaves or cinnamon bark in hot water. Carbonated beverages are also popular, especially fruit-flavored ones, which often are taken at lunch. *Chocolate* (made with cocoa, sugar, and milk) is also consumed. *Manzanita* (an apple-flavored carbonated beverage) is preferred by mothers when they are sick.

Lard and cottonseed oil are the main types of fat used for cooking. *Nata* or *crema* (milk cream) is sometimes consumed, but butter is infrequently used. During one study people reported buying and using butter only once a year, in November, when they traditionally prepare elaborate dishes and special cakes that they take to the cemetery as offering to their dead relatives. This is a symbolic offering only; the prepared dishes are later brought back home and eaten by the family.

Slight variations in these meal patterns, particularly with respect to the *desayuno* and the *comida* and the frequent consumption of soft drinks, have been recently reported by Kaiser and Dewey in the state of Guanajuato.[3] Reportedly, children sometimes have milk with oatmeal, rice, or cornflakes for the *desayuno*. In addition to tortillas, the *comida* consists of a *sopa* of pasta or rice and a sweetened fruit drink or soda. The meal may also include beans (boiled or fried) or meat (beef, pork, or chicken in a chile sauce or broth with vegetables). Many families eat beef or pork only on Sundays or special holidays. Fruit, candy, and sodas are consumed between meals.

Food Preparation and Preservation

In many rural areas simple and routine food preparation takes a great part of the mother's time compared with her other tasks, such as child care and housekeeping. An older daughter usually helps with food shopping, cooking, and serving meals, but the mother decides what foods to buy and eat each day. When young wives live with in-laws, the mothers-in-law may make these decisions.

Generally, foods are boiled or fried. A few foods are roasted or charcoal-broiled. Baking is rare because few families own ovens. Drying is the most common method of food preservation in rural villages, particularly corn. Beef, pork, fish, and *chiles* are commonly dried by hanging them up in the kitchen.

The kitchen may be simply an area of a one-room home or a separate room apart from the living quarters. People eat in the kitchen. Food is served on metal or glass plates, and beverages in mugs. Tortillas often take the place of forks or spoons. This way of eating is called *sopear* by the villagers.

Kitchen tools   There are several common pieces of kitchen equipment and utensils. *Tortilleras* (tortilla presses) are used to shape tortillas that are then baked directly on a *comal* (clay, iron, or metal griddle) over the fire. A *molcajete* (clay or stone mortar), and *tejolote* (stone pestle) are used to grind *chilies, jitomates,* and other condiments for sauces.

Utensils may differ in quantity among families but usually not in kind. *Ollas* (deep pots) of pottery or metal are used to hold and cook liquids. Many housewives pride themselves in having a large collection of the pottery *ollas* in different shapes and sizes. A *sartén* (metal skillet) is used for frying. Cooking is done primarily over a wood fire in a *tlecuitl* (an open clay fireplace). Although some families own bottled gas stoves, they still prefer the *tlecuitl* for baking the tortillas.

Food Consumption of Adults and Children

Tables 3.1 and 3.2 show typical diets for adults and children, respectively. The tables are based on various publications by the National Institute of Nutrition in Mexico, in particular from its 1987 publication that reported on 12 years (1976–87) of research and programming. For validation purposes, all typical diets shown in this chapter for the central/southern and northern regions of Mexico were developed and reviewed by various Mexican nutritionists with work experience in both areas.

Adults' Diets   Studied over three typical days, adults' diets appear high in complex carbohydrates and low in animal protein. Small amounts of meat, eaten as *carnitas* (beef or pork meat), or eggs are the major sources of protein. Intakes of animal protein are low compared to Western intakes. The major portion of kilocalories is consumed in the first two meals of the day, with the third meal being lighter. It is worth noting, however, that alcoholic beverages such as *pulque* are frequently consumed by adults (and sometimes even children). *Pulque* contributes a significant amount of some vitamins and minerals. One liter (430 calories) contains 60 milligrams of vitamin C, 4 mg of niacin, 7 mg of iron, and 120 mg of calcium. In the northern region, *pulque* is often replaced by beer.

Children's Diets   Children's diets follow a pattern similar to adults', with variations in the beverages and in the amounts consumed (Table 3.2). For example, when children drink coffee, it has fresh, dried, or evaporated milk added to it. *Licuados* (fresh fruit drinks with water or milk) are more often served to children.

As with adults, children do not eat much animal protein, except for the small amount of egg mixed with rice soup. Children also eat fried eggs at breakfast or raw eggs beaten into the *licuados*. Fruits and vegetables also seem limited in the diets of children.

TABLE 3.1 Typical Diets of Adults from Central/Southern Mexico

	Day 1	Day 2	Day 3
Breakfast (almuerzo) 8–10 a.m.	1 cooking tsp. of fried beans 3 corn tortillas 1 cup of black coffee 1 tsp. of sauce, with red or green hot pepper, onion, tomato, and coriander	1 cup of corn atole (gruel) 1 piece of white bread 1/2 cooking tsp. of fried beans 1 tsp. of sauce	1 medium glass of licuado (mixture of milk, fruit, usually banana, and sugar)
Dinner (comida) 1–3 p.m.	1 plate of pasta soup, with tomato, onion, and dry bouillon 1 cooking tsp. of fried beans 3 corn tortillas 1 tsp. of sauce 1 big glass of lemonade	1/3 cooking tsp. of rice soup (dry), with tomato, onion, dry bouillon 1/4 cooked egg 3 corn tortillas 1 tsp. of sauce 1/4 small glass of pulque	2 tacos of pork (carnitas) with corn tortillas 2 tsp. of sauce 1 medium bottle of soft drink
Supper (cena) 6–9 p.m.	1 cup of corn atole (gruel) with milk and sugar 1 piece of sweet bread	1/2 tsp. of fried beans 3 corn tortillas 1 cup of black coffee 1 tsp. of sauce	1 cup of tea (mint, cinnamon, chamomile, or lime leaves) 1/2 cooking tsp. of fried beans 3 corn tortillas
Snacks (entre comidas)	1 medium bottle of soft drink	1 small bag of corn chips or potato chips	1 medium bottle of soft drink

SOURCE: M.I. Ortega and A. Castañeda, personal communication (CIAD, AC), Hermosillo, Sonora, Mexico, 1992.

Table 3.3 shows the foods that mothers and their toddlers ate during a day. These longitudinal data come from the Solis Valley population in the government region of Temascalcingo, in the central highlands of Mexico, and include six communities. The major sources of animal protein are beef and eggs; the major source of energy is the carbohydrate-rich tortillas for adults and *atole* and tortillas for children.

Pulque Consumption by Adults and Older Children In central Mexico, consumption of the locally brewed *pulque* (a beerlike beverage, about 2% alcohol, 43 kilocalories per 100 grams) is accepted as the norm for adults, including pregnant and lactating women and older children. The custom of fermenting *agave* juice may have had "survival value" in times of food scarcity

TABLE 3.2   Typical Diets of Children from Central/Southern Mexico

	Day 1	Day 2	Day 3
Breakfast (*almuerzo*) 8–10 a.m.	1 medium glass of *licuado* (milk, sugar, and fruit, usually banana) 1/2 cup of fried beans or bean broth 1–2 corn tortillas	1/2 cooking tsp. of fried beans or bean broth 1 piece of salted bread 1 cup of coffee with milk	1 plate of pasta soup (watery), with garlic, tomato, onion, and dry bouillon 1–2 corn tortillas 1 tsp. of sauce, with red or green hot pepper, onion, garlic, tomato, and coriander
Dinner (*comida*) 1–3 p.m.	1 plate of pasta soup 1 tsp. of fried beans or bean broth 1–2 corn tortillas 1 cup of tea	1 plate of chicken soup, with chicken meat, carrots, squash, and rice 1 tsp. of fried beans or bean broth 1–2 corn tortillas 1 tsp. of sauce	1/3 cooking tsp. of rice soup (dry), with egg, tomato, onion, garlic, and dry bouillon 1 tsp. of fried beans or bean broth 1–2 corn tortillas 1/2 small glass of soft drink
Supper (*cena*) 6–9 p.m.	1/2 cooking tsp. of fried beans or bean broth 1 piece of white bread 1 cup of coffee with milk	1/2 cooking tsp. of fried beans or bean broth 1–2 corn tortillas 1 tsp. of sauce 1/2 small glass of milk	1 cup of corn *atole* (gruel), with milk and sugar 1 piece of sweet bread
Snacks (*entre comidas*)	1/2 small glass of soft drink	1 small bag of corn chips or potato chips	1 popsicle

SOURCE: M.I. Ortega and A. Castañeda, personal communication (CIAD, AC), Hermosillo, Sonora, Mexico, 1992.

because this processing allows consumption of an otherwise nonutilizable substance that is available in the environment. Calloway et al. found that *pulque* contributed 12% of dietary energy for men and 6% for women. Men usually drank between 500 ml and 1 liter (500 to 1,000 g), but some men reported drinking 3 to 5 liters per day. So, although *pulque* appears regularly in the study's food intake records, consumption may still be somewhat higher than the reported mean figures.[4]

According to Calloway et al., for the Mexican population studied, the total food energy supply appears to be adequate, but food quality is less reli-

TABLE 3.3 Sample Diets of Mothers and Toddlers in Central Mexico

	(Ounces of Food Consumed in One Day)	
	Mother	*Toddler*
Coffee with sugar	8	—
Atole de harina, made of rice, flour, water, and sugar	—	17
Tortillas	28	10
Huevo (egg), with tomato, onions, oil, and salt	2	2
Calabacitas (squash), with onions and oil	3	2
Carne guisada, made of beef, tomatoes, onions, and salt	7	0.3

SOURCE: Based on data from D. H. Calloway, S. P. Murphy, and G. H. Beaton, *Food intake function: A cross-project perspective of the collaborative research support program in Egypt, Kenya and Mexico*, research monograph, University of California, Berkeley, August 1988.

ably assured. Preliminary evidence suggests that the situation would be improved by increasing the proportion of animal protein, the source of vitamin B_{12}, and a major contributor of other vitamins and trace minerals. Energy derived from *pulque* might well be replaced by more nutritious foods with benefit to health.

Infant Feeding Practices

In reading this discussion of infant feeding practices, it is wise to remember that variations do exist and take place from community to community.

Breast Feeding In rural areas most mothers do nothing special to prepare their breasts for nursing. Neonates are not nursed until the second or third day because mothers consider colostrum unfit for the child or, more commonly, "because the milk does not come down until after the third day." Consequently, sweetened herbal teas (boiled water with sugar) are given to infants in the first few days after birth. These teas, thought to have remedial effects, are recommended by midwives, mothers-in-law, and grandmothers to cure *cólico* (stomachache) until the infant is several months old.

Breast feeding usually begins by the third day, but if lactation has not started by then, women may resort to traditional techniques that are thought to ensure an abundant flow of milk. Favorite methods include drinking liquids, eating seafood, and taking yeast pills. Permanent lactation failures are rarely reported.

The initiation of breast feeding is simple, with mothers washing their nipples with water and alcohol; as the baby gets older this practice is dropped. The infant is generally allowed to suck for an unlimited time from both breasts at each feeding. Some mothers fear that if the child is fed from only one breast, this breast will get smaller and the milk will dry up. More traditionally oriented mothers, especially those who gave birth in a hospital, practice rigid scheduled feeding.

Maternal Caloric Intake during Lactation   Calloway et al. report that Mexican women increased their food intakes by about only 200 kilocalories per day during the first six months of lactation.[5] This is far below the required 700 kilocalories per day needed for infants to achieve ideal growth. In addition, the energy cost of producing milk adds another 100 to 150 kilocalories per day to the maternal requirements. The deficit in maternal energy intake to meet lactational needs is of nutritional concern, particularly because women's usual activity patterns range from moderate to heavy. These investigators conclude that mothers were unlikely to have enough dietary energy to produce enough milk to meet the needs of their infants. Negative relationships between lactation or pregnancy status and maternal intake, when expressed as a percentage of the Mexican recommended daily intakes, have also been reported by Kaiser and Dewey in their study of 178 households in central Mexico.[6]

Supplementary Feeding   In central Mexico, supplementary foods are usually introduced gradually to infants after 3 months of age. Herbal teas with sugar provide about 12% and dairy products about 18% of the supplementary food energy. Various types of milk given to a baby include cow's milk, either fresh, powdered, or evaporated, and, less often, goat's milk. Often this milk is combined with cereal, in a gruel (*atole*). Other supplementary foods are often introduced by the fourth month. *Caldo de frijol* (bean soup) is usually given mashed as a watery soup. Whole red beans, on the other hand, are considered too "heavy" for young children. (The "goodness" of a food is judged by its digestibility and according to whether or not the baby thrives on it. This belief holds true not only for the young infant but for some preschool children as well.) A wide variety of fruits, mostly tropical, are given to babies, commonly bananas, oranges, apples, and papayas.

Soft drinks, especially fruit-flavored ones, are often given to children. When children are sick with diarrhea or fever, mothers usually give them soft drinks. For young children, *tortillas* are usually mixed with bean soup, in order to soften their texture. Bread and crackers, *sopa aguada* (watery soup), and eggs are also offered to infants. The age at which children eat the family's diet and are offered table foods varies widely, usually somewhere between one and two years.

DIETS AND MEALS IN NORTHERN MEXICO

Changing Food Patterns

The northern region of Mexico is quite different from the central and southern regions. Various historical, cultural, and economic reasons account for these differences. The northern region, first of all, was able to resist the conquest of the Spaniards, given the rough topography, hard weather of the region, and the difficulties to make the land productive. Because it is adjacent to the United States, this region's economy is in many ways dependent on the state of the U.S. economy. Many Mexicans in this region work in the United States but still live in Mexico. As a consequence, the dietary pattern of Mexicans in the northern region has been influenced by the American diet. In fact, many families buy their food in American supermarkets.

Special characteristics of the northern region are exemplified by the state of Sonora, located in the northwest part of the country. For many years, Sonora's main economic activities were cattle raising and subsistence agriculture that provided such staple foods as corn, beans, and wheat. In addition, vegetables such as squashes, hot green peppers, and string beans and watermelons and cantaloupes were cultivated in the *parcela* (portion of cultivable land near the rivers) between the summer crops of corn and beans. Other legumes were grown in small quantities to be used when fresh vegetables were not available or in dishes cooked for special occasions. The legumes included lentils, chickpeas, peas, and lima beans. Also, a variety of fruits, such as lemons, oranges, grapefruits, and limes, were grown on a portion of the *parcela*, referred to as *huertas*, or patios. Vegetables grown included tomatoes, onions, and garlic. In addition, wild plants and animals were an important part of the diet. Commonly eaten wild plants included *quelites* (a leafy vegetable like spinach) and such fruits as *tunas* (fruit of *nopal*, a cactus plant), *pithayas* (cactus fruit), and *manzanita del campo* (wild apple). In many of the rural communities, men hunted for deer and wild pork. To preserve them, these meats were dried and salted.[7]

Foods derived from cattle raising included milk, meat, cheese, and butter—mainly produced for personal consumption. Cattle raising provided a

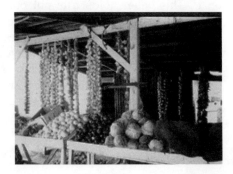

A road stand in Northern Mexico showing strings of garlic, cabbages, and onion.

steady source of food and income. Usually people sold cattle only to meet se-rious economic emergencies.

With the "green revolution" of the 1950s, agricultural production changed in Sonora. At the beginning of the century much of the grain pro-duced was sold, but a large portion of land was designated for cultivation of grain for self-consumption. With increased technological modernization, the cultivation of grain became more efficient, and grain production shifted from self-consumption to the marketplace.

In the early 1950s, Sonora's economy began to change in response to an increasing demand for beef by the American middle class. As a consequence, the food production of the region changed. The land reserved for production of grain for human consumption was used to produce forage and forage grains for cattle. Staple grains (corn, beans, and wheat) disappeared. Also, vegetables and fruits were no longer grown in the *parcela*. In addition, vari-ous foods derived from animals decreased. A substantial portion of the corn produced was used to feed animals such as pigs and chickens (for eggs pro-duction and for human consumption). As a large portion of milk was shifted to feed calves, the production of cheese and butter decreased.

In accordance with the economic changes, the dietary pattern in rural regions changed. The dietary pattern that originally depended on personal food production slowly was transformed to one with greater reliance on store-bought foods. In the 1950s, when these economic and dietary changes began, access to and availability of commercial foods was limited. However, with in-creased economic development, roadways were improved to allow foods to be transported to and from cities such as Hermosillo City. As a consequence, by the 1970s and 1980s, the dietary pattern of rural communities became more urbanized.

Although there is still some home food production, it is relatively little compared to earlier periods. The diet in many rural communities has become almost completely urban, as indicated by the consumption of pastas, lun-cheon meats, soft drinks, chips, and candies. Components of the traditional diet that still remain are some wild plants and fruits in the summer. However, some traditional foods that used to be very popular are now eaten only in the poorest communities.[8]

The "Food Consumption Basket" for Rural Sonora

Among government policymakers, the concept of a "food consumption bas-ket" is of special interest relative to improving nutrition for poor sectors of the population. Valencia et al.[9] carried out a nutrition survey in 26 rural com-munities in Sonora. The 20 most commonly consumed foods or groups of foods, corresponding to 69% of the total quantity of food consumed, are:

1. Wheat and wheat products
2. Pinto beans

3. Corn and corn products

4. Coffee

5. Meats

6. Sugar

7. Whole milk

8. Eggs

9. Potatoes

10. Soft drinks

11. Cheese

12. Tomatoes

13. Coffee-milk-sugar

14. Onions

15. Oranges

16. Shortening

17. Apples

18. Bananas

19. Candies and other sweets

20. Chile

Wheat products (mostly flour tortillas), pinto beans, and corn products (mostly corn tortillas) constitute the staple diet in 26 rural Sonoran communities. Of the 20 basic food items, soft drinks occupy position number 10 in the food consumption basket. This corresponds to 387 ml of soft drink per person, and approximately 6% of the per capita consumption of kilocalories.[10] The 20 foods provide adequate amounts of essential nutrients. However, Valencia et al. note that this does not mean that all families surveyed receive an adequate diet. What it does show is that, theoretically, the food consumption basket for this region meets the nutrient needs of the population.

Food Consumption of Adults and Children

Following is a description of the contemporary dietary patterns of most low- and medium-low-income Sonoran families. Numerous longitudinal and cross-sectional studies, including food consumption baskets, have been used to derive these descriptions.

Adults' Diets   In the northwest region of Mexico, most adults (with low- and medium-low incomes) eat three meals a day and some snacks between meals. Before the *desayuno* (breakfast), eaten between 8 and 10 a.m., most adults drink a cup of coffee with sugar (Table 3.4). Often, when the head of the family (father or mother) has to go to work early, he or she has a cup of

TABLE 3.4 **Typical Diets of Adults from Northwest Mexico**

	Day 1	Day 2	Day 3
Breakfast (*almuenzo*) 8–10 a.m.	2 scrambled eggs with tomato, onion, green hot pepper	2 cooking tsp. of fried potatoes with onion, green hot pepper	2 scrambled eggs with 1 pork sausage
	2 cooking tsp. of fried beans	2 cooking tsp. of fried beans	2 cooking tsp. of fried beans
	3–4 corn or flour tortillas	3–4 corn or flour tortillas	3–4 corn or flour tortillas
	1 cup of coffee with sugar	1 cup of coffee with sugar	1 cup of coffee with sugar
Lunch (*comida*) 1–3 p.m.	1 medium fried beefsteak with tomato, onion, and green hot pepper	2 cooking tsp. of fried potatoes with onion and green hot pepper	2–5 *tacos* of grilled beef with lettuce, tomato, onion, and *salsa* (tomato, garlic, onion, and green or red hot peppers)
	2 cooking tsp. of fried beans	2 cooking tsp. of fried beans	
	3–4 corn or flour tortillas	red hot pepper	
	1 big glass of lemonade	3–4 corn or flour tortillas	2 beers
		1 big glass of Kool-Aid (with sugar)	
Dinner (*cena*) 6–9 p.m.	2 cooking tsp. of fried potatoes	2 cooking tsp. of fried beans with fresh cheese	2 cooking tsp. of fried potatoes with pork *chorizo*
	2 cooking tsp. of fried beans	3–4 corn or flour tortillas	2 cooking tsp. of fried beans
	3–4 corn or flour tortillas	1 cup of coffee with sugar	3–4 corn or flour tortillas
	1 cup of coffee with sugar		1 cup of coffee with sugar
Between meals (*entre comidas*) 5–6 a.m. 3–4 p.m.	coffee with sugar coffee with sugar 1 corn or flour tortilla	coffee with sugar coffee with sugar 1 small sweet bread (*concha o cuerno*)	coffee with sugar coffee with sugar

SOURCE: M. I. Ortega and A. Castañeda, personal communication (CIAD/AC), Hermosillo, Sonora, Mexico, 1992.

coffee at home and then a *desayuno* at work. This *desayuno* is usually tortillas (corn or wheat), eggs (scrambled), fried beans, fried potatoes, pork sausage, and coffee. Members of the family who stay at home eat the same foods in their *desayuno*.

The second meal is the *comida* (dinner), eaten between 1 and 4 p.m. The *comida* almost always includes tortillas and fried beans and a main dish of fried, grilled, or boiled beef (beefsteak, *taco* of grilled beef, or *cocido* or *albóndigas*), pasta soup, fried potatoes, or rice. The main dish is sometimes cooked with such vegetables as tomatoes, onions, garlic, and green hot peppers. Often the meal is accompanied by small quantities of fresh vegetables, such as lettuce, tomatoes, onions, and *salsa* (tomato, green or red hot pepper, onion, and garlic). The *comida* usually includes lemonade, Kool-Aid, a soft drink, or water. Some men drink beer. They may drink beer once a week, at the minimum, usually when they eat away from home.

The last meal, the *cena* (supper), is usually a light one, eaten between 6 and 9 p.m. This meal again includes tortillas, beans, coffee, and sometimes fried potatoes, cheese, and fried pork or beef spiced sausage (*chorizo*). Between the *comida* and the *cena,* most adults drink coffee, sometimes accompanied by tortillas or sweet bread.

Children's Diets   Children who eat table foods eat at basically the same times as adults do (Table 3.5). The main difference between children's and adults' diet is in the number of servings and in some types of food. For example, children drink coffee, with milk added, only at the *desayuno* and *cena*. Also, unlike adults, children may eat cereal at the *desayuno*. The cereal can be corn (cornflakes), oat, or wheat (cream of wheat) with milk and sugar added. Fruit, usually banana, is eaten with the cereal. Also, the *desayuno* can include eggs (scrambled), accompanied by fried beans, tortilla, and milk or coffee with milk.

For children, the *comida* often includes a pasta (watery) or rice (dry) soup as a main dish. When the *comida* contains beef, it is in small portions or in a dish with potatoes as the main ingredient. Although consumption of grilled beef is common, children's *tacos* are made from ground beef and potatoes. *Tacos* for men are usually made from grilled beef when they are eaten away from home. *Cena* for children often includes *atole* (cereal gruel), in addition to tortilla, fried beans, cheese, and coffee with milk. Children often eat candies, corn chips, and sweet bread between meals at home or at school.

In short, the dietary pattern of people of the northwest region of Mexico is changing as the consumption of cheaper animal foods such as luncheon meats increases. This is especially true for low-income families as prices of foods increase and household incomes decline.

Nutrient Contribution of Regional Northern Dishes   The significant nutrient contribution by typical dishes was illustrated by Jardines et al.[11] (See the glossary at the end of this chapter for a detailed description of main ingredients and caloric value of some of these typical regional dishes.) Analyses of 15 dishes from six regions of Sonora revealed that a serving of *gallina pinta* contributed more than 25% of the daily recommended amount of energy, protein, iron, and niacin; 24% of thiamin; and 21% of calcium for an adult man. The *chivichangas de queso* contributed 45% of the calcium requirement, and the *tamales de carne* 36% of the iron requirement. *Ejotes con chile* provided 5.2% of the vitamin A requirement. But, according to these investigators, the vitamin A contribution of all of the remaining dishes studied was below 2%

TABLE 3.5 Typical Diets of Children from Northwest Mexico

	Day 1	Day 2	Day 3
Breakfast (almuenzo) 8–10 a.m.	1 scrambled egg 1 cooking tsp. of fried beans 1–2 corn or flour tortillas 1 cup of coffee with milk	1–2 cooking tsp. of fried beans 1–2 corn or flour tortillas 1 cup of coffee with milk	1 medium plate of cereal (oat, corn, or wheat) with milk 1 medium banana
Lunch (comida) 1–3 p.m.	1 medium plate of pasta soup 1 cooking tsp. of fried beans 1–2 corn or flour tortillas 1 medium glass of "Kool-Aid"	1 serving of fried beef, with potatoes, tomato, onion, garlic, and green hot pepper 1 cooking tsp. of fried beans 1–2 corn or flour tortillas 1 medium glass of lemonade	2 tacos of ground beef, with potatoes, tomato, and lettuce 1 medium glass of soda
Supper (cena) 6–9 p.m	1 cup of atole (a drink made with cornstarch, milk, and sugar) 1–2 corn or flour tortillas	1 cooking tsp. of fried potatoes 1–2 corn or flour tortillas 1 cup of coffee with milk	1 cooking tsp. of fried beans 1 small piece of fresh cheese 1–2 corn or flour tortillas 1 cup of coffee with milk
Between meals	1 candy Rolly Pop	1 small bag of corn chips	1 sweet bread

SOURCE: M.I. Ortega and A. Castañeda, personal communication (CIAD/AC), Hermosillo, Sonora, Mexico, 1992.

of the daily recommendation. These data are important because they show that traditional foods provide essential nutrients as well as energy. Because of the frequency of their consumption, these foods can and do make important contributions to the diet.

Eating Out   As noted earlier, proximity to the United States has influenced the dietary pattern of the northern population of Mexico in different ways. One of the most evident influences is the "eating-out" patterns. Baer describes a wide array of fast foods that are available from foodstands and restaurants in Hermosillo, Sonora.[12] American-style establishments that sell fried chicken, pizza, and hamburgers and Mexican-style stands that sell *tacos* and *tortas* are quite popular.

Infant Feeding Practices

Breast Feeding   It has been argued that in Mexico the duration of breast feeding differs significantly between the border and nonborder states. However, Campbell, in her study of poor urban neighborhoods in Hermosillo, Sonora, reports that the mean weaning age was later than 6 months, a figure quite close to the weaning age reported in the south central region.[13] Other surveys of rural and of 23 urban poor *colonias* (neighborhoods) conducted by Valencia et al. at the Centro de Investigación en Alimentación y Desarrollo (CIAD) in Sonora also found that infants were not receiving breast milk after 6 months of age.[14] As with a previous investigation among low-income women, Campbell found a negative association between maternal work and the initiation of breast feeding. Clearly, there is an issue of trade-offs between breast feeding and women's employment that should be reexamined as greater numbers of rural and urban women join the labor force in many parts of the world. Baer's findings in Hermosillo and Arroyo Lindo, in northern Mexico, suggest the importance of women's employment on household food consumption patterns.[15] Wives tended to use a high percentage of their earnings for household expenses. Thus the effect of women's work on the rest of family activities is an important underlying issue that must be considered as one examines infant feeding practices among low-income households.

A recent study by Saucedo del Socorro on infant feeding practices in Chihuahua found that almost all women (about 94%) breast-fed their infants at birth, but by the end of the first year, only 21% were still breast-feeding.[16] The author also found that supplementary feedings were common. Over half (54%) of the breast-feeding mothers gave their infants a supplementary bottle during the first month. The most common reasons for giving supplementary bottles to breast-feeding infants were because the baby seemed hungry and because mothers were working. During the first year, infants were offered fruits, most often apples, bananas, mangoes, oranges, and grapes. Infants were also offered vegetables, including carrots, squash, potatoes, *chayote,* and avocado, and legumes such as beans, lentils, and, less often, peas.

Cereals appear to provide the highest source of food energy for infants, with pasta soups, *avena,* tortilla, and rice gruels normally introduced by about the third month. *Caldos,* mostly made of chicken, beef, and beans, are thought to be of high nutritive value for infants. However, a large number of processed baby foods are also fed to infants. It is not surprising, given the number of working mothers in the north, that some rely on convenient commercial baby foods.

Food Preparation and Preservation

Most cooking is done from scratch. Canned food makes up only 10% of the total food, and mixes 1 percent.[17] In the north, the main food preparation methods are frying and grilling. Although soups or *caldos* (broths) are boiled, the ingredients are often fried first. When frying, cooks may use safflower or corn oil. Traditionally, lard (pork and beef) and vegetable shortening were used to make tortillas. Some families continue to use butter for making tortillas, but many others have switched to margarine. Grilling is one of the most popular methods used to cook beef. However, most people only eat grilled beef on special occasions or when they eat outside the home.

Drying of cow or deer meat, a traditional method of food preservation, has decreased over the years. Now most drying of meat from cows is done commercially. People use dried meat to make *cazuela*, a watery dish that also includes potato, tomato, onion, and green hot pepper. Although *cazuela* was more popular when cattle raising for self-consumption was prevalent, it is still occasionally eaten by most Sonorans.

Fried beans are common and are prepared and served in many ways— *frijoles aguaditos* (watery fried beans), *frijoles sequitos* (dry fried beans), *frijoles refritos* (fried beans with 25% more fat than regular fried beans), *frijoles de la olla* (boiled beans), and *frijoles puercos* (fried beans with chorizo, red hot pepper, and cheese). *Frijoles de la olla* can be mixed with tomato, onion, and green hot pepper to make *frijoles rancheros*. Also, fresh cheese can be included in almost all types of bean preparation. Different methods of preparation affect the concentrations of certain nutrients, even when the same ingredients are used.

Ingredients used to prepare tortillas remain constant (flour, water, cow's milk or margarine, sometimes baking powder, milk, whey, or fresh cheese), but their quantities change. *Tortillas de agua* are made with very small quantities of fat and are usually about 30 centimeters (cm) in diameter. *Tortilla mediana* or *intermedia* is smaller than *tortilla de agua* (about 12 cm in diameter). *Tortilla de manteca* is smaller than *tortilla intermedia* and has a lot of butter. In rural communities *tortilla de manteca* and *tortilla de agua* are more common; in urban communities *tortilla mediana* is more common because of its commercial production.

Kitchen Utensils Common kitchen utensils are made of a metal called *peltre*. These utensils include *ollas* (deep pots), *sartenes* (skillets), and *cucharas*

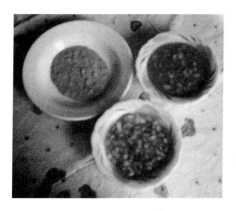

Three different preparations of beans: refritos *(refried),* puercos *(fried with sausage, hot peppers, and cheese), and* aguaditos *(watery).*

(cooking spoons). Urban families and some rural families have bottled gas stoves. However, rural families make their tortillas in a *comal* (piece of hot metal), using wood as a fuel source. Often, rural families have a *estufa de leña* (wood combustible stove), but it is mainly used to cook during the winter season.

OVERVIEW OF MEXICAN DIETS

Differential Patterns in Northern and Southern Diets

As has been stated earlier, in Mexico, foods, mixed dishes, and methods of cooking are as varied and numerous as the country's states. However, the main ingredients used in all regions are corn, beans, wheat, and various types of *chiles*. Each region has its own ingredients, based on its food production and cooking traditions. In spite of these variations, in order to highlight differences in eating patterns, one can divide the country into two large regions, based on geographic and economic considerations: north and south. The different dietary patterns in these regions are influenced by local food production and food availability, rural or urban characteristics, and geographic location, among others.

Historically, corn and beans were the basis of the Mexican diet. Later, during the Spanish conquest, wheat was introduced by the Spaniards, and it was mainly adopted by people in the northern region. Other important components of the traditional diet were squash, hot peppers of various kinds, *quelites, nopales* (cactus), tomatoes, and onions.

In 1976, researchers at the National Institute of Nutrition (INN-SZ) studied the different types of foods consumed and the nutritional adequacy of the diet nationwide.[18] Among the main findings were that high levels of animal

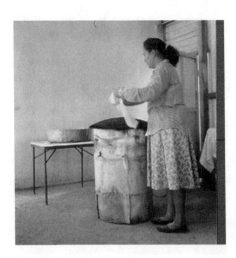

A traditional way of preparing flour tortillas over a comal.

protein and low levels of vegetables and fruits were consumed in the northern region. As a result, inadequate intakes of vitamins A and C, riboflavin, and minerals such as iron were common. In contrast, in the southern region, intakes of animal protein were low. In the south, where traditional vegetarian diets were more common, the researchers found that there was a greater consumption of corn, beans, and some vegetables such as squash, *nopales, quelites,* and potatoes. In addition, fruits were consumed, mostly as a drink called *aguas frescas,* but this drink was seasonal and not commonly consumed by the poorest families in the region. As a result, the southern diet was deficient in vitamins and minerals as well as in protein and kilocalories.

In contrast to the common stereotype, Baer notes that northern Mexicans use very little *chile.*[19] The elaborate *chile*-based sauces common in southern and central Mexico are not used in Sonora, where canned *mole* sauce is more commonly used. *Mole* is homemade on rare occasions. As stated earlier, in the north, flour tortillas are preferred over corn. Meat and egg intake are also higher in the north than in the south. Vegetable use is quite limited in the north. Also used extensively are *queso regional* (similar to cottage cheese) and limes, which are used in soups and on vegetables, fruits, and even Chinese food. But Baer makes a very central point when she argues that in spite of the observed American influence on the northern food habits because of proximity to the United States, Sonoran lives and food use patterns remain distinctly Mexican.

Differential Patterns in Rural and Urban Diets

There is little current information on dietary patterns within the different zones of Mexico. However, cross-sectional studies conducted in some marginal regions of the country provide new information about food consumption. Avila and Ysunza compared the information reported by the National Institute of Nutrition of Mexico (INN) at three different times—1962, 1971, and 1979—with their own investigation in the state of Oaxaca during 1988.[20] In 1979, INN reported a higher consumption of corn in the south and southeast zones and a higher consumption of animal products in the northern states and Mexico City. Avila and Ysunza strongly argue that these differences reflect differences in rural/urban as opposed to northern/southern consumption patterns.

These investigators also reported on the observations of other studies. On one side is the Mexican traditional rural diet, with corn and beans as staple foods, complemented by fruits, vegetables, and limited amounts of animal products (if these were sufficient in quantity and variety, diets could be adequate). On the other side is the urban diet that substitutes wheat for corn and animal products for beans. As a result, the urban diet is higher in saturated fats and in commercially produced and processed foods with low nutrient density. Between the rural and urban diets is the "transitional diet," where the urban diet is gradually replacing the rural diet. This occurs when

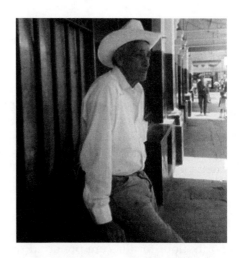

Rural migrants are assimilated into their urban environments in Northern Mexico.

rural areas become more urbanized or when people migrate from rural to urban areas.

Avila and Ysunza also found that recent migrants to urban areas had better nutrition than did long-term urban residents. Migrants tended to eat some processed foods, but due to their generally low incomes, they also continued to eat most of their traditional foods. Many foods, such as animal products, were unaffordable to the migrants. Consequently, the authors reported that migrants had diets that were deficient in protein, calories, vitamins A and C, riboflavin, and iron. These deficiencies were similar to those found by INN in 1976. The modernization or urbanization of the diet was accompanied by increased overweight in certain segments of the population. Interestingly, problems of undernutrition were concurrently found in the same population, as reported by Suárez and Hernández.[21]

In contrast, studies conducted in the north, specifically in the northwest, have found that the most important change in the dietary pattern of this region has been the increased consumption of processed foods as a consequence of modernization and urbanization. Another dietary change among the poorer families was the substitution of beef for luncheon meat or chicken, fish, or eggs.

Lastly, besides the factors discussed above, differences in agricultural technology help explain differences between diets and nutritional trends in the northern and southern regions of Mexico. In 1983, for example, the northern region possessed 71% of the irrigated land, owned 49% of the tractors, and produced 35% of the agricultural crops. In contrast, the southern region had 5 percent of the irrigated land, owned 11% of the tractors, and produced 14% of the agricultural crops.[22] These dramatic differences illustrate the north's greater economic resources that allow its population to buy larger quantities of nutritious foods.

The southern region includes central and southern portions of Mexico. It is important to highlight other distinctive differences within this region. For example, the central region, which includes the state of Mexico and Mexico City, has easy access to foods from other regions of the country at relatively low prices. Food products converge in Mexico City, and their supply is abundant. Available foods include vegetables, fruits, fish, eggs, milk, chicken, and pork. However, animal products are still unaffordable for most of the people.[23]

The south and southeast region have the poorest states in the country, Oaxaca and Michoacán. In this region diets, as the studies by INN-SZ indicate, are poor in both quantity and quality. Even the commonly eaten meal of corn, beans, and *salsa* may be limited in quantity and may not satisfy basic caloric needs.

DIETARY TRENDS AND NUTRITIONAL STATUS OF MEXICAN-AMERICANS IN THE UNITED STATES

Breast-Feeding Trends

The analysis by John and Martorell of the Mexican-American component of the Hispanic Health and Nutrition Examination Survey (HHANES-MA) is the best profile of breast-feeding behavior, covering a large sample of 2,402 infants born between 1970 and 1982.[24] Since the 1970s, considerable data on breast feeding and its economic, nutritional, and health consequences have been gathered. However, few of these studies have been conducted among Mexican-Americans in the United States.[25] These, like many other cross sectional studies, suffer from small and geographically limited samples, where even "self-selection" (low-income program participants vis-à-vis non-program participants) might play an important role in the outcome of study variables. Large variations among practices—sample characteristics, including socioeconomic differences, research sites (hospital versus home), as well as significant differences in methodologies employed—can add up, thereby imposing great limitations relative to the inferences and conclusions that can be made from these data.

These cross-sectional studies, however, do provide insights into the process of breast feeding, and they generate hypotheses that can be tested in more extensive investigations. For example, cross-sectional studies can investigate reasons why working mothers decide to continue to breast feed or how ethnicity, maternal rural versus urban origin, or mother's age or education influence duration of breast feeding.

John and Martorell found that the proportion of Mexican-American infants ever breast-fed has increased substantially in recent years. Weighted proportions of breast-fed infants were 30.7% for 1970–74, 38.1% for 1975–78, and 47.6% for 1979–82. Children born into families with a college-educated head of household were more likely to be breast-fed than were other children. Breast feeding was also positively associated with birth weight. John and Martorell also found that infants in households for which the preferred interview language was Spanish were more likely to be breast-fed than were infants living in households for which the interview was conducted in English. Analysis and in-depth examination of other factors influencing the distribution of weaning times among infants were less definitive because reported weaning times are heaped on multiples of three months. These investigators recommend that in future studies researchers gather current status, or status quo, information on infant feeding.

Food Group Contributions to Total Nutrients

Administering a 24-hour dietary recall to 431 whites, blacks, and Mexican-Americans (98 were Mexican-Americans of whom 77 were women) living in two counties in southeast Texas, Borrud and coworkers examined their food consumption patterns and nutrient intake.[26] The following information focuses on the Mexican-American component of the sample, although attention will be directed when appropriate to a comparative analysis with the other two ethnic groups.

Mexican-Americans ate traditional or familiar Mexican foods, such as beans and tortillas, and preferred foods not previously reported to be commonly consumed by this ethnic group, specifically beef. Table 3.6 shows the nutrients provided by 12 food groups.

Results relative to food groups and nutrient intake can be summarized as follows:

> Mexican-Americans consumed a greater percentage of their saturated fat and cholesterol intake from meats than did whites or blacks, a result of the greater use of beef and organ meats by this ethnic group. The reported use of pork and pork products was also high.
>
> Within the grain and grain products group, breads, rolls, and tortillas were the primary sources of dietary fiber for Mexican-Americans.
>
> Vitamin A has been reported to be a limited nutrient in the diet of Mexican-Americans. In the Borrud et al. study, green beans, summer squash, and corn were consumed more frequently than were carrots or dark green leafy vegetables. However, mixed vegetables, sweet potatoes, lettuce salads, vegetable soup, and dishes containing tomatoes were important contributors to total vitamin A for Mexican-Americans. The vitamin A contribution from liver was considerably greater for Mexican-Americans than for whites and blacks, as was the consumption of legumes.
>
> Enriched fruit-flavored beverages were the primary contributor to vitamin C intake by Mexican-Americans in the study. The Mexican-American preference for desserts and other sweets was also evident. Chili sauces, an important source of vitamins A and C, were also found to contribute significantly to the intake of these two nutrients.

TABLE 3.6 Percent Contribution of Food Groups to Total Nutrients among Mexican-Americans in Texas

						Food Groups					
Nutrient	Meat, Fish, and Poultry	Eggs	Milk and Milk Products	Fat and Oils	Grains and Grain Products	Vege-tables	Legumes	Mixed Dishes and Sandwiches	Soups	Fruits and Fruit Products	Bever-ages	Desserts/ Sugars and Sweets
1. Energy	25.2	2.3	6.7	1.8	18.3	7.6	3.2	9.0	0.9	5.1	7.0	11.1
2. Carbohydrates	1.3	0.2	4.9	0.1	29.7	8.7	5.1	8.1	1.0	10.2	13.6	16.0
3. Protein	49.9	3.7	8.5	0.1	11.5	4.1	5.0	10.0	1.5	1.0	0.2	3.2
4. Total fat	42.3	4.1	8.2	4.5	7.2	8.6	0.4	9.7	0.7	1.6	0.1	9.4
5. Saturated fat	49.5	5.2	17.2	4.3	4.4	3.7	0.1	4.6	0.6	0.9	—	8.2
6. Cholesterol	41.0	38.6	6.8	1.0	1.8	3.4	0.0	2.1	0.8	0.0	—	4.4
7. Dietary fiber	0.5	—	0.4	0.0	21.2	20.1	28.8	7.7	0.8	9.4	0.0	7.8
8. Calcium	6.4	3.7	39.5	0.2	16.9	7.5	5.5	6.9	0.9	3.1	1.3	6.4
9. Vitamin A	35.3	3.1	7.0	2.1	4.7	25.3	0.5	10.3	2.8	1.7	0.2	1.7
10. Vitamin C	3.5	—	1.2	—	2.3	21.0	0.8	6.7	0.3	38.3	22.1	0.7

SOURCE: Adapted from L.G. Borrud et al., Food group contributions to nutrient intake in whites, blacks, and Mexican-Americans in Texas. *Journal of American Dietetic Association*, 89(8) (August 1989), 1061–1069.

Borrud and coworkers also note that it is important to consider cultural frameworks when attempting to effect dietary change. The need to be aware of factors affecting clients' food choices is illustrated by Day and coworkers, who investigated the frequency with which foods were used by Spanish-speaking New Mexicans.[27] Reasons most often given for why certain foods were eaten included easy to prepare, appeals to senses, inexpensive, available, and good for health. Diet modification, to be effective, needs to be compatible with habitual behavior; it also needs to recognize the value in current practices.

Dietary Intakes of Essential Nutrients

The San Antonio Heart Study   In what is now commonly called the San Antonio Heart Study, dietary intakes of essential nutrients were measured using a 24-hour recall, as part of a population-based investigation of diabetes and cardiovascular risk factors. Subjects included 2,134 individuals (25 to 64 years of age) who lived in San Antonio, Texas.[28] They were both Mexican-Americans (MAs) and Anglo-Americans (AAs) selected from three socioeconomically distinct neighborhoods: a low-income, exclusively Mexican-American section in which traditional MA cultural orientation was maintained (barrio); a middle-income, ethnically balanced (transitional neighborhood); and an upper-income, predominantly Anglo neighborhood (suburb). In the barrio only MAs were sampled (the number of AAs living in the barrio was negligible); in the other two neighborhoods approximately equal numbers of both ethnic groups were sampled.

This group of investigators previously reported that MAs, especially in low socioeconomic neighborhoods, are more obese and have a higher prevalence of non-insulin-dependent diabetes mellitus than do AAs.[29] Higher rates of diabetes among Latino populations, particularly Mexican-Americans and Puerto Ricans (together accounting for 75% of all U.S. Latinos), have also been reported by Davidson.[30] Similarly, the data from the San Antonio Heart Study on obesity agree with the 1982–84 Hispanic HANES, in which 29.6% Mexican-American men and 30.1% Mexican-American women were classified as overweight.[31]

Mean Nutrient Intakes as Percentage of the Recommended Dietary Allowance   Knapp et al. found that dietary intakes of calcium, vitamin A, vitamin C, niacin, and phosphorus were significantly lower for MAs than AAs of both sexes.[32] Mean calcium intakes in women were strikingly low, with intakes of 55% and 67% of the recommended dietary allowance (RDA) observed in MA and AA women, respectively. Dietary intakes of vitamin A were also relatively low for both ethnic groups, ranging from 61% to 52% of the RDA in MA men and women, respectively. Overall, dietary iron intake exceeded the RDA for men, whereas for women of both ethnic groups, it averaged 71% of the RDA. Dietary intakes of the B vitamins and phosphorus met or exceeded the RDA for men and women from both ethnic groups. Dietary intakes of riboflavin were significantly greater among MAs than AAs. The investigators were surprised by this finding, given the results for calcium intakes. However, they argue that other foods which are good sources of riboflavin but not of calcium—enriched bread, flour tortillas, pinto beans—may make a greater contribution than dairy products to riboflavin intakes in MAs.

One important objective of the Knapp report was to determine how ethnicity and socioeconomic status (SES), alone and together, influenced dietary intakes of MAs and AAs. However, because there was no low-income AA population, it was impossible to measure the effect of SES independent of ethnicity. Nevertheless, Knapp and coworkers report that dietary intakes of calcium were influenced primarily by ethnicity and, to a lesser extent, by SES. In every neighborhood, MAs consumed less calcium than AAs. Among MAs, higher intakes of calcium were associated with higher SES. The authors acknowledge that lactase deficiency may be partly responsible for the lower consumption of milk products among MAs.

Dietary Intake of Macronutrients   Haffner et al. found that dietary intakes of macronutrients for MAs and AAs were similar to intakes found in the National Health and Nutrition Examination Survey (NHANES). Men in both ethnic groups consumed similar amounts of kilocalories, but MA women consumed more calories than did AA women. MAs of both sexes consumed less protein than did AAs, although the difference was significant only for women. Carbohydrate consumption was higher in MAs than AAs, and there were no ethnic differences in total fat consumption. MA men consumed more saturated fat than did AA men. Both MA men and women consumed less linoleic acid and more cholesterol per 1,000 kilocalories than did their AA counterparts.

Avoidance of Saturated Fat and Cholesterol   Knapp et al. also analyzed avoidance of saturated fat and cholesterol among individuals who participated in the San Antonio Heart Study.[34] Women of both ethnic groups were more likely than were men to avoid saturated fat and cholesterol. Women scored higher on a scale used to determine whether individuals avoided six dietary sources of saturated fat and cholesterol, measured by the following questions:

1. When you eat chicken, how often do you remove the skin?
2. What type of milk do you usually use?
3. Which type of hamburger meat do you usually use?
4. What type of fat/oil do you use most often in cooking?
5. How often do you trim the fat off your meat before you eat it?
6. How often do you eat eggs (times per month)?

Although there were no ethnic differences in overall avoidance of saturated fat and cholesterol, more AAs then MAs recognized milk, eggs, and visible fat on meat as food sources to avoid.

The San Antonio Heart Study is the first population-based study of Mexican-Americans that measured lipids, lipoproteins, and dietary intakes at different socioeconomic levels. The data from Haffner et al. suggest that within a socioeconomic strata there is little ethnic difference in the consumption of macronutrients.[35] In contrast, Knapp et al., from the same research group, suggest that Mexican-Americans have lower intakes of vitamin A and calcium than do Anglo-Americans within the same socioeconomic stratum.[36]

The fat/cholesterol avoidance scale is practical and easy to administer. With further revision and validation, it may become a very useful tool for research and nutrition education. The public health significance of the research findings of the San Antonio Heart Study cannot be overemphasized.

Children's Diets

Limited information is available to aid researchers in assessing the diets of children from birth to preschool age. Thus investigators must depend largely on dietary surveys conducted in adult populations. Both the National Food Consumption Survey (NFCS) and the first National Health and Nutrition Examination Survey (NHANES) relied on a responsible adult for data on food consumption of young children. Though there have been various cross-sectional studies of food consumption patterns among teenage and adult populations, limited information is available on the dietary intake of children under two years of age, especially Hispanic children.

The lack of information on the nutritional status of Hispanic persons in general and of young children in particular has long been recognized.[37] A few studies suggest that Hispanic children tend to consume low amounts of selected nutrients (iron, calcium, vitamin A, vitamin C) in relation to recommended allowances, whereas other studies indicate that their diets are adequate.[38]

With regard to determinants of dietary quality among U.S. Hispanics, a review paper ascertained the significant effects of selected economic and sociodemographic variables on the nutritional quality of their diets.[39] Nutrient intake increased as income increased, but there was little variation in nutrient intake among individuals at higher income levels. There was a positive association between the educational level of women heads of households and their families' nutrient intake and dietary quality. Hispanic persons consumed relatively higher amounts of calcium, iron, and vitamin B_{12} than did other ethnic groups. In summary, the review paper reported that economic and sociodemographic variables had a consistent impact on caloric intakes.

Food Intake of Toddlers   From birth to 24 months is a critical period when toddlers begin to eat the same foods as other family members do. Therefore, examining the food practices of toddlers would be helpful and perhaps reflect family food intakes as well.

Our discussion reviews dietary data collected from 793 food records of 90 toddlers, aged 1 to 2 years, who were predominantly U.S. Hispanics living in low-income households in Denver, Colorado.[40] Although the sample of toddlers was predominantly of Hispanic origin (the remainder were Anglos), there was no significant difference in the age and sex of the toddlers by ethnicity. These data represent a serial examination of nine days of food intakes of very young children collected over a six-month period at many individual observation data points. Although the dietary analysis was done at Cornell University, the study was part of a larger investigation undertaken by the University of Colorado Health Science Center. The main objectives were to evaluate the efficacy of vitamin and mineral supplements for very young children.

Table 3.7 outlines two meal patterns for breakfast, lunch, dinner, and snacks. Meal patterns were developed on the basis of two criteria: according

TABLE. 3.7 Two Meal Patterns of Foods Most Frequently Consumed by Toddlers

Pattern A	Pattern B
Breakfast	*Breakfast*
Milk (whole, 2% low-fat milk)	Milk (whole, 2% low-fat milk)
Cereal (toasted oats, oatmeal)	Bread (white, wheat)
Bread (white, wheat)	Eggs (scrambled)
Fats (butter, margarine)	Meats (bacon, sausage)
Concentrated sugar (sugar, jelly)	Fats (butter, margarine)
Fruit juice (orange, apple)	Concentrated sugars (sugar, jelly)
	Fresh fruit (apple, orange)
Lunch	*Lunch*
Meat (ground beef, cold cuts, frankfurter)	Soups (chicken noodle, vegetable)
Bread (white, wheat, rolls)	Dairy products (American cheese)
Beverage (soda, sweetened fruitade)	Bread (white, wheat)
Concentrated sugar (jelly)	Beverage (soda, sweetened fruitade)
Fresh fruit (apple, orange, banana)	Fresh fruit (apple, orange, banana)
	Concentrated sugars (gelatin dessert)
Dinner	*Dinner*
Meat (ground beef)	Meat (chicken, pork)
Dairy products (American cheese, cheddar cheese)	Vegetables (tomato, green beans)
Pasta (spaghetti)	Potato (mashed potato)
Sauce and gravies (tomato sauce)	Pasta or rice
Vegetables (corn, tomato)	Milk (whole, 2% low-fat)
Potatoes (boiled, french fries)	Fruits (peach, apple, pear)
Beverage (soda, sweetened fruitade)	Beverage (soda, sweetened fruitade)
Bread (white, wheat, tortilla)	Fruits (peaches, apple)
Snack	*Snack*
Cookies and cakes	Fruits (apple, orange, banana)
Milk (whole)	

SOURCE: D. Sanjur, R. Aquilar, R. Furomoto, A. García, and M. Mort, *Socioeconomic profile, dietary patterns and mutrient intake of Mexican-American and Anglo children (1–2 years) living in Denver, Colorado.* Research report, Cornell University, Ithaca, NY, 1988.

to the frequency of food consumption and according to the common ways in which different combinations of foods were eaten by the children at each meal (i.e., milk and cookies, soup and crackers). Combination dishes were recorded as separate foods (e.g., burritos were recorded as a wheat tortilla, cheddar cheese, and refried beans). For breakfast, meal pattern A shows that milk and cereal were the main sources of protein. In pattern B, the main sources of protein were milk, eggs, and meat. The primary source of vitamin C was fruit juices in pattern A and fresh fruits in pattern B. At lunchtime, the children consumed protein from meat (in pattern A) or cheese (in pattern B). Breads and fresh fruits were consistently observed in both patterns. Soft drinks were the preferred beverage in both patterns.

The food combinations in the dinner meal patterns show that the toddlers had been exposed to a variety of food flavors, textures, and colors. Early exposure to a variety of foods has a central influence on the formation of food preferences and choices as children grow older. For snacks, the toddlers ate milk and cookies (or chips or cakes) in pattern A and fruits in pattern B.

Based on the meal patterns, an example of a child's one-day menu, including energy values, was constructed, as shown in Table 3.8. The menu's total energy content adequately met the RDA at 88%. Dinner contributed the largest percentage of total energy (31%), followed by lunch (27%) and breakfast (21%). Snacks contributed 10% of total energy.

When the mean intakes of energy and 14 nutrients were examined by Murphy and colleagues, the following findings were reported:

> Consumption of energy and all the examined nutrients met at least 75% of the 1989 RDAs. Protein intake was particularly high, exceeding the RDA at 278%. Mean sodium intake (which did not include discretionary salt) was greater than the estimated minimum requirement for healthy persons of 225 mg and 300 mg sodium for 1-year-old children and 2-to-5-year old children respectively. For potassium, the mean intake approximated the estimated minimum requirements of 1,000 mg for 1-year-old and 1,400 mg for 2-to-5-year-old children.[41]

Interesting issues relative to sodium intake by children merit further discussion here. The hypothesis that the sodium content of infant foods contributes to hypertension in later life has not been confirmed.[42] Infant foods, even those with salt added, do not contribute as much sodium to the diet as do whole milk or table foods. Studies of infants fed diets that were either high or low in sodium from age 3 to 8 months showed no correlation between salt intake during infancy and blood pressure at 1 and 8 years of age.[43] However, it has been recommended that because high sodium intakes are unnecessary, parents and children should have the opportunity to avoid inapparent sources of sodium in the food supply.[44]

Whole milk contributed 24% of the total sodium intake in the toddlers' diets; 82% of the toddlers drank whole milk and 34% of the toddlers drank low-fat milk. Snacks such as potato chips, hamburgers, and pizza contributed

TABLE 3.8   Example of Toddler One-Day Diet and Its Energy Value

Meal	Measure	Energy (kcal)	% RDA
Breakfast			
Toasted oat cereal	1/2 cup	37	
Whole milk	4 oz	75	
Sugar	1 tsp	14	
White bread toast	1 slice	70	
Margarine	1 tsp	33	
Grape jelly	1 tsp	17	
Orange juice	2 oz	30	
Subtotal		276	21
Lunch			
Chicken noodle soup	1/2 cup	31	
American cheese	1 oz	104	
White bread	1 slice	70	
Grape drink	4 oz	56	
Banana	1/2	50	
Orange gelatin dessert	1/4 c	35	
Subtotal		346	27
Dinner			
Meatloaf	1 oz	60	
Spaghetti	1/2 cup	78	
Tomato sauce	1 tbsp	6	
Corn	1 ear	120	
Soda	4 oz	48	
Tortilla (corn)	1/2	66	
Peaches (raw)	1/2	20	
Subtotal			31
Snacks			
Chocolate chip cookies	1	50	
Whole milk	4 oz	75	
Subtotal		125	10
Total		1,145	88

SOURCE: D. Sanjur, R. Aguilar, R. Furomato, A. García, and M. Moto, *Socioeconomic profile, dietary patterns and nutrient intake of Mexican-American and Anglo children (1–2 years) living in Denver, Colorado.* Research report, Cornell University, Ithaca, NY, 1988.

33% of the toddlers' sodium intake. On the average, the toddlers' diets consisted of 15.3% protein, 34.3% carbohydrate, and 50.4% fat.

Table 3.9 shows the distribution of the toddlers' mean energy and nutrient intakes examined as percentages of the 1989 RDAs. Most toddlers met at least two-thirds of the RDA for energy and for the ten nutrients. Mean intakes of protein, riboflavin, and thiamin were high, with most toddlers exceeding the RDA for these nutrients. However, mean iron intake was 51% of the RDA. A major portion of the iron was provided by cereals and one-fifth of it by meat

TABLE 3.9   Toddler Nutrient Intakes, by Percentage of the 1989 RDAs

Energy or Nutrient	1989 RDAs	<34% RDAs	34%–66% RDAs	67%–110% RDAs	>110% RDAs
Energy	1,300 kcal	0	18.5	66.6	14.9
Protein	16 g	0	0	0.9	99.1
Calcium	800 mg	5.6	33.3	37.8	22.2
Iron	10 mg	2.8	34.3	50.9	12.0
Vitamin A	2,000 IU	2.2	15.6	33.3	48.9
Thiamin	0.7 mg	0	5.6	32.2	62.2
Riboflavin	0.8 mg	0	2.2	17.8	80
Niacin	9 mg	1.1	14.4	42.2	42.2
Vitamin C	40 mg	5.6	28.7	20.3	45.4
Phosphorus	800 mg	1.1	12.2	53.3	33.3
Magnesium	80 mg	3.7	16.7	37	42.6

SOURCE: D. Sanjur, R. Aguilar, R. Furomoto, A. Garciá, and M. Mort, *Socioeconomic profile, dietary patterns and nutrient intake of Mexican-American and Anglo children (1–2 years) living in Denver, Colorado.* Research report, Cornell University, Ithaca, NY, 1988.

and eggs. The RDA for iron for toddlers is problematic because of the iron density needed to meet the RDA. The low percentage adequacy of iron intake in this study is consistent with national survey results that have reported mean intakes for 1- to 3-year-olds ranging from 52% to 70% of the RDA.

On the basis of prior dietary and nutrient findings, toddlers should eat more foods that are good sources of iron and magnesium (e.g., liver, meats, egg yolk, nuts, legumes, and whole grains) and fewer foods that are high in sodium (snacks such as potato chips, hamburgers, and pizza). A nutrition education program emphasizing the importance of childhood eating patterns for shaping adult food choices might be beneficial in future intervention programs aimed at Hispanic families. The mothers, however, should be commended for the many positive things they are doing, given their economic circumstances. Furthermore, constructive suggestions should be made within the Hispanic cultural and economic framework.

Food Group Intake of Children and Teenagers   The Hispanic Health and Nutrition Examination Survey (HHANES) offered a unique opportunity to examine in detail the food intake patterns of a large sample of Mexican-American children.

Murphy et al.[45] looked at the food group daily servings for 3,436 children (four age groups: 1 to 2 years, 3 to 5 years, 6 to 11 years, and 12 to 17 years) who participated in the Mexican-American portion of the 1982–83 HHANES and who lived in five states in the southwestern United States (California, Arizona, New Mexico, Texas, and Colorado). This segment of the HHANES reported by Murphy et al. corresponds to the food frequency data only, with questions about intakes of 57 foods and food groups during the previous three months.

On average, Mexican-American children in all age categories consumed more than the recommended two daily servings of meat. Mean servings of

FIGURE 3.1 **Percentage of Mexican-American children who consumed fewer than the recommended number of food group servings**

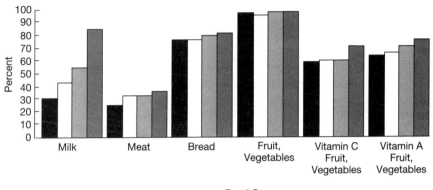

Age Group

1-2	years	
3-5	years	
6-11	years	
12-17	years	

SOURCE: Adapted from S. P. Murphy, R. O. Castillo, R. Martorell, and F. S. Mendoza, An evaluation of food group intakes by Mexican-American children. *Journal of the American Dietetic Association, 90* (1988), 388–390.

milk met the recommendations for children 1 to 11 years, but teenagers' intake was much less than the recommended four servings. Bread intakes were approximately one serving per day short of the recommended four servings for all ages. Fruit and vegetables servings were less than half (33% to 47%) of the recommended four servings per day.

The percentage of children who reported eating less than the recommended number of servings of foods from each of the groups is shown in Figure 3.1. USDA, Daily Food Guide "standard serving" is based on 1 cup of milk, 2 to 3 ounces of meat, 1 slice of bread, and 1/2 cup of fruit/vegetables. However, culture-specific data relative to children's portion sizes are an important and unresolved issue in dietary assessment; future research on this and other issues such as nutrient data bases for specific ethnic foods merit further investigation.) Murphy et al. found that a substantial number (75% and 95%) had fewer than the recommended four servings from the fruit and vegetable groups each day. Over half of the children over age 5 had low intakes of milk.[46]

Both the food frequency questionnaire used during HHANES I (1971–74), as well as the one used during HHANES II (1982–83) appear to suggest that Mexican-American children have particularly low intakes of fruits and vegetables. The data from Murphy et al. are of nutritional concern, given the large numbers of Mexican-American children, particularly teenagers, who consume well below recommended levels of milk and fruits and vegetables while consuming large amounts of relatively nonnutritious high-fat, high-sugar foods. Creative and interesting educational efforts to reach parents and children would be useful to address these issues.

Elderly Mexican-Americans

Information is very limited about the dietary and nutritional habits of elderly Hispanics. The population of older Hispanics is estimated to be increasing three and one-half times faster than that of older African-Americans and five times faster than that of older non-Hispanic whites.[47]

A food frequency survey of 254 low-income, elderly (age 60 to 96) Mexican-Americans and non-Hispanic whites was conducted by Bartholomew et al. as part of a larger health study of elderly persons living in a San Antonio, Texas, barrio.[48] Weekly intakes of selected foods were assessed using the food frequency questionnaire from HHANES. Previous research had shown that elderly persons, particularly Mexican-Americans, have low intakes of calcium, vitamin A, vitamin C, protein, iron, and riboflavin. Therefore, the researchers collected information on the consumption of 30 foods that were considered common, good sources of these nutrients. The selected foods included 10 foods, 10 beverages, 4 dessert/snack foods, and 3 condiments. Three fats were also included in order to compare consumption patterns with patterns identified in other studies. The variance in food consumption was estimated by using multiple regression analysis for the independent socioeconomic variables of age, sex, income, education, and ethnicity. Of these, ethnicity was the major variable influencing food intake. (See Chapter 2 for a discussion of the pivotal influence of ethnicity on food intake.)

There were significant differences between Mexican-Americans and non-Hispanic whites. Elderly Mexican-Americans consumed eggs, poultry, legumes, organ meats, avocados/olives, flour tortillas, and sugar more frequently than did non-Hispanic whites; they also used saturated fats in cooking more frequently. Conversely, elderly Mexican-Americans consumed skim milk, ice cream/ice milk, beef, all fruits or juice, all vegetables, breads, and oil/margarine less frequently than did non-Hispanic whites. In view of their findings, Bartholomew et al. conclude that ethnicity plays a major role in predicting dietary patterns. This may be true not only for low-income Mexican-American elderly populations but for other income and ethnic groups as well.

These investigators also suggest that ethnicity may be a factor contributing to ethnically related food choices, which in turn could affect health status and the promotion of health or prevalence of disease. Previous work by investigators in the San Antonio Heart Study also revealed nutrition-related health differences between Mexican-Americans and non-Hispanic whites age 25 to 64 years. Specifically, Bartholomew et al. found that Mexican-Americans "had higher rates of obesity and diabetes; consumed greater quantities of high-cholesterol foods, saturated fats, and carbohydrates; and had lower intakes of calcium, vitamins A and C, and linoleic acid" than did non-Hispanic whites.[49]

Finally, Marks et al. investigated the health behavior of 603 elderly Hispanic women residing in Los Angeles to evaluate the usefulness of cultural factors as predictors of preventive health behavior (e.g., physical exam, screening for breast cancer).[50] Factor analysis of responses yielded four dimensions of cultural assimilation: language preference, country of birth, contact with homeland, and attitudes about children's friends. After controlling for education and age, no dimension of assimilation associated strongly or consistently with health behavior. Of the four dimensions, use of English language associated most closely with increased screening.

Dietary Changes among Mexican-American Families

Migrant families of Mexican descent, like many other newcomers, hold tenaciously to their traditional food preferences and language. However, the pervasive force of the dominant culture, coupled with the unavailability and high cost of some of the traditional foods, cause families to abandon some of their traditional food habits. Thus substitutions occur and dietary changes take place. As children of migrant families explore and observe the world around them, they often help interpret and promote the new culture, particularly as it relates to family food choices. As children learn about new foods, they talk their parents into buying them.[51]

Measuring Dietary Change An important issue in nutrition research beyond specific dietary changes is how to measure such changes. There are a number of ways to measure dietary change, particularly among societies in transition and immigrant groups. Such indicators of change as retention, loss, addition, substitution, or integration of food items have been examined. Retention or continuity of traditional ethnic patterns is conditioned by geographic distance from country of origin, as well as by the availability of ethnic foods (supply) and population density of that particular subcultural group (demand) in the host country. This is an important issue, for example, in the case of Mexican, Cuban, or Puerto Rican migrant families where proximity to the countries of origin, as well as population concentration in specific areas, may make it easier to keep alive their traditional cultural heritage through foods.

In measuring dietary change, it is also important to examine changes in meal patterns and frequency of eating ("Before, I ate two main meals; now I eat three meals and a snack"); dietary diversity ("I now usually eat six different foods at dinner; before, I usually ate three); and food preparation methods ("I do more boiling and baking now, rather than frying").

Another significant variable sometimes appears to work independently of the degree or rate of dietary change. Length of residence is not always related to the degree of dietary change. There are conflicting findings in the migration/acculturation literature confirming some of the observations relative to the influence of length of residence on dietary change.

Some of the most commonly used measurement techniques, as well as factors influencing the dietary changes, and reasons for them, are:

1. One conventional approach for measuring dietary change is to study changes relative to the "core," secondary, and peripheral food items. By measuring the number of food items in the core diet eaten per week, investigators can assess the continuity or change of specific food items, as well as evaluate which of the core items stayed the same in the host environment.

2. Dietary change can also be measured by using food scales that are designed to assess dietary complexity. On a scale food items range from simple and monotonous to the most varied. In this case, it is assumed that a complex diet, in terms of number of food items consumed, is a proxy for dietary change.

3. Measurement of loss or retention of traditional foods, addition of new foods characteristic of the host society, and addition or loss of basic foods and processed foods in both cultures is also a common technique. This approach is a slight modification of measuring changes in the core, secondary, or peripheral food items.

4. Another way in which some investigators have examined dietary change has been through the examination of continuity or rate of disappearance of folk food beliefs. Although to some extent it may indirectly reflect certain changes relative to food, it may better reflect trends toward modernization and urban attitudes.

Dewey et al. studied 140 migrant and nonmigrant families of Mexican descent in California.[52] These researchers observed that traditional food avoidances were not related to the length of time that respondents lived in the United States, their level of education, their ability to speak English, or their knowledge of nutrition. These observations support the contention that food beliefs are pervasive and less subject to change than patterns of food consumption. Therefore, from a methodological point of view, adherence to folk food beliefs as an indicator of dietary change may not be valid.

The limited research on dietary change among Mexican-American families suggests a persistence of traditional cultural eating patterns, concurrent with the adoption of new foods and dishes. Some of these changing trends similarly reflect nutritional benefits as well as drawbacks among Mexican-American diets.[53]

In studying any type of dietary change among migrating populations, the following key points are important:

1. For the majority of the families, almost all food acquisition occurs through purchasing rather than growing it. In the United States, studies have shown that migrant families purchase their food in large supermarkets, primarily because of availability and lower cost. However, a small segment of the population purchases food at small local stores that carry some indigenous foods not found in the large supermarkets.

2. Processed foods displayed in large supermarkets may be unfamiliar yet attractive. In California, for example, when migrant children accompany their parents during food shopping, the children often ask for specific foods, such as candy, cookies, ice cream, snack chips, soft drinks, and cakes.[54] The mothers' eagerness to please their children and grant their requests outright must be evaluated in light of some children's preference for sweet foods.

Changes in Children's Diets In 1984, Dewey et al. observed that Mexican-American migrant children in California had a high consumption of such foods as breakfast cereals and peanut butter and a low consumption of some traditional Mexican foods such as *atole* (milk-based hot cereal gruel).[55] Consumption of sweet foods varied. Most children ate few desserts, such as pie or cake; a moderate to large amount of candy, cookies, and ice cream; and a large quantity of soft drinks.

When parents were asked what they thought about their diets, 71% of the migrant parents stated that their diets had improved, and many said that they had more money to buy food in the United States. As an indicator of affluence, mothers were asked how often they used to eat meat in Mexico and ate meat now in the United States. Mothers reported an average consumption in Mexico of 3.6 times per week and in the United States of 4.4 times per week. Specifically, mothers reported eating more canned foods, frozen foods, and fruits and vegetables in the United States than in Mexico.

A slightly different but related issue relative to children's food intake concerns their frequency of eating and snacking patterns. Garcia et al. conducted a study in the state of Guanajuato.[56] (An overwhelming number of Mexican migrants to the United States come from central Mexico, particularly from the states of Jalisco, Michoacán, and Guanajuato, with substantial numbers also coming from northern Mexico.) The researchers noted that preschool-age children ate much more frequently (on the average 13.5 times per day) than did their parents and older siblings, whose schedules are influenced by work or school. When preschoolers asked for food, 76% of their requests were granted outright. Whether or not the requests were granted was not associated with the age or gender of the child or with the socioeconomic status of the household. Sometimes when mothers first denied requests because of concerns about nutritional value, or of eating snacks before meals, they later granted the requests.

Changes in Adults' Diets   Interesting changes in maternal diets were found in the California study.[57] In general, consumption of basic foods increased or stayed the same, consumption of traditional foods decreased or stayed the same, and consumption of new (processed) foods increased or were not consumed at all. When women were asked why they had increased consumption of the basic or new categories of food, they explained that the foods were more available in the United States, they had more money for food, or the foods cost less than in Mexico. A major reason for eating fewer of the traditional foods was because they were less available. However, this was only true for certain traditional foods because Mexican staples of tortillas and beans were available.

Of the foods categorized by Dewey et al. as basic, there was a maximum consumption of 13 foods (mean 5.9). Among these were various meats and dairy products, eggs, vegetables, and pasta. Among the traditional foods consumed was a maximum of 21 foods (mean 6.9). These included tortillas, beans, chili peppers, sweet rolls, avocado, and various traditional vegetables and dishes such as tacos, *moles,* and *chiles rellenos.* Their last category of new foods consumed (maximum 18 foods; mean 8.2) included mainly processed foods (canned and frozen items), soft drinks, cake mixes, and chips.

Romero-Gwynn and Gwynn conducted a recent study of dietary changes and acculturation in California among 266 women of Mexican descent.[58] These authors suggest that changes in dietary patterns may have an important role in the development of obesity. They report significant dietary changes, with beneficial as well as detrimental nutritional consequences, as a result of their migration to the United States. Decreased consumption of lard and cream and a moderate increased consumption of vegetables, fruits, and milk were considered positive changes. Conversely, an increased consumption of salad dressing, mayonnaise, margarine or butter, oil, and sour cream were negative changes. Another negative change was the substitution of highly sugared commercial beverages for traditional *aguas frescas de frutas* and *atole.*

Romero-Gwynn and Gwynn note that an increased consumption of vegetables among these migrant families should be viewed with some caution, as it does not truly reflect a large increase in total vegetable consumption. Rather, the change is more a reflection of the *way* vegetables are eaten, as well as the *types* of vegetables being consumed. For example, soups, stews, and tortilla-based dishes, which are usually prepared with vegetables, are disappearing from the diet. Instead, vegetable salads and vegetables are now consumed as side dishes. One potentially negative nutritional consequence of this change is that individuals have begun to consume new sources of fat in the form of salad dressing and margarine/butter. Furthermore, whereas salads are mainly made of lettuce, the traditional dishes contain *chiles,* coriander, and tomatoes, better sources of vitamins A and C.

Another change in vegetable consumption concerns the consumption of rice. Traditional Mexican rice is cooked with substantial amounts of tomatoes or other vegetables, and this is being replaced with plain white rice.

SUMMARY

This chapter has reviewed typical diets and meal patterns of Mexicans living in central/southern Mexico and northern Mexico. The nutritional strengths and weaknesses of Mexican diets were highlighted, as well as the nutrient contributions of selected typical regional dishes and a "food consumption basket" for northern Mexico. In-depth detail was provided about cultural ways of eating, with particular emphasis on diets and meal patterns of adults and children, food preferences, food preparation methods, and kitchen utensils of northern/southern regions of Mexico. A contrasting perspective of diets in these two regions, or rather what some investigators view as urban/rural differentials, was discussed. Breast-feeding trends, using data from the Hispanic HANES, among Mexican-Americans in the United States were reviewed, along with infant feeding practices and some food ideologies.

Assuming that dietary patterns in the United States are heavily influenced by diets observed in Mexico, as well as by other factors (cost, availability) in the U.S. environment, this chapter reviewed contemporary dietary trends and nutritional status of Mexican-Americans in the United States.

Selected data relative to dietary changes, including measurement techniques, among adults and children of Mexican descent were also reviewed. Lastly, a glossary of Mexican food items and mixed dishes, developed from a wide variety of sources and validated by Mexican nutritionists, is included.

GLOSSARY OF MEXICAN FOODS*

agave	plant with spiny margined leaves and flowers; also used to make tequila
aguamiel	sweet beverage obtained from *agave* before making *pulque*
alverjón	green peas
bisque	type of salted white bread
bolillo o birote	type of bread similar to a French roll
buñuelo	deep-fat-fried flour tortilla served with syrup
café con leche	coffee with milk
café negro	plain black coffee
cajeta	candy made from sweetened milk

* Instituto Nacional de la Nutrición (INN), *Valor nutritivo de los alimentos*, Tabla de Uso Práctico, Mexico (1979). Centro de Investigación en Alimentación y Desarrollo, A.C. (C.I.A.D., A.C.), *Tablas de composición de alimentos regionales*, unpublished data, Sonora, Mexico (1992). R. P. Jardines, M. C. Bérmudez, P. Wong, and G. Leon, Platillos tipicos consumidos en Sonora: Regionalización y aporte de nutrientes, *Archivos Latinoamericanos de Nutrición*, 35 (4) (1985), 595. I. Ortega, and A. Castañeda (C.I.A.D., A.C.), personal communication, October 1992. E. Romero-Gwynn and D. Gwynn. *Food and dietary patterns of Latinos of Mexican descent*. Monograph, University of California, Cooperative Extension, Department of Nutrition, Davis, CA, October 1990.

calabacita	small, round, green squash native to Mexico
caldo	soup or stew with a clear broth base
camote	yellow sweet potato
ceviche	raw fish, marinated in lemon juice with some vegetables
champurrado	chocolate-flavored *atole*
chayote	cactuslike fruit with a fleshy texture
chicharrones	fried strips of pork rind, commonly eaten as snack
chile	any of a variety of hot peppers used raw or in sauces
chirimoya	a fruit with a rough green outer skin
chongos	desserts made of cooked milk curds and sugar
chorizo	highly seasoned sausage of chopped beef or pork with red sweet peppers
churros	mexican crullers made of heavy dough
cilantro	fresh coriander, a popular herb used to flavor salsas, meat dishes, and soups
cocido o puchero	stew
consomate	bouillon with tomato flavor
consomé	chicken broth or bouillon
fideo	thin noodle
flor de calabaza	squash flower used to fill *quesadillas* or make *caldos*
frijoles	beans, usually pinto or black
guayaba	sweet, juicy fruit with tiny seeds that has a green or yellow skin and red or yellow flesh
jicama	jam bean
longaniza	pork sausage
maizoro	cornflakes
manteca	lard
masa	dough of dried corn to which water is added to make corn tortillas and other corn-based foods
molletes	*bolillo* topped with fried beans, cheese, and *salsa*
moronga	dried beef or pork blood
pancita	soup made of tripe
pan dulce	sweet bread
picadillo	minced or ground meat
piloncillo o panocha	dark brown sugarcane
pinole	type of cornmeal eaten with *piloncillo* and water or milk
pithaya	red and sweet fruit from a type of cactus
plátano	among Mexicans, the banana is called *plátano*. In the Caribbean and Central America, the plantain, a starchy vegetable that looks like a large banana (could be greenish or fully ripe), is also called *plátano*, and is never eaten raw but is usually pan-fried
pozol	beverage made with a mixture of corn and cocoa with water

queso blanco, fresco or mexicano	soft, white cheese made of part-skim milk, similar to cottage cheese in nutrient value
romeritos	type of herb cooked and seasoned with a red *salsa*
salsa	raw or cooked mixture of tomato, onions, garlic, any kind of *chiles* (hot peppers) and sometimes coriander
sesos con huevo	brains with eggs
sopa aguada	watery soup, usually made of thin spaghetti, rice, or vegetables only
sopa seca	dry soup, usually made of rice (*sopa de arroz*) or noodles (*sopa de coditos*)
sopes	small corn cakes filled with beans, beef or chicken, vegetables, (lettuce, tomato, onion, cucumbers) and cheese
torta	Mexican version of a submarine sandwich, prepared on a *bolillo*
totopos	corn chips
tripas de leche	small intestines of beef
tuna	green or red fruit of *nopales*
uchepo	sweet *tamal*
verdolagas	green leaves used in salads; tender leaves and young stalks can also be cooked like spinach
viznaga	a cactus plant from which a type of candy is made
zapote	apple-sized fruit with green skin and black flesh

NOTES

1. J. A. Bustamante and W. A. Cornelius, eds., *Flujos migratorios Mexicanos hacia Estados Unidos, Comisión sobre el Futuro de las Relaciones Mexico-Estados Unidos*, Fondo de Cultura Económica, México, 1989.

2. S. M. Haffner, J. A. Knapp, H. P. Hazuda, M. P. Stern, and E. A. Young, Dietary intakes of macronutrients among Mexican Americans: The San Antonio Heart Study. *American Journal of Clinical Nutrition, 42* (1985), 1266–1275.

3. L. L. Kaiser and K. G. Dewey, Household economic strategies, food resource allocation, and intrahousehold patterns of dietary intake in rural Mexico. *Ecology of Food and Nutrition, 25* (1991), 123–145.

4. D. H. Calloway, S. P. Murphy, and G. H. Beaton, *Food intake function: A cross-project perspective of the collaborative research support program in Egypt, Kenya and Mexico.* Research Monograph, University of California, Berkeley, August 1988.

5. Ibid.

6. Kaiser and Dewey, Household economic strategies.

7. M. I. Ortega and L. Pérez, *Tendencias de la nutrición en la mujer y cambios agropecuarios en la Sierra Norte de Sonora.* (Mexico: Fundación Friedrich-Naumann, 1988).

8. M. N. Ballesteros, *Valor proteínico de la dieta Sonorense.* Thesis, Centro de Investigación en Alimentación y Desarrollo, C.I.A.D., A.C., Hermosillo, Sonora, Mexico, 1989.

9. M. E. Valencia, R. P. Jardines, E. Noriega, R. Cruz, I. Grijalva, C. E. Peña, The use of 24-hour recall from nutrition surveys to determine food preference, availability and food consumption baskets in popu-

lations. *Nutr. Rep. Int.*, *28*(4) (1983), 815–823.

10. Ibid.

11. R. P. Jardines, M. C. Bermúdez, P. Wong, and G. León, Platillos típicos consumidos en Sonora: Regionalización y aporte de nutrientes. *Archivos Latinoamecanos de Nutrición, 35*(4)(1985).

12. D. R. Baer, The interactions of social and cultural factors affecting dietary patterns in rural and urban Sonora, Mexico. Ph.D. thesis, University of Arizona, 1984.

13. Carolyn E. Campbell, The effects of migration on women's roles and infant feeding, growth and morbidity among migrant squatters in Hermosillo, Sonora, Mexico. Ph.D. Thesis, Cornell University, Ithaca, NY, August 1986.

14. M. Valencia, R. Jardines, E. Noriega, I. Higuera, J. Lozano, P. Wong, and I. Grijalva, *Estudio nutricional en centros urbanos marginados*. Reporte Técnico, C.I.A.D., A.C., Hermosillo, Sonora, Mexico, 1981.

15. Baer, The interactions.

16. T. Saucedo M. del Socorro, Efectos de la lactancia y ablactación sobre el crecimiento físico en infantes de un año de edad que acuden a consulta externa al Hospital Infantil del Estado de Sonora. Thesis, Universidad Autónoma de Chihuahua, April 1989.

17. M. Valencia, R. Jardines, E. Noriega, and I. Higuera, *Estudio Nutricional en la Zona Serrana de Sonora*. Reporte Técnico, C.I.A.D., A.C., Hermosillo, Sonora, Mexico, 1980.

18. Instituto Nacional de la Nutrición (INN), *Encuestas nutricionales en México*. Publicación L-21, División de Nutrición, I.N.N. Departamento de Epidemiología de la Nutrición, Grupo de Nutrición CONACYT-PRONAL, Mexico.

19. Baer, the Interactions.

20. A. Avila Curiel, and A. Ysunza, Las tendencias nacionales de la nutrición en el México Rural, *Producir para la Desnutrición?* Centro de Ecodesarrollo-Fundación Friedrich Naumann, Mexico (1988), pp. 35–57.

21. B. Suárez, and M. Hernández, La sustitución de granos y su impacto en la nutrición: Evidencia en una zona rural del estado de puebla, *Producir para la Desnutrición?* Centro de Ecodesarrollo-Fundación Friedrich Naumann, Mexico (1989), pp. 167–194.

22. Avila and Ysunza, *Las tendencias*.

23. *Instituto Nacional*, Encuestas.

24. A. M. John and R. Martorell, Incidence and duration of breast-feeding in Mexican-American infants, 1970–1982. *American Journal of Clinical Nutrition, 50* (1989), 868–874.

25. M. Kokinos and K. G. Dewey, Infant feeding practices of migrant Mexican-American families in Northern California. *Ecology of Food and Nutrition, 18* (1986), 209–220; S. C. M. Scrimshaw, P. L. Engle, and A. L. Haynes, Factors affecting breast-feeding among women of Mexican origin or descent in Los Angeles. *American Journal of Public Health, 77* (1987), 467–470; J. C. Smith, C. G. Mhango, C. W. Warren, R. W. Rochat, and S. L. Huffman, Trends in the incidence of breast-feeding for Hispanics of Mexican origin and anglos on the USA-Mexican Border. *American Journal of Public Health, 72* (1982), 59–61; E. Romero-Gwynn and L. Carias, Breast-feeding intentions and practice among Hispanic mothers in Southern California. *Pediatrics, 84* (4): (1989), 626-632.

26. L. G. Borrud et al., Food group contributions to nutrient intake in whites, blacks, and Mexican-Americans in Texas. *Journal of American Dietetic Association, 89*(8) (August 1989), 1061–1069.

27. M. L. Day, M. Lentner, and S. Jaquez, Food acceptance patterns of Spanish-speaking New Mexicans, *Journal of Nutrition Education, 10*(3) (1978), 121–123.

28. J. Knapp, S. M. Haffner, E. A. Young, H. P. Hazuda, L. Gardner, and M. P. Stern, Dietary intakes of essential nutrients among Mexican-Americans and Anglo-Americans: The San Antonio Heart Study, *American Journal of Clinical Nutrition, 42* (August 1985), 307–316.

29. Haffner et al., Dietary intakes; J. A. Knapp, H. P. Hazuda, S. M. Haffner, E. A. Young, and M. P. Stern, A Saturated fat/cholesterol avoidance scale: Sex and ethnic differences in a biethnic population. *Journal of the American Dietetic Association, 88* (1988), 172.

30. J. A. Davidson, Diabetes in Hispanics, *Diabetes Care and Education, 11*(6) (1978), 121–123.

31. National Center for Health Statistics, *Hispanic Health and Nutrition Examination Survey*, DHHS Publication no. (PHS) 89-1689, Hyattsville, MD, 1988.

32. Knapp et al., Dietary intakes.

33. Haffner et al., Dietary intakes.

34. Knapp et al., Dietary intakes.

35. Haffner et al., Dietary intakes.

36. Knapp et al., Dietary intakes.

37. L. B. Larson, J. M. Dodds, D. M. Massoth, and H. P. Chase, Nutritional status of children of Mexican-American migrant families. *Journal of the American Dietetic Association, 64* (1974), 29; P. B. Acosta and R. G. Aranda, Cultural determinants of food habits in children of Mexican descent in California, *Practices of low-income families in feeding infants and small children.* HEW Pub. 75-5605, Washington, DC, 1975.

38. S. P. Murphy, R. O. Castillo, R. Martorell, and F. S. Mendoza, An evaluation of food group intakes by Mexican American children. *Journal of the American Dietetic Association, 90* (1990), 388–393; K. G. Dewey, M. A. Strode, and Y. R. Fitch, Dietary change among migrant and nonmigrant Mexican-American families in Northern California. *Ecology of Food and Nutrition, 14* (1984), 11–24; N. Cross, M. B. Korbs, and R. Olson, Nutritional status of Hispanic Head-Start children in Chicago. *Nutrition Reports International, 29* (1984), 1, 67; D. Sanjur, A. García, R. Aguilar, R. Furumoto, and M. Mort, Dietary patterns and nutrient intake of toddlers from low-income families in Denver, Colorado. *Journal of the American Dietetic Association, 90* (1990), 823–829.

39. J. M. Hihn and S. Lane, *Economic and sociodemographic variables affecting nutritional quality of diets: A review.* Working Paper No. 395 (Berkeley, Department of Agricultural and Resource Economics, Division of Agriculture and Natural Resources, University of California, 1986).

40. D. Sanjur, R. Aguilar, R. Furumoto, A. García, and M. Mort, *Socioeconomic profile, dietary patterns and nutrient intake of Mexican-American and anglo children (1–2 years) living in Denver, Colorado.* Research Report, Cornell University, Ithaca, NY, 1988.

41. Murphy et al., An evaluation.

42. G. C. Frank, L. S. Webber, T. A. Nicklas, and G. S. Berenson, Sodium, potassium, calcium, magnesium, and phosphorus intakes of infants and children: Bogalusa Heart Study. *Journal of the American Dietetic Association, 88* (1988), 801; C. F. Whitten and R. A. Stewart, The effect of dietary sodium in infancy and blood pressure and related factors: Studies of infants fed salted and unsalted diets for 5 months, 8 months, and 8 years of age. *Acta Paediatr. Scand. Suppl, 279* (1980), 3.

43. Whitten and Stewart, The effect of dietary sodium.

44. *Pediatric nutrition handbook, Recommendations of the Committee on Nutrition* (Elk Grove Village, IL: American Academy of Pediatrics, 1985).

45. Murphy et al., An evaluation.

46. Ibid.

47. *Demographic characteristics of the older Hispanic population.* A Report by the Select Committee on Aging, Comm. Publ. no. 100–696 (Washington, DC: U.S. Government Printing Office, 1989).

48. A. M. Bartholomew, E. A. Young, H. W. Martin, and H. P. Hazuda, Food frequency intakes and sociodemographic factors of elderly Mexican Americans and non-Hispanic whites. *Journal of the American Dietetic Association, 90* (1990), 1693–1696.

49. Ibid.

50. G. Marks, J. Solís, J. L. Richardson, L. M. Collins, L. Birba, and J. C. Hisserich, Health behavior of elderly Hispanic women: Does cultural assimilation make a difference? *American Journal of Public Health, 77* (1987), 10, 1315.

51. Dewey et al., Dietary change.

52. Ibid.

53. E. Romero-Gwynn, D. Gwynn, L. Griveti, R. McDonald, G. Stanford, B. Turner, M. A. E. West, and E. Williamson, Dietary acculturation among Latinos of Mexican descent. *Nutrition Today* (July/August 1993).

54. Dewey et al., Dietary changes.

55. Ibid.

56. S. García, L. Kaiser, and K. G. Dewey, Self-regulation of food intake among rural Mexican preschool children, *European Journal of Clinical Nutrition, 44* (1990), 371–380.

57. Dewey et al., Dietary changes.

58. E. Romero-Gwynn and D. Gwynn, Changes in dietary patterns of immigrant groups predispose them to obesity: Focus on Mexican-Americans. Paper presented at the Obesity Update: Assessment and Treatment of the Patient with Medically Significant Obesity. Sacramento, California, October 18–20, 1991.

4

Puerto Rican Diets
and Nutrient Intake

**From Island to Mainland to Island:
Influencing Each Other's Lifestyles and Eating Patterns**
Understanding *Puertorriqueños*
Background
Macroenvironmental Factors Affecting Diet Patterns

**The Puerto Rican Food Guide
and USDA Food Guide Pyramid**

Puerto Rican Diets and Meals
The Basic Puerto Rican Diet
A Historical Review of Food Consumption Trends
Puerto Rico and New York: Differential Intake in
Food and Meal Patterns
Typical Meal Patterns in Puerto Rico and New York

**Changes in Dietary Practices Among Puerto Rican Families in
Puerto Rico and in the United States**
The Effects of Environmental and Socioeconomic
Changes on Food Intake
Intergenerational Differences in Food Choices
Dietary Changes over Time: Typical Menus in
the South Bronx and East Harlem
Changes in Food Consumption
Differences in Food Prices
A Comparison of 1946 and 1980 Diets
Changes in Milk Consumption
Nutritional Consequences of U.S. Migration
Migration Status and Macronutrient Profile: A Comparison
with the U.S. Dietary Goals

**Contemporary Hispanic Dietary
and Nutrient Intake in New York State**
Food Consumption Patterns
Vitamin and Mineral Intake
Fat, Saturated Fat, Cholesterol, and Sodium Intake
Food-related Practices
Weight Loss Practices

FROM ISLAND TO MAINLAND TO ISLAND: INFLUENCING EACH OTHER'S LIFESTYLES AND EATING PATTERNS

Understanding *Puertorriqueños* (Puerto Ricans)

According to Sonia Badillo, Puerto Ricans represent

> all shades of the racial spectrum from blond and blue eyed to olive-skinned cinnamon shade to deep black; Puerto Ricans have two languages, two flags, two citizenships, and two basic philosophies of life, which in turn has created difficulties for them in dealing with this ambivalence in the U.S. environment. The language difficulty encountered by Puerto Ricans has meant that children, who often know English better than their parents, have had to interpret and negotiate with the authorities. This role reversal causes loss of face to parents. Thus, it is important to maintain a deferential attitude toward the father as the head of the family, especially in the presence of outside observers. . . .[1]

Badillo's experience as a social worker in the South Bronx, New York City, brings home the point that health workers and nutritionists, regardless of their own ethnic backgrounds, should appreciate the traditions and culture of Puerto Ricans in order to work effectively with them. Her article invites readers to challenge any stereotypes and racist attitudes regarding Puerto Ricans, and she urges sensitivity toward language difficulties. A very high proportion of Puerto Ricans (91%) still speak Spanish at home. This is a higher percentage than for any other Hispanic origin group in New York City; for Cubans and other Hispanics, the figure is 90%, for Mexicans, it is 64%.[2] Badillo stresses the need to become familiar with the emotional significance and nutritional value of indigenous foods of Puerto Ricans before making judgments. Understanding Puerto Ricans requires familiarity with their unique bicultural background. The value of knowing and respecting clients' social milieux and cultural attitudes relative to nutrition and health before attempting "intervention" is a major goal of this book.

Dietary patterns are intimately linked to cultural behavior that is learned, patterned, and shared with other members of a social group, as well as to individual behavior that is unique and internalized. The critical role of culture in influencing and determining food habits was discussed in Chapter 2. Because food is specifically and distinctively tied to culture, and because food habits are emotionally based and culturally bound, nutrition workers must consider cultural variables in order to counsel clients effectively.

This chapter considers Puerto Rican diets and nutrient intake in the context of changing socioeconomic patterns, changing maternal work patterns, and changing health values and attitudes. Specifically, this chapter provides background on Puerto Ricans, and information about the diets of adults, children, and the elderly, meal patterns, and nutrient intake. There is particular emphasis on documented dietary changes over time, both in Puerto Rico and in the United States.

Background

For the *Taíno* Indians who called it home, the island of Puerto Rico was *Borinquén*, "the land of the brave lord."[3] The island, half the size of New Jersey, is approximately 110 miles long and 35 miles wide. Puerto Rico's total area of 3,435 square miles includes its adjacent islands of which Vieques, Culebra, and Mona are the largest.[4] The interior of the island is rugged and mountainous. The coastal areas are densely populated, with about 3.5 million inhabitants, 71% of whom, according to the 1992 U.S. Bureau of the Census, live in urban areas (2.508 million). Puerto Ricans blend cherished Spanish traditions and American ways with their own distinctive characteristics; they put a high value on human dignity and self-respect and have a special feeling for *la patria* (the motherland).[5]

Patria is the Puerto Rican environment, with its changing seasons, palm-fringed sandy beaches, vivid green mountains and El Yunque rain forest, the ancient fortress of El Morro, modern factories, fast-food establishments, and fancy resort hotels. *Patria* is also traditional ways of preparing foods rooted in Spanish, Taíno, and African customs. Even more important, Puerto Rican *patria* is the people and their spirit. Hospitality is a way of life for Puerto Ricans. Puerto Ricans really mean it when they say *"mi casa es su casa"* (my house is your house).

Family ties are very strong in Puerto Rico. These ties extend beyond the nuclear family to include grandparents, aunts, uncles, nieces, nephews, cousins, and *compadres* and *comadres* (godfathers and godmothers). Families often get together, especially at holidays, birthdays, and weddings.

Puerto Ricans live in every section of the United States, but the largest concentration is in New York City. Because Puerto Rico is a self-governing commonwealth of the United States, Puerto Rico is American in its citizenship, currency, postal service, armed forces, and applicable federal laws. However, although politically they are U.S. citizens, culturally Puerto Ricans are profoundly different from citizens of the mainland. Puerto Ricans' deep pride in their island and heritage cannot be overemphasized.

In the last four decades, Puerto Rico has seen dramatic development of its industries, broadening of its public education system, and improvement in its public health programs. The island's natural beauty and climate, as well as affordable airfares, have helped make tourism a key industry. On the other hand, agriculture, formerly the most important economic activity, has given way to a rapidly increasing industrial sector, with manufacturing and construction as its major components.

Due to special economic incentives by the Puerto Rican government, many industries have been established, providing more jobs and higher incomes for residents. At the same time, production of the main crop of sugarcane has decreased substantially. Although the dairy industry has been widely developed and now provides for most local needs, the majority of the staple foods, such as rice, beans, and codfish, are imported. Fresh fruits, fresh

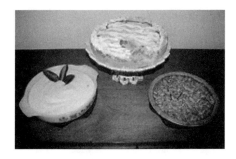

Puerto Rican desserts (pecan pie, apple strudel, and mafarete) *illustrate both the American and Spanish influence.*

milk, and sugar are some of the few foods produced locally in considerable amounts. According to Vicéns de Sánchez, the Puerto Rican diet is becoming "Americanized," and almost 70% of foods available are imported, the majority from the United States.[6]

Activities in streets, restaurants, offices, and supermarkets reflect both the island's ancient Spanish heritage and its newer ties with America. Thus Puerto Ricans in the United States are faced with the dilemma of preserving their Spanish cultural heritage while trying to absorb the newer American culture.

Macroenvironmental Factors Affecting Diet Patterns

The U.S. mainland and Puerto Rico represent quite different macroenvironments. Puerto Ricans have been traveling back and forth to the mainland since the beginning of the twentieth century. Therefore it is reasonable to expect that Puerto Ricans' present-day dietary patterns reflect their traditional habits and their increased per capita income, as well as their exposure to the U.S. environment. Per capita income in Puerto Rico increased from $317 in 1950, to $2,126 in 1980, to $4,177 in 1990.[7]

Macroenvironmental factors that may affect food consumption patterns of Puerto Rican migrants include food prices, physical availability of specific foods, accessibility to supplementary feeding programs, social prestige values of different foods, and lifestyles that necessitate changes in food preparation practices. Some of these factors may have a more immediate impact on food intake patterns than others. For example, food prices usually have a greater effect than the social prestige of foods. Because Puerto Rico imports a substantial amount of its food supply, mainly from the United States, the U.S. food system has a strong impact on everyday eating patterns on the island. (In the early 1950s, Puerto Rico passed a law where all flour and rice consumed on the island must be enriched with various micronutrients.)

In the early 1950s, large numbers of Puerto Ricans came to the United States in search of employment and a better life. There is the possibility that migrants may differ from nonmigrants in socioeconomic characteristics and exposure to different macrolevel variables. These differences may in turn produce further adjustments in dietary intake patterns.[8]

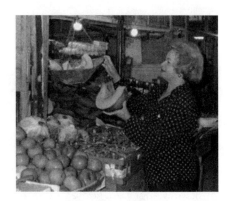

Puerto Ricans often buy their traditional foods from small grocery stores.

Coming primarily from an agrarian lifestyle, with a different language and traditions, Puerto Rican migrants have had to adjust to the different environment of the United States. This adjustment has produced many conflicts. Tirado notes that early Puerto Rican migrants responded, as had other migrant groups before them, by setting up systems to continue their cultural traditions.[9] *El barrio latino* (Spanish Harlem), *la marketa* (the Park Avenue market), and *la bodega* (the small grocery store) became links for supporting dietary traditions. Throughout New York City, areas like *la marketa* that sell tropical produce, rice, beans, herbs, and spices allow for continuation of cultural traditions.

Changing Trends in U.S. Food Availability   One of the major factors affecting food intake is food availability. Changes in U.S. food availability, particularly in the last three decades, have resulted in some changes in nutrient intake. Consequently, there is growing concern, both here and in Puerto Rico, about the health aspects of some contemporary eating patterns. One major change has been the increased consumption of fats, partly reflecting the greater availability of vegetable oils and the increased consumption of poultry, beef, and dairy products. Figures for the last decade show that the per capita consumption of fats and oils in the United States increased by 6%, with all of the increase accounted for by vegetable oils (Figure 4.1A). Approximately 17% of the fat consumed in 1989 was derived from animal sources and 83% from vegetable sources.[10]

Protein intake, on the other hand, remained relatively constant over the last three decades. However, interesting trends were observed between 1980 and 1990. Although beef had been the meat consumed in greatest quantity, its consumption peaked in 1975, at 75 pounds per capita. Since then, its consumption has decreased by 14%, to 64 pounds per capita in 1990 (Figure 4.1B). Between 1980 and 1990, pork consumption decreased by 11%, to 46 pounds per capita. Over the same period, chicken consumption increased 44%, from 34 to 49 pounds per capita. As of 1990, per capita consumption of chicken had surpassed that of pork. Although fish consumption also increased by 23%, to

FIGURE 4.1   Per capita consumption of fat and animal protein in the United States

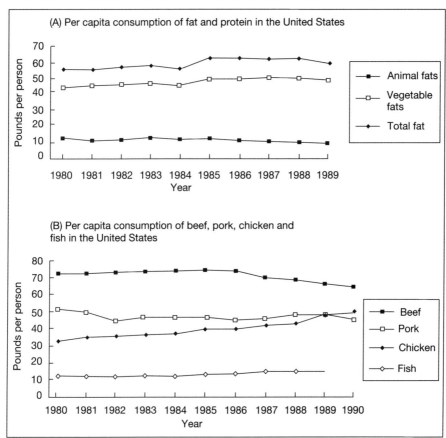

SOURCE: J. J. Putman and J. E. Allshouse, *Food consumption, price, and expenditures, 1968–1969,* Statistical Bulletin 825 (Washington, DC: U.S. Department of Agriculture, 1991).

16 pounds per capita in 1990, consumption of fish lags far behind beef, pork, and chicken.[11]

Over the same years, carbohydrate intake declined, with an increased intake of sugar not making up for a decreased intake of cereals. Interestingly enough, between 1980 and 1988, consumption of fresh, frozen, and canned vegetables increased 6%, to 190 pounds per capita, and per capita consumption of potatoes increased 7%, to 71 pounds.[12]

Food Purchasing Establishments   Another factor that affects the food intake of migrating populations is where they live and where they purchase their food. According to Green et al., access to grocery stores for New York City residents varies depending on where they live.[13] In 1990, low-income neighborhoods in Manhattan, the Bronx, and Brooklyn had significantly fewer supermarkets per person than did middle-class and affluent neighborhoods. The supermarkets in low-income neighborhoods were also smaller, offered less variety, and had higher prices; the greatest difference in prices was found in fresh fruits and vegetables. A market basket of foods purchased in poor neighborhoods cost 9% more than the same foods purchased in middle-income or affluent areas. Even more important, Green et al. noted that sanitary conditions of stores were also worse in low-income neighborhoods, with 54% of stores in poorer areas failing New York State sanitary inspections. Somewhat ironically, the researchers found that in low-income neighborhoods in New York City, "those who can least afford it may have to pay more for poorer quality food, or pay for transportation to neighborhoods where the food supply is better and less expensive. . . ."[14]

Given that many Puerto Ricans, Dominicans, and other Central American and Latino families live below the poverty line in New York City, these data have significant health and social implications. The nutritional implications of changing national food consumption trends have been the subject of concern and debate among nutritional scientists. A few argue that there is no evidence that diet modification will alter the morbidity or mortality from any of the "killer" diseases. Many others strongly argue that substantial epidemiological data justify the need for dietary modification. The recently issued U.S. Department of Agriculture (USDA) Food Guide Pyramid and the U.S. Department of Health and Human Services (DHHS)/Public Health Service Report Healthy People 2000 support the need for dietary modification.

Living in a society that values newness and variety also presents problems for some Puerto Rican families. Shopping in a supermarket that carries more than 10,000 food items and reading unit price or nutritional labels can baffle any homemaker in a new environment. Increased variety requires making more informed decisions, and thus a modern supermarket requires more decision making by consumers than does a small *colmado* or *bodega* (small grocery store). In this respect, Tirado notes that some purchase decisions are based on the heavily advertised convenience factor.[15] She argues that Puerto Rican families often purchase high-priced convenience foods instead of or in addition to traditional foods. Considering that approximately one-third of the Puerto Rican population in New York City lives below the poverty level, purchase of these food items can use a large percentage of the total food budget. (According to Rodríguez, when compared to whites, African-Americans, or other Hispanic groups, Puerto Rican families in New York City have the highest poverty rates.[16] Regardless of whether they are headed by women, by men, or by couples, they are still disproportionately represented below the poverty line.) Although Puerto Rican homemakers should be afforded the opportunity to select convenience items, nonetheless homemakers need information and tools to make wise decisions.

The impact of mass media advertising, particularly on television, on health and food intake has long been recognized. This effect is conceivably more considerable for low-income populations that lack resources to purchase even small amounts of foods advertised on television. Placing food providers in the position of having to say no to their children's food requests can lead to feelings of inadequacy.[17] Another issue of concern relates to children watching television for prolonged periods of time, snacking on high-calorie foods and getting very little exercise. The lack of safe recreational facilities in low-income urban areas may contribute to this unhealthy habit.

Lastly, another major determinant of food intake is available income. Studies have shown that as income decreases, the proportion of income spent for food also increases. However, more is at stake than just percentages. For well-off people, spending 15% of a monthly income of $5,000 on food is quite different from spending 50% of a monthly income of $1,000 for poor people. Because a significant proportion of the Puerto Rican population living in the United States is below the poverty level, limited income often affects their ability to purchase an adequate quantity and variety of food.

THE PUERTO RICAN FOOD GUIDE
AND USDA FOOD GUIDE PYRAMID*

The first Food Guide for Puerto Rico was developed in 1946 and used until 1988. It was prepared by the Puerto Rico Nutrition Committee, a professional group organized in 1940 to deal with the nutritional problems of Puerto Rico, which were aggravated by World War II. Dr. Lydia J. Roberts was at the helm of this effort. The objective of the Food Guide was to encourage Puerto Ricans to add "protective foods" to their basic food pattern in order to alleviate nutritional deficiencies. Over the years, the committee has also:

> Played a decisive role in establishing laws to enrich flour and flour products and rice, to import skim milk, and to prohibit the adding of sugar and talc to polished rice
>
> Conducted many nutrition education projects that included promoting skim milk, tropical fruits, and yellow vegetables
>
> Gathered data and determined the nutritional value of foods produced and consumed in Puerto Rico

Many years after the publication of the original Food Guide, the Nutrition Committee set up an ad hoc group of about 12 food and nutrition specialists to study and recommend changes in the Food Guide. Recommendations were requested and received from all governmental agencies, universities, and programs involved in foods and nutrition. In a joint effort with the Department of Health of Puerto Rico, and after many years of work,

* The section on the Puerto Rican Food Guide was written by Dr. Carmín E. Bueso, Professor at the University of Puerto Rico and one of the Nutrition Committee's contributors to the guide.

a revised version of the Food Guide for Puerto Rico was published and officially issued in March 1988. The main objectives of the new guide are, as before, to help people select foods to achieve and maintain optimal health. This objective was designed mainly to prevent nutrition-related deficiencies, as the major causes of mortality in Puerto Rico are presumed to be nutritionally related.

The Puerto Rican Food Guide emphasizes the importance of selecting adequate quantities of foods from among the five food groups and of drinking six to eight glasses of water per day. It is directed mainly toward healthy adults, although some specific guidance is given for children.

Figure 4.2 compares the Puerto Rican Food Guide and the USDA Food Guide Pyramid. The food groups are presented in a circle, with the word "water" in the center. At the top is the title, "Food Guide for Puerto Rico," and at the bottom are the single message "Eat foods from each group everyday" and a map of Puerto Rico. The circle is divided into five sections of different sizes. The food groups, the percentage of space occupied by each group, photographs of relevant raw and processed foods included are:

FOOD GROUP	SPACE ALLOWED (%)	FOODS PHOTOGRAPHED
Cereals, legumes, starches	31	Spaghetti, bread, rice, potatoes, plantains, tanniers, sweet potatoes, chick-peas, red kidney beans, pigeon peas
Milk and milk products	18	Pasteurized, UHT, dry, evaporated, low-fat yogurt, Edam cheese
Fruits	14	Fresh pineapple, guava, papaya, banana, orange, lime, grapefruit, mango, West Indian cherry; canned orange juice
Vegetables	15	Pumpkin (squash), carrots, cabbage, tomatoes, green beans, green and red peppers, broccoli
Meat, poultry, fish, eggs	19	Steak, ground beef, chicken, pork fish

The relative size of the sections is not exactly related to the number of servings or to the caloric contribution of the group. However, the category cereals, legumes, and starches occupies about one-third of the total area, and together with fruits and vegetables takes around 60% of the space.

A booklet that accompanies the illustration of the Food Guide presents the serving size for all foods and recommends the following servings per day:

FIGURE 4.2 Comparison of the USDA Food Guide Pyramid and the Puerto Rican Food Guide

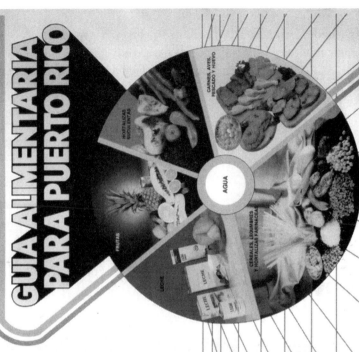

CONSUMA ALIMENTOS DE CADA
GRUPO TODOS LOS DÍAS

Departamento de Salud y Comité de Nutrición de Puerto Rico 1988

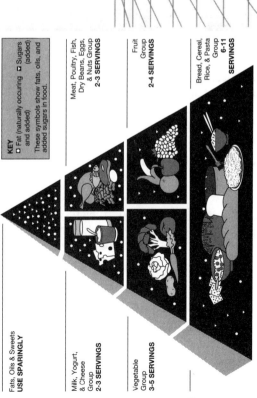

Food Guide Pyramid
A Guide to Daily Food Choices

Fats, Oils & Sweets
USE SPARINGLY

KEY
☐ Fat (naturally occuring   ◪ Sugars
   and added)   (added)
These symbols show fats, oils, and
added sugars in food.

Milk, Yogurt,
& Cheese
Group
2-3 SERVINGS

Meat, Poultry, Fish,
Dry Beans, Eggs,
& Nuts Group
2-3 SERVINGS

Vegetable
Group
3-5 SERVINGS

Fruit
Group
2-4 SERVINGS

Bread, Cereal,
Rice, & Pasta
Group
6-11
SERVINGS

Since May 1994 a new *Piramide Alimentaria para Puerto Rico* (Food Guide Pyramid for Puerto Rico) has been in use.

FOOD GROUP	PUERTO RICO	USDA
Cereals, legumes, starches	None (serving size for each is specified)	2–11
Milk, milk products	2–4 glasses (8 oz) according to age and status	2–5
Fruits	2 (serving sizes given for 6 different fruits)	2–4
Vegetables	2 (1/2 cup/serving)	3–5
Meat, poultry, fish, eggs	2 (meat, poultry, fish) 2 oz./serving 1 egg/serving	2–3

The booklet devotes one page to fats and sugar, explaining their importance and the need for moderation in their use; it also indicates that these do not have to be totally avoided. The fats pictured are bacon, salt pork fat, mayonnaise, butter, margarine, and fat. Sugars pictured are caramels, brown sugar, white sugar, and honey. The booklet also indicates the need to read and use food labels and gives information about water, recommending six to eight glasses per day.

The Puerto Rico Food Guide and the USDA Food Guide Pyramid differ in the following ways:

Water is central to the Puerto Rican Guide; it is not included in the USDA Food Guide Pyramid.

Fats, oils, and sweets are the top food group in the Pyramid. Although they are not a separate group in the Puerto Rican Guide, they are briefly discussed in the Puerto Rican booklet.

Legumes (which are commonly eaten in Puerto Rico) are grouped with cereals and starches in the Puerto Rican Guide. Their major nutritional contribution is considered to be energy. In contrast, in the USDA Pyramid, legumes are grouped with meat, poultry, fish, dry beans, eggs, and nuts.

Nuts, peanut butter, and tofu are included in the USDA Food Pyramid but not in the Puerto Rican Guide.

Although the USDA Pyramid and Puerto Rican Guide give similar serving sizes for different foods, they recommend different numbers of servings per day of foods from different groups. For example, the Puerto Rican Guide does not recommend servings for cereals, legumes, or starches; the USDA Pyramid recommends 6 to 11 servings.

PUERTO RICAN DIETS AND MEALS

The Basic Puerto Rican Diet

The Puerto Rican Nutrition Committee, after an islandwide survey taken several decades ago, found that the basic dietary pattern included rice, beans, *viandas* (starchy tubers), *bacalao* (dried codfish), sugar, lard, and coffee. Regardless of economic level, Puerto Ricans ate these basic foods. This staple diet provides sufficient calories, iron, thiamine, and niacin but is limited in calcium, high-quality protein, vitamin A, vitamin C, and riboflavin.[18]

According to Cabanillas, Puerto Rican food habits are strongly influenced by three major ethnic groups who lived on the island before and after the discovery of America, the Taíno Indians, the Spaniards and the Africans.[19]

The traditional diet of dried fish, rice, and lard of the plantation workers in Puerto Rico was influenced partly by the New England companies that controlled the sugar plantations. It also reflected the types of products brought to the Caribbean islands by the British West India Company in colonial times. Some of the preferred starchy *viandas* and coffee also reflect the tropical environment in which these foodstuffs grow.[20]

The basic food pattern observed in Puerto Rico in the mid-1940s—a light breakfast, heavy lunch, afternoon snack, and light dinner—directly reflected an agrarian lifestyle. Meals were eaten as a family. The food preparation methods showed the influence of the African, Spanish, and American Indian heritages. Most foods were fried or stewed, using wood fuel and native cooking utensils. Food was not baked because most people did not own ovens. However, baked foods were purchased and highly valued.

Traditionally, *viandas* (starchy vegetables) are boiled whole or in large pieces and served hot with boiled dry codfish, oil, and vinegar. The most popular *viandas* are green bananas and green plantains. *Calabaza* (yellow squash) is also very popular and used in soups, bean dishes, and fritters. Other *viandas* are *batata amarilla* (sweet potatoes), *batata blanca* (white sweet potato), *ñame, yautía blanca o amarilla* (white or yellow tanier), *panapén* (breadfruit), and yucca or cassava.

When eaten in quantities, *viandas* supply adequate B vitamins and iron. They are generally low in protein and vitamin A, with the exception of plantain, which is a fairly good source of vitamin A. When 1,000 or more kilocalories are consumed in a day, as is not uncommon, *viandas* supply adequate amounts of thiamine, niacin, riboflavin, and even vitamin C. *Viandas*, how-

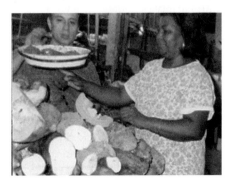

Viandas *(starchy tubers) reflect the tropical environment in which they grow.*

ever, have substantially increased in price in recent years, both in Puerto Rico and in the United States, and this may have affected their consumption.

Rice and beans, extremely popular foods, are eaten once or twice a day. The daily per capita consumption is 7 ounces of rice and 3 to 4 ounces of beans. Rice, enriched by Puerto Rican law, is usually the short-grain variety. It is cooked in small amounts of salted water with added lard or vegetable oil. In addition to being combined with beans, rice is eaten with Vienna sausages, pork sausages, dry codfish, or chicken. Rice is colored with *achiote* (annato seeds), a yellow coloring.

Cornmeal mush, also popular, is prepared with water or milk. Cornmeal, used occasionally as a substitute for rice, may be eaten with beans and codfish. Oatmeal may be cooked in thin gruel for breakfast, especially for children. Imported Cream of Wheat and other cereals, as well as wheat bread, noodles, and spaghetti, are also widely used. Wheat flour in the form of bread, noodles, *pastelillos* (thin turnovers), and spaghetti are used extensively.

Granos (legumes), including chick-peas, navy beans, *rosita* (pink) beans, white beans, pigeon peas, and dried peas, are eaten almost daily, but red kidney beans are most preferred. Beans are boiled until tender and then stewed and dressed with *sofrito* (a mixture of tomatoes, green pepper, onion, garlic, salt pork, lard, and cooking herbs).[21]

Milk is well liked and often used, and nonfat dry milk is well accepted. Most milk is consumed in *café con leche* (coffee with milk), which is drunk for breakfast, in the middle of the afternoon, and at other meals. Coffee for Puerto Ricans is mocha, never a blend, and is very strong; American coffee is considered very weak and is not well liked. A cup of *café con leche* contains 2 to 5 ounces of milk.[22] Other favorite drinks are chocolate and cocoa made with milk and sugar.

Fruits and vegetables are used in limited quantities and tend to be expensive and imported. Greens, other than watercress, are not often used. Beets and eggplant are commonly eaten vegetables. Green beans, tomatoes, cabbage, carrots, and lettuce are also frequently consumed. Spinach and chard are used occasionally. However, in general, Puerto Ricans consume insufficient amounts of green vegetables. Of the yellow vegetables, *batata mameya* (sweet potato), carrots, and *calabaza* (a Puerto Rican variety of squash) are well liked.

Tropical fruits, such as *acerola* (West Indian cherry), one of the best sources of vitamin C, pineapples, bananas, guavas, *quenepas*, mangoes, *chinas* (oranges), papayas, *pajuil* (cashew nut fruit), grapefruit, and *guanábanas* (soursop) are among the favorites. Fruits are usually eaten between meals as snacks rather than during meals. Consumption of fruits, however, is affected by seasonality as well as cost. Again, as with the *viandas*, tropical fruits, even when grown locally, have become quite expensive in Puerto Rico. Canned or frozen juices providing vitamin C are also consumed. *Pastas* (fruits cooked in syrup) are made from a variety of fruits and are especially well liked and eaten as dessert. For example, *pasta de guayaba* (guava paste) is often served with Puerto Rican white cheese as dessert.

Among the protein sources, chicken and pork are well liked, particularly chicken.[23] Chicken is eaten fried, stewed, or cooked with rice, as in *arroz con pollo*, or as *asopao* (soupy rice), or with spaghetti. Pork is consumed either as *chuletas* (pork chops), which are fried, or stewed *pernil* (fresh cooked ham), or as *lechón asado* (young pig roasted), or as *cuchifrito* (fried pig intestines). Codfish, as mentioned earlier, is frequently served with *viandas*. Recent steep increases in the price of codfish, however, have limited its consumption somewhat. Canned tuna fish, sardines, or salmon are also consumed to a lesser extent. Of the shellfish, *jueyes* (crabs) are a favorite. (A full description of various foods and mixed dishes, including main ingredients, serving portions, weight in grams, and caloric value, is provided in the glossary at the end of the chapter.).

As do Mexican-Americans, Puerto Ricans prefer high-fat meats, and frying is a popular method of cooking. Any nutrition education material developed for Puerto Ricans should reinforce the strengths of the basic diet (for example, high complex carbohydrates) and encourage the addition of foods that contribute other nutrients. Consumption of foods high in simple sugars and fats should be monitored so that dietary counseling can be given whenever necessary.

Rice and beans, basic staples of the Puerto Rican diet, contain complementary proteins. Eating them together increases the quality of the protein they provide. Rice and beans also contribute substantially to meeting calorie needs. Rice has one of the best amino acid patterns of all vegetable proteins. In rice, lysine is the only essential amino acid that is limited. Conversely, methionine and cystine are the most limiting amino acids in beans. However, beans have an advantage over rice, because beans contain three times as much total protein as rice. Therefore, eating rice and beans together is better than eating each alone. When eaten together, the lysine deficiency of rice completely disappears because lysine is contributed by the bean protein. Conversely, the amounts of available methionine and cystine also increase (relative to the amount found in beans alone) because of the contribution of lysine by the bean protein.

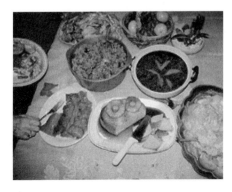

Puerto Rican holidays are marked by plentiful consumption of traditional and American dishes.

A Historical Review of Food Consumption Trends

It has long been recognized that the population in Puerto Rico has experienced marked changes in lifestyle, in household and per capita income, and in both the quality and quantity of foods consumed. These changes are illustrated by four dietary and nutritional surveys done in Puerto Rico over four decades. Further information comes from cross-sectional dietary studies among migrant Puerto Rican families in New York City and in Puerto Rico over 20 years. These studies provide an opportunity to study historical changes in food consumption and in the nutritional status of the Puerto Rican population. Finally, recent Hispanic dietary data from New York State are provided.

Patterns of Living in Puerto Rican Families In 1946, Roberts and Stefani conducted a survey as an outgrowth of work on curriculum revision in the Department of Home Economics at the University of Puerto Rico.[24] Prior to this survey, there was no published evidence available in Puerto Rico on many aspects of family life. A random sample of 1,044 families reflecting various demographic and socioeconomic characteristics was selected. This sample included about 5,670 people; 63% of them lived in rural and 37% in urban areas. Findings from this survey revealed the following serious problems:

Inadequate incomes: three-fourths of all Puerto Rican families had annual incomes below $1,000

Poor and insufficient housing: overcrowding in urban areas and remoteness from roads in rural areas; meager or no facilities within the home

Insufficient, unsafe, or inaccessible water supply

Unsanitary waste disposal

Inadequate provisions for prenatal and infant care: 91% of rural and 72% of urban women gave birth to babies at home with no prenatal care

Diets deficient in most essential nutrients: about 75% of the families consumed markedly inadequate diets

Poor educational facilities, particularly among the poor in rural areas

This landmark study revealed extreme poverty, particularly in rural areas. Interestingly enough, family income was the most important determining factor for the frequency with which different kinds of foods were included in the diet. Families with higher incomes ate fruit more often and ate more kinds of fruits than did families with lower incomes.

This classic study served as the basis for governmental agencies to address the needs and living conditions of the Puerto Rican people, especially those residing in isolated mountain communities. One of the major problems recognized was the need for better coordination of efforts by community service agencies. It was established that intensive nutrition education efforts based on the perceived needs of the people would be necessary to correct the existing nutritional problems and to avoid imminent deterioration of the nutritional status of the Puerto Rican population.

One of the major programs developed in response to the survey became known as the Doña Elena Rural Development Project.[25] This pilot program was designed to improve standards of living in isolated rural communities by maximizing use of local resources and practical agricultural techniques and by employing home economics and extension personnel to teach the *jíbaros* (rural highlanders) how to solve their own problems. These isolated communities were also used as "living laboratories" where students from the University of Puerto Rico were trained in learning by doing.

Nutritional Status of the Puerto Rican Population: Master Sample Survey A second study, conducted in 1966 by Fernández, collected information about socioeconomic, dietary, clinical, and biochemical parameters; 827 families were interviewed at their homes in order to collect in-depth data about general dietary intake, frequency of consumption of various foods, and availability of cooking appliances and kitchen facilities.[26] The study revealed great improvements in dietary intakes since the 1946 study, and interesting information regarding patterns of food consumption among different socioeconomic levels and between the urban-rural population was obtained. Higher incomes were not necessarily associated with more nutritious diets. People from remote rural communities had better intakes of several nutrients than did urban people from slums.

The Puerto Rican Department of Health Study The third major nutritional survey was conducted by the Puerto Rican Department of Health in 1977.[27] Researchers collected dietary, clinical, and anthropometric data from a sample of 1,737 families, 59% from urban and 41% from rural areas. Internal migration, with a shift of population from rural to urban areas, was beginning to take place at the time of the survey. Dietary data consisted of a frequency list of foods consumed during the previous week and a 24-hour recall.

The study findings revealed that traditional staple Puerto Rican foods were still consumed, but that there were also marked increases in consumption of other foods, including meats (mainly beef and chicken) and processed meats, milk, eggs, legumes, and fruit juices. Although there was an increased consumption of fruits and vegetables, their overall consumption was still low. This study also found that income transfer programs, such as the Food Stamp Program, contributed significantly to improvement of the diets and may even have eliminated previous differential food intakes between rural and urban or low- or high-income families. Interestingly enough, this investigation also found that some population groups were consuming excessive amounts of food. This was the first time that overconsumption of foods became an area of concern. For the first time, malnutrition was occurring because of excess rather than insufficient food intake.

Food Consumption and Dietary Levels of Puerto Rican Households
The fourth major islandwide study was carried out in conjunction with the 1977–78 U.S. Department of Agriculture Nationwide Food Consumption Survey.[28] Trained interviewers used an "aided record schedule" to collect data on the kind, form, quantity used, and cost of each food and beverage consumed in each household during the seven days prior to the interview. The methodology used to collect the information was the same as that used in the National Food Consumption Survey, 1977–78, for the mainland states. However, the Puerto Rican segment of this survey was in Spanish and included foods common in Puerto Rico.

The results of the survey indicated that household diets in Puerto Rico supplied the recommended dietary allowances (RDAs) for the 10 nutrients studied (protein, calcium, iron, magnesium, phosphorus, vitamin A, thiamine, vitamin B_6, vitamin B_{12}, and vitamin C) as often as did diets in the United States (49% compared to 47%, respectively). However, compared to U.S. diets, Puerto Rican diets were notably less likely to meet the RDA for vitamin A and more likely to meet the RDA for calcium.

Puerto Rico and New York: Differential Intake in Food and Meal Patterns

Sanjur et al. conducted an investigation in four communities in Puerto Rico and in the South Bronx, New York City. The total sample of 526 Puerto Rican households included 2,434 persons.[29] Because the study included a large sample and the interviews were conducted in Spanish at home over several months, they captured more of the day-to-day variation sometimes lost in large data sets. To ensure validity and reliability of the dietary survey data, data on food purchasing and food preferences were simultaneously collected from these families, and great efforts went into training interviewers to standardize methods and minimize biases in data collection.

This investigation attempted to examine nutritional problems caused by migration of Puerto Ricans from low-income rural to urban areas, as nutritional and dietary information about Puerto Rican families who migrated to the United States was quite scanty. Specifically, researchers measured and compared the nutritional status of 200 families residing in the South Bronx with that of 326 families residing in the four communities of Puerto Rico: the three coastal communities of Luquillo, Río Grande, and Fajardo and Naranjito, in the highlands. The four communities were a blend of rural, semirural, and semiurban. The urban counterpart was represented by 200 Puerto Rican families living in the South Bronx.

Table 4.1 illustrates the consumption of 23 food groups by the different families. Differences in food consumption between families in the South Bronx and Puerto Rico can be summarized as follows:

1. The families in the South Bronx consumed a more varied diet. Of the 23 food groups, 12 were consumed by 50% or more of families in the South Bronx sample. In contrast, only 8 groups were consumed by 50% or more of the families in Puerto Rico.

TABLE 4.1 **Differential Intake of 23 Food Groups in the South Bronx and Puerto Rico**

(Based on a 24-hour recall method)

Food Group	South Bronx		Puerto Rico		Percent Differences	
	(N)	%	(N)	%	South Bronx	Puerto Rico
Milk	200	100	283	87	+ 13	—
Leafy raw and other vegetables	186	93	178	55	+ 38	—
Coffee	179	90	247	76	+ 14	—
Fats and oils	175	88	217	67	+ 21	—
Breads (mostly white)	168	84	150	46	+ 38	—
Rice	158	79	265	81	—	+ 2
Fruit juices	144	72	101	31	+ 41	—
Starchy vegetables	135	68	265	81	—	+ 13
Fruits	134	67	51	16	+ 51	—
Legumes	131	66	192	59	+ 7	—
Eggs	118	59	103	32	+ 27	—
Beef	105	53	88	27	+ 26	—
Sugar	83	42	261	80	—	+ 38
Chicken	75	38	147	45	—	+ 7
Cheese	70	35	66	20	+ 15	—
Fish, tuna fish, codfish	61	31	78	24	+ 7	—
Cooked and dry cereal	52	26	52	16	+ 10	—
Canned fruits	39	20	4	1	+ 19	—
Cold cuts	39	20	97	31	—	+ 11
Pork	39	20	82	25	—	+ 5
Pasta	37	19	32	10	+ 9	—
Crackers	33	17	77	24	—	+ 7
Soft drinks	8	4	103	31	—	+ 27

SOURCE: D. Sanjur, M.D.C Immink, M. Burgos, and S. Alicea, Trends and differentials in dietary patterns and nutrient intake among Puerto Rican families. *Archivos Latinoamericanos de Nutrición,* 36(4) (December 1986), pp. 625–641.

2. Mothers in the South Bronx consumed higher intakes of 15 different food groupings and lower intakes of the remaining 8 food groupings.

3. There were substantially higher intakes (of 25% or more) in the South Bronx for the following groups:

Fresh fruits	+ 518
Fruit juices	+ 41%
Leafy raw and other vegetables	+ 38%
White bread	+ 38%
Eggs	+ 27%
Beef	+ 26%

Conversely, there were higher intakes (of 25% or more) in Puerto Rico for the following groups:

Sugar	+ 38%
Soft drinks	+ 27%

4. Milk was a favorite food among Puerto Ricans, thus making it the highest ranked food consumed among the 23 food groups (100% in the South Bronx and 87% in Puerto Rico). Its preferred form of consumption was in combination with coffee. The second ranked food consumed was leafy raw and other vegetables (93%) for the Bronx and starchy vegetables and rice (81% each) for Puerto Rico.

In general, this study found an overconsumption of certain food groups, particularly of foods high in protein in both locations, and of sugar and soft drinks in Puerto Rico. Overconsumption of certain foods appeared consistent with anthropometric measurements showing a tendency for overweight, as well as of obesity, among the women.

The increased use of fresh fruits, juices, and leafy raw vegetables reported by South Bronx mothers was very encouraging. Conversely, the increased use of sugar and soft drinks by the mothers in Puerto Rico was somewhat disturbing. These findings have implications for nutrition education programs.

Typical Meal Patterns in Puerto Rico and New York

Table 4.2 compares sample menus showing the typical meal patterns of 200 families residing in the South Bronx and 209 families living in two communities in Puerto Rico, Rió Grande (95 families) and Naranjito (109 families).

Breakfast In Sample Menu 1, Puerto Rican mothers in the South Bronx consumed a more diverse breakfast than did mothers in Puerto Rico, although *café con leche* was always included in both places. In Sample Menu 2, in the South Bronx, oatmeal (which in the Puerto Rican tradition is prepared with milk and sugar rather than water only) replaced the boiled egg or American cheese that was consumed in both communities in Puerto Rico. Orange juice

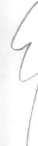

TABLE 4.2   Comparative Analysis of Typical Meal Patterns in the South Bronx and Puerto Rico

		South Bronx (1981)	Naranjito (1981)	Rio Grande (1981)
Sample Menu 1	Breakfast	Coffee w/milk White bread Boiled eggs Orange juice	Coffee w/milk and sugar	Coffee w/milk and sugar
	Lunch	Sandwich Milk or juice Fresh fruit	Boiled codfish w/vegetable oil Vianda (Starchy vegetable) Coffee w/milk and sugar	Fried or stewed chicken Rice Stewed kidney beans Rice
	Dinner:	Rice Beans Stewed or fried chicken Lettuce and tomato salad	Rice Stewed red kidney beans Fried chicken Avocado	Stewed red kidney beans Fried pork chops Soft drink or milk
	Before bed snack	Milk Cakes, cookies	Coffee w/milk and sugar	Coffee w/milk and sugar
Sample Menu 2	Breakfast	Coffee w/milk White bread Oatmeal w/milk Orange juice	Coffee w/milk and sugar Pan criollo (french bread) or white bread American cheese or eggs	Coffee w/milk and sugar Boiled eggs or cheese
	Lunch	Sandwich Lettuce and tomato salad Coffee w/milk	Boiled codfish w/vegetable oil Vianda (Starchy vegetable) Milk	Fried or stewed chicken Vianda Soft drink or water Lettuce and tomato salad
	Dinner	A. Rice Beans Pernil or chuleta Watercress, lettuce and tomato salad B. Rice Beans Steak w/onions or beef stew Lettuce and tomato salad	Rice Stewed red kidney beans Fried chicken Avocado	Stewed rice w/beans Beefsteak w/onions Lettuce and tomato salad Milk
	Before bed snack	Milk Coffee w/milk Crackers, cookies	Coffee w/milk and sugar	Coffee w/milk and sugar Soda crackers

SOURCE: D. Sanjur, M.D.C. Immink, M. Burgos, and S. Alicea, Trends and differentials in dietary patterns and nutrient intake among Puecto Rican families. *Archivos Latinoamericanos de Nutrición*, 36(4) (December 1986), pp. 625–641.

was included in both menus in the South Bronx, but not in menus for either community in Puerto Rico.

Lunch   In the South Bronx the mothers consumed a light lunch, whereas in both communities in Puerto Rico, the majority of the mothers consumed a heavy lunch. Specifically, in the South Bronx there was a marked preference for sandwiches (mainly hot dogs, bologna, or other processed meats), a beverage, and a fruit. In Puerto Rico, the traditional *serenata* of codfish and starchy vegetables or of rice and beans with chicken prevailed in both menus.

Dinner   It is interesting to note that three communities so environmentally different and distant consumed such similar foods for dinner. The continuity of traditional habits is evidenced by the consumption of rice and stewed kidney beans. In Sample Menu 1, all three communities had similar dinner patterns, with the exception of the types of salad (lettuce and tomato or avocado or watercress). In addition, in Sample Menu 2, the South Bronx and Río Grande included a beverage, in this case, milk or a soft drink.

Merienda or Snack   In the South Bronx, 114 mothers (57%), in Río Grande, 59 mothers (62%), and in Naranjito, 52 mothers (48%), had a snack before bed. In all three communities the most common snack was *café con leche* (coffee with milk).

CHANGES IN DIETARY PRACTICES AMONG PUERTO RICAN FAMILIES IN PUERTO RICO AND IN THE UNITED STATES

The Effects of Environmental and Socioeconomic Changes on Food Intake

Modification of eating patterns occurs as newcomers come in contact with various environmental forces, but the rate of change varies from family to family. It is not clear why some families cling tenaciously to traditional patterns, regardless of cost, time, or food availability, while other families modify, add to, or give up their family food heritage in favor of new food patterns and individual preferences. Sanjur et al. studied factors influencing the development of food habits of preschool children in East Harlem[30] and in upstate New York.[31] They found that the food patterns practiced by mothers, such as beliefs about withholding or giving foods during illness, strongly reflected Puerto Rican traditions. Parker and Bowering also found strong cultural influences in the development of food habits of infants in East Harlem.[32] Such practices as giving cleansing teas before changing formulas, following the "hot-cold belief system" described by Harwood,[33] giving coffee to children, weaning late, and the cultural norm of a fat baby all reflected these traditions.

Dietary recalls of Puerto Rican women enrolled in nutrition education programs in New York City also showed high consumption of traditional foods. Approximately 80% of the homemakers reported that they had eaten at least one meal that included a traditional dish on the day that the recall was taken.[34] In contrast, a study by Duyff et al. of Puerto Rican teenagers in Chicago showed changes in food patterns related to outside influences.[35] In this instance, the negative influence of frequent snacking was associated with increased intakes of low-nutrient-density foods. Experiences of nutritionists in working with Puerto Rican women in the East Harlem Nutrition Education Program found that mothers expressed interest in learning how to cope with the nontraditional food preferences of their children.

Tirado notes that changing patterns can also be observed in the number of children who do not eat such typical foods as beans, *mondongo* (tripe), *asopao* (soupy rice/chicken), codfish, and even homemade soup. Many Puerto Rican children prefer hamburgers, hot dogs, canned spaghetti, cold cereals, and pizza. This may result in a narrow selection of foods given to children if mothers are not familiar with different food preparation methods and therefore depend on convenience foods. Because the new preferred foods do not fit the Puerto Rican traditional meal pattern, food providers are less able to plan balanced diets. These observations are extremely important from a health and nutrition viewpoint, because the Puerto Rican population is quite young.

Studies of children of migrant groups in Hawaii and in California also found that modification of food habits occurred rapidly as contact with outside forces increased. Therefore a significant proportion of the Puerto Rican population is exposed to and susceptible to different socioeconomic forces and environmental stimuli that can have a strong impact in modifying their food habits.

Intergenerational Differences in Food Choices

With increased advertising of food items, increased eating out in restaurants, school cafeterias, and fast-food establishments, increased snacking, and so on, many Puerto Rican youth are abandoning the traditional diets of their parents. Tirado, working with Puerto Ricans in New York City, has observed that "the typical mainland Puerto Rican adult was born in Puerto Rico, while the typical Puerto Rican child is U.S. reared. . . ."[36] As a result, an intergenerational dietary conflict often develops, with the mother preparing mainland types of foods requested by her children as well as traditional dishes for herself and other adults. While maintaining the Puerto Rican diet for adults in the home, the Puerto Rican mother often replaces the traditional foods with those that are requested by her children.

In the upstate New York study,[37] it was observed that Puerto Rican children refused the traditional lunch because it was easier to carry a bologna sandwich to school than any traditional dish, and by taking an "American" lunch, kids were then able to "swap" the foods with other kids and thus have more fun!

This author has studied Puerto Rican dietary patterns over two decades. Together with my graduate students, I have examined and analyzed dietary continuity and change among this population. From an epidemiological perspective, these data can show the relationship of diet changes to disease, as opposed to cross-sectional data, which show food intake at only one point.

Dietary Changes over Time: Typical Menus Consumed in the South Bronx and East Harlem

Typical menus consumed in the South Bronx and East Harlem collected during 1980 and 1972, respectively, are presented in Table 4.3. These data are considered not only on the basis of the dietary *changes* (substitutions, additions of new foods, or loss of core foods) in Puerto Rican diets over the years but also in terms of *stability or retention* of cultural dietaries and traditional foods. (See Chapter 3 for a review of methodological issues relative to measuring dietary changes.)

Breakfast Two major changes were observed in the breakfast patterns of Sample Menu 1. First, white bread was substituted for unsalted soda crackers, and second, boiled eggs replaced Gouda cheese. In Sample Menu 2, oatmeal, prepared with milk, sometimes replaced boiled eggs. The beverage pattern of orange juice and coffee with milk showed continuity in both locations, over time.

Lunch Major changes had taken place in the lunch patterns as well. First, the 1980 South Bronx data showed a light lunch pattern for both sample menus, whereas the 1972 data for East Harlem revealed a heavy lunch that included traditional dishes such as *serenata* (starchy vegetables with codfish) or ripe plantains with fried eggs. Two new trends seemed to emerge from the more recent data, namely, fresh fruit juices and sandwiches were eaten at lunch. Although not specified in the menus shown, sandwiches were not prepared at home, but purchased from fast-food establishments.

Dinner Traditional Puerto Rican foods for dinner still prevailed among these families, as reflected by their consumption of rice and beans and in their preparation of *biftec* (beefsteak) in Puerto Rican style, as thin slices of fried beef with lots of onions. Thus dinner has changed the least of the three meals. This finding agrees with previous research on dietary changes among immigrants that found that dinner was the least likely meal to change. This may be because dinner is usually eaten in the privacy and comfort of home, with most family members present, where foods with emotional significance can be prepared and enjoyed.

In 1980, as in 1972, rice and beans continued as traditional foods of the Puerto Rican diet. Many varieties of beans were mentioned in the 1980 study, particularly red kidney beans, perhaps substituting the *rosita* (pink) beans reported earlier for East Harlem. In addition to traditional preferences for lettuce and tomato salad, watercress was often mentioned as a favorite leafy vegetable in the South Bronx.

TABLE 4.3 Changes in Meal Patterns — East Harlem and South Bronx

		South Bronx (1980)	East Harlem (1972)
Sample Menu 1	Breakfast	Orange juice White bread Boiled eggs Coffee w/milk	Orange juice Unsalted crackers Gouda cheese Coffee w/milk
	Lunch	Milk or juice Sandwich Fresh fruit	Coffee w/milk Serenata Vianda
	Dinner	Rice Beans Stewed or fried chicken Lettuce and tomato salad	Rice Beans Fried pork chops Canned peas and carrots Coffee w/milk
	Before bed snack	Milk Cakes, cookies	None
Sample Menu 2	Breakfast	Orange juice White bread Oatmeal w/milk Coffee w/milk	Orange juice Unsalted crackers Gouda cheese Coffee w/milk
	Lunch	Sandwich Lettuce and tomato salad Coffee w/milk	Fried eggs Ripe plantain (plátano) Canned vegetables & lettuce Coffee w/milk
	Dinner	A. Rice Beans Steak w/onions or beef stew Lettuce and tomato salad	a. Rice Rosita (pink) beans Steak w/onions Lettuce and tomato salad w/ oil and vinegar
		B. Rice Beans Biftec w/onions or beef stew Lettuce and tomato salad	b. Rice w/pidgeon peas Biftec w/onions Tostones Coffee w/milk
	Before bed snack	Milk Coffee w/milk Crackers, cookies	None

NOTE: See the glossary for a description of traditional foods and mixed dishes.

SOURCE: D. Sanjur, M.D.C. Immink, M. Colón, L. Bentz Rivera, L. B. Collachi, S. Alicea, and M. Burgos, *The effect of environmental changes on food consumption and nutrient intake among Puerto Rican families: South Bronx and Puerto Rico.* Research report, Division of Nutrition Sciences, Cornell University, Ithaca, NY, December 1981. D. Sanjur, E. Romero, and G. Neville, *A community study of food habits and socioeconomic factors of families participating in the East Harlem nutrition education program.* Research report, New York State College of Human Ecology, Cornell University, Ithaca, NY, 1972.

Snack   A major change in 1980 was the addition of a snack. Of the 200 women studied in the South Bronx, 114 (57%) reported eating some kind of snack. Of these, 51% liked to drink fresh whole milk before bed, and 49% liked to drink coffee with milk. Thirty-one percent of the women who drank milk or coffee also had cake, cookies, and/or crackers.

Changes in Food Consumption

This section assesses recent and past changes in dietary patterns of the 200 Puerto Rican mothers living in the South Bronx and the reasons given for such changes. All mothers who participated in the study reported changing their diets during the year prior to the interview and also during the previous five years. For both periods, the reasons given for changes were primarily of a personal and family nature, followed by health reasons.

Table 4.4 shows specific changes that occurred during the last year and the last five years. In the last year, the most outstanding change was an increased consumption of vegetables, reported by 45%. This reported change was validated by food consumption data collected using a 24-hour recall method. Women also reported an increased consumption of fruits (34%), three

TABLE 4.4 Specific Dietary Changes Reported by 200 Women in the South Bronx During the Past Year and Last Five Years

	Last Year		Past Five Years	
Type of Change	Foods	%	Foods	%
Consumed less	Fried foods, fat greasy foods, stop using lard	31	Salt	16
			Fried foods, fat greasy foods	14
	Salt	21	Sugar and sweets	14
	"All foods"	8	Do not buy any more sodas and *maltas*	11
	Sugar	4		
	Stopped buying sodas and *maltas*	4		
	Bread	3		
	Rice	3		
Consumed more	Vegetables	45	Vegetables	28
	Fruits	34	Fruits	23
	Powdered milk, whole milk, and skim milk	23	Whole milk, skim milk, and powdered milk	14
	Fruit juices	23	Fish	10
	"All foods"	10	"All foods"	6
	Fish	6	Eggs	3
	Eggs	5	Chicken and beef	3
	Cereal/whole wheat	5		

SOURCE: D. Sanjur, E. Romero, and G. Neville, *A community study of food habits and sociocultural factors of families participating in the East Harlem nutrition education program.* Research report, New York State College of Human Ecology, Cornell University, Ithaca, NY, 1972.

TABLE 4.5 Mothers' Reasons for Changing Dietary Patterns, South Bronx

English Version	Spanish Version
"I eat more fruits, more strawberries, apples and peaches, and I give more importance now to the green vegetables."	"Como más frutas tales como fresas, manzanas y melocotones, y le doy más importancia a los vegetales verdes."
"Because of my health and my child's health, I have learned to make different dishes. Now I eat carrots and spinach, and use less fat."	"Por mi salud y la de mi nene yo he aprendido a hacer platos diferentes ahora como zanahorias y espinacas, y uso menos grasa."
"I drink skim milk now, I bake meats, I eat more vegetables and less starchy vegetables because I need to lose weight."	"Tomo leche descremada, aso las carnes; como más vegetales y menos cantidad de viandas, pues tengo que bajar de peso."
"Before I did not have breakfast, but now I do; besides, now I eat more vegetables like cabbage, carrots, and broccoli.	"Antes yo no acostumbraba a desayunar y ahora sí; además vegetales como repollo, zanahoria y brécol."
"Since I began participating in this Nutrition Program, I have learned to eat vegetables like spinach and carrots."	"Desde que participé en este Programa he aprendido a comer vegetales como espinaca y zanahoria."
"I do not put salt in my food, I learned about it in the Nutrition Program; now I eat more vegetables and fruits."	"No le echo sal a la comida, lo aprendí en el Programa de Nutrición, ahora como más vegetales y frutas."
"Now I do not fry food so much; I'll rather bake it, particularly the meat because it is more healthy."	"Ahora no frío tanto y hago la carne al horno porque es más sano."
"I use the oven more often and I use less fat. I eat more vegetables now and I have learned to prepare them in different ways."	"Uso más el horno, uso menos grasa. Como más vegetales ahora y he aprendido a prepararlos en distintas formas."

SOURCE: D. Sanjur, M.D.C. Immink, M. Colón, L. Bentz Rivera, L. B. Collachi, S. Alicea, and M. Burgos, *The effect of environmental changes on food consumption and nutrient intake among Puerto Rican families: South Bronx and Puerto Rico.* Research report, Division of Nutrition Sciences, Cornell University, Ithaca, NY, December 1981.

types of milk (23%), fruit juices (23%), "all foods" (10%), and fish, eggs, and cereal/whole wheat, with 6, 5, and 5%, respectively. Decreased consumption was reported for the following: fried foods and fat greasy foods (31%), salt (21%), "all foods" (8%), sugar (4%), and sodas and *maltas* (Puerto Rican malt beverage, viewed as having high nutritive value) (4%). Decreased consumption of bread and rice was also mentioned.

Direct quotations of the mothers' reasons for their dietary changes are shown, in Spanish and English, in Table 4.5. Most of the reasons appear to be in a positive nutritional direction. Many mothers attributed changing their diets because of their participation in the federally funded Expanded Food and Nutrition Education Program (EFNEP).

Differences in Food Prices

Major differences in food prices were also found between the South Bronx and Puerto Rico. For example, cereals (bread, rice), meat (beef, pork), fish (codfish), and starchy vegetables (potato, green plantain, tannier) were more expensive in the South Bronx. Eggs, fat and oils, leafy vegetables (cabbage, lettuce), and fruits tended to be higher priced in the four communities in Puerto Rico. It would be interesting to explore how differences in food prices and the dynamics of other environmental changes interact with household income levels to influence food intake patterns of migrating populations.[38]

Factors Fostering Dietary Change The dynamics behind dietary changes and the factors that encourage or discourage shifts away from traditional dietary patterns are not well understood. Why, for example, do some Puerto Rican families maintain their ethnic food patterns, even after living on the mainland for several decades, while others rapidly abandon traditional practices? Researchers continue to study dietary change in attempts to unravel these questions, but some potential influential factors have been identified.

In this study women's responses suggested that their participation in the Expanded Food and Nutrition Education Program (EFNEP) made them aware of dietary modifications that could help them reduce weight and live a healthier life. Furthermore, they alluded that the program coordinator and nutrition aides all spoke Spanish, tested and developed the Spanish-language nutrition education materials among the program's participants, and had a history of good rapport with the mothers. Additional factors, such as exposure to new and convenient foods and their children's food preferences, also contributed to the observed dietary changes. Bilingual children can have a major role in promoting dietary modifications within societal groups in transition.[39]

A Comparison of 1946 and 1980 Diets

Table 4.6 shows the variation in food consumption in terms of two ecologically different *municipios* (municipalities) in Puerto Rico and at two different times (1946 and 1980): Naranjito, a highland community located southwest of San Juan, and Río Grande, a coastal community in the extreme northeastern part of Puerto Rico. Overall, the basic food patterns in both communities were quite similar, although people in Naranjito had higher preferences for *viandas,* and people in Río Grande preferred rice and beans. In both communities, a light breakfast, a heavy lunch and supper, and a before bed snack were prevailing patterns. A comparison of the diets in 1980 with those in 1946 showed:

1. Traditional patterns of food consumption persisted across time and across communities.

2. Diets consumed in 1980 were more varied than those in 1946.

3. Diets in 1980 were better in nutritional quality and quantity than in 1946.

TABLE 4.6 Comparative Analysis of Typical Meal Patterns

Puerto Rico			Naranjito (highland community)	Rio Grande (coastal community)
Sample Menu 1	Breakfast	Coffee w/milk or black coffee	Coffee w/milk and sugar	Coffee w/milk and sugar
	Lunch:	Vianda (starchy vegetable)	Boiled codfish w/vegetable oil Vianda Coffee w/milk and sugar	Fried or stewed chicken Rice Stewed red kidney beans
	Supper	Vianda	Fried chicken Rice Stewed red kidney beans Avocado	Fried pork chops Rice Stewed red kidney beans Soft drink or milk
	Before bed snack	None	Coffee w/milk and sugar	Coffee w/milk and sugar
Sample Menu 2	Breakfast	Coffee w/milk or black coffee Bread, cereal, or vianda	Coffee w/milk and sugar American cheese or boiled eggs Pan criollo (french bread) or white bread, soda crackers	Coffee w/milk and sugar Boiled eggs or American cheese
	Lunch	Rice and beans or rice, beans, and viandas	Boiled codfish w/vegetable oil Vianda Milk	Fried or stewed chicken Vianda Soft drink or water Lettuce and tomato
	Supper	Rice and beans or rice, beans, and vianda	Fried chicken Rice Stewed red kidney beans Avocado	Beefsteak (Puerto Rican style) Stewed rice and beans Lettuce and tomato Milk
	Before bed snack	None	Coffee w/milk and sugar	Coffee w/milk and sugar Soda crackers

sources: Raw data for Puerto Rico: from L.J. Roberts and L. Stefani, *Patterns of living of Puerto Rican families* (Rio Piedras: University of Puerto Rico, 1949). Raw data for Naranjito: from Mirta Colón, Home food production and household income as predictors of nutritional status of Puerto Rican preschool children and their mothers. M.S. thesis, University of Puerto Rico, June 1981. Raw data for Rio Grande: from Laura Bentz Rivera, Patrones de consumo de alimentos e ingestion de nutrientes en Rio Grande, Puerto Rico: Un enforque sociocultural. M.S. thesis, University of Puerto Rico, June 1981.

There were many similarities between meal patterns in 1946 and 1980. For example, the traditional staple foods of rice, beans, *viandas,* and coffee remained consistent. Likewise, no fruits or desserts were served during the meals. In 1946, when Roberts and Stefani asked why some families avoided fruits, general responses were "fruits are dangerous, they cause indigestion, or they are "cold." Other reasons were specific to the fruit itself, such as "*Mamey* is poisonous or is heavy on the stomach; *mamey* when eaten with pineapple causes colic; or guava causes appendicitis."[40]

In 1946, canned fruit cocktail, peaches, pears, pear nectar, and pineapple juice were popular but expensive. Offering canned fruit cocktail to a visitor conveyed status and hospitality. In 1946, desserts played a minor role in the Puerto Rican diet and were only affordable for people with higher incomes. The most popular desserts in 1946 for families who could afford them were guava paste, *casquitos de guayaba* (guava in syrup), green papaya preserve, and *pasta de batata* (sweet potato preserve). In contrast, in 1980, cookies, soda crackers, and cakes were commonly eaten as desserts.

There was also more variation in the diets of 1980 than of 1946. In 1946, few vegetables were consumed; in 1980, vegetables (mostly lettuce and tomato) were eaten at least once a day. And there was nutritional improvement in the diets from 1946 to 1980. In 1980, in both Naranjito and Río Grande, meat, mostly fried or stewed, was served twice a day. In 1946, on the other hand, protein intake was low and codfish was the main source of it. Overall, diets in 1980 appeared to provide more calories and protein than diets in 1946.

Breakfast   For years, the most popular breakfast among Puerto Ricans has been *café con leche* (coffee with milk) or black coffee. In 1946, the most common combination was coffee with bread, cereal, or *vianda,* whereas in 1980, for both communities, it was coffee accompanied by a source of protein (eggs or cheese). In 1946, eggs were considered a luxury that only high-income families could afford daily. In Naranjito, in 1980, mothers also ate either white bread or *pan criollo* (French-type bread) for breakfast.

Lunch   In 1946, the bulk of the diet for many families, especially poor rural families, was starchy vegetables or *viandas.* At that time, the most favored *viandas* were green plantain, green banana, white tannier, ripe plantain, and white sweet potato. In Naranjito the most commonly used *viandas* were green plantain, ripe plantain, tannier, green banana, and breadfruit; in Río Grande they were breadfruit, green banana, *malanga, ñame,* and green plantain. The higher consumption of *viandas* in Naranjito was not surprising, as 66% of the families there grew at least one food crop, with *viandas* (62%) being the most common.[41]

In 1946, very few families could afford to have meat every day, and a high percentage of families had it very rarely or never.[42] In contrast, in 1980, meat was served at lunch and at dinner in both communities. Similarly, in 1946, poultry was the meat most frequently consumed in both communities either at lunch or supper (Naranjito, 54%; Río Grande, 44%), followed by pork (25%).

Dinner   Rice and beans continued as the backbone of the typical Puerto Rican diet. In 1946 families consumed rice and beans at least once a day, mostly during the evening meal. This same pattern persisted in 1980. The use of *viandas*, however, was less common in 1980 because they were less available and prices had increased. People no longer grow *viandas* as commonly they used to.

Snack   In 1946, snacking was not common. Only 16% of the families studied reported having a snack. In contrast, in 1980, 48% of the families in Naranjito and 62% of the families in Río Grande had snacks before bed.

Changes in Milk Consumption

Figure 4.3 shows a comparative analysis of milk consumption among Puerto Rican families. Data from studies by Roberts and Stefani,[43] Colón,[44] and Sanjur et al.[45] were compiled in order to examine patterns of milk consumption over time in terms of the types and amounts of milk consumed and the most popular forms of consumption.

According to Roberts and Stefani, in 1946, when milk was consumed it was consumed as fresh milk by 74% of the mothers, as evaporated milk by 14.6%, and as powered milk by 6.4%. None of these families reported using skim milk. In Naranjito, in 1981, the preferred form of milk was still fresh milk, consumed by 88% of the mothers. In 1980, only 1% of the mothers drank powdered milk, and none reported consuming evaporated or skim milk.

Figure 4.3 shows the different ways in which milk was consumed. In all three time periods the most popular way that mothers consumed milk was as *café con leche* (coffee with milk). The frequency of consumption was as follows: in 1946, 55%; in 1971, 50%; and in 1981, 82%—thus reflecting rural milk consumption patterns among Puerto Rican families. (Note that the three data sets cited here reflect milk consumption behavior among poor Puerto Rican rural families, with the 1946 and 1981 data collected in Puerto Rico. The 1971 data represent newly arrived Puerto Rican migrant families settled in rural upstate New York.)

In Puerto Rico the amount of milk usually recommended to meet the nutritional needs of an adult is 16 ounces per day. Although consumption of milk increased between 1946 and 1981, overall consumption was still low for many women in 1981. For example, Figure 4.3B shows that three-fourths of the mothers had an intake of less than 16 ounces of milk per day: 79.8% in 1946; 76% in 1971, and 75% in 1981. Similarly, in 1946 and 1971, more than half of the mothers had less than 8 ounces of milk or none at all, and in 1981 the figure was reduced to 33%. The data, however, suggest a trend toward increased consumption of milk. In 1946, the mean intake was 7.6 ounces (229 g); in 1971, it was 9.5 ounces (269 g); and in 1981, it was 11.9 ounces (357 g) of milk, per person, per day.

FIGURE 4.3   Milk consumption trends among Puerto Ricans

A. Ways in Which Milk Is Consumed

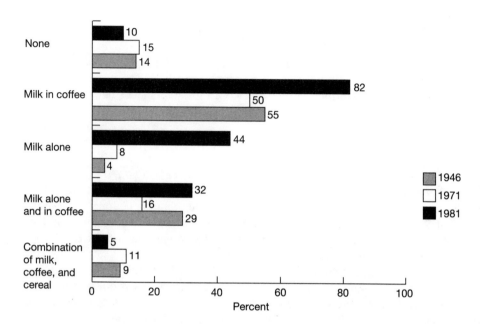

B.   Per Capita Milk Consumption per Day

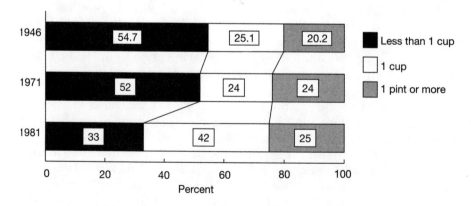

SOURCE: L.J. Roberts and R. Stefani, *Patterns of living of Purerto Rican families* (Rio Piedras: University of Puerto Rico, 1949). D. Sanjur, E. Romero, and M. Kira, Milk consumption patterns of Puerto Rican preschool children in rural New York. *American Journal of Clinical Nutrition, 24* (1971), 1320. Mirta Colón, Home food production and household income as predictors of nutritional status of Puerto Rican preschool children and their mothers. M.S. thesis, University of Puerto Rico, June 1981.

Nutritional Consequences of U.S. Migration

Data from a 1980 study by Immink et al. of 326 families illustrate the nutritional consequences of U.S. migration among Puerto Rican women.[46]

Homemakers' Migration Status   Three groups of Puerto Rico-born, adult females with different migration patterns were compared. Of the 326 homemakers residing in Puerto Rico, a large majority, 253 (78%), had never migrated to the United States, and this group was labeled "nonmigrants." The remaining homemakers, 73, had moved at least once to the United States and thus labeled "return migrants." The remaining South Bronx homemakers were labeled "forward migrants."

Fifty-three percent of the nonmigrants were still living in the community in which they were born, and 12% had moved within Puerto Rico three times or more. Forty-four percent of the return migrants had only moved once to the United States and once back to Puerto Rico, with half of these having returned to Puerto Rico within the past eight years. For almost 58% of the forward migrants, their first move to the United States was their only move during their lifetime. Thirty-eight percent migrated once or twice; in addition, thirty-nine homemakers (21.1%) had moved at least once within Puerto Rico before departing for the United States. Most of the forward migrants were long-term U.S. residents, with half of them having arrived more than 19 years ago. Immink et al. compared the repeat migration status of the Puerto Rican homemakers in the three groups and found significant differences between the return migrants, who exhibited the most repeat migration, and the forward migrant group, the least.

Migration Status and Socioeconomic Attributes   One-way analysis of variance showed that the three groups of migrant women differed in age, formal schooling, use of mass media, and per capita income. The nonmigrants tended to be younger than the return migrants, who in turn were younger than the forward migrants. Return migrants tended to have completed more schooling than the homemakers in the other two groups. The same pattern of educational selectivity associated with the U.S. migration status of Puerto Rico women has been reported by Sandis.[47] Forward migrants generally made use of more mass media than return and nonmigrants. Significant differences among the three groups were found in per capita income, but the income differentials between the groups in Puerto Rico and in the South Bronx were not adjusted for differences in the cost of living. Per capita income, however, was the only socioeconomic variable that was significantly correlated with the length of U.S. residence by return and forward migrants.

Energy and Micronutrient Intake   One-way analysis of variance showed that the forward migrants generally had a more adequate intake of energy and nutrients than either the nonmigrants or return migrants (Table 4.7). With the exception of iron intake, the return migrants tended to have a more adequate energy and nutrient intake than the nonmigrants. Energy, cal-

TABLE 4.7 Percentage of Adequate Energy and Nutrient Intakes of Puerto Rican Women Grouped by U.S.-Puerto Rican Migration Status.

Percent of Recommended Daily Allowance	Non-migrants (N = 253)	Return migrants (N = 73)	Forward migrants (N = 189)	F	P > F
	Mean (± S.E.)				
Energy	79	85	101	27.11	0.001
	(2)	(4)	(2)		
Protein	136	148	211	74.77	0.001
	(4)	(8)	(4)		
Calcium	70	83	115	68.32	0.001
	(3)	(5)	(3)		
Iron	52	52	91	96.92	0.001
	(2)	(3)	(3)		
Vitamin A	104	120	402	41.07	0.001
	(10)	(7)	(40)		
Riboflavin	111	122	211	80.73	0.001
	(4)	(8)	(8)		
Vitamin C	94	152	315	182.18	0.001
	(6)	(17)	(10)		

SOURCE: M.D.C. Immink, D. Sanjur, and M. Burgos, Nutritional consequences of U.S. migration patterns among Puerto Rican women. *Ecology of Food and Nutrition, 13* (1983), 139–148.

cium, and iron intakes were the least adequate among both nonmigrants and return migrants. Vitamin C intakes of the nonmigrants and iron intake of the forward migrants also tended to be low. There appears to be a significant migration status effect on the adequacy of energy and nutrient intakes, with the largest differences between the forward migrants and the nonmigrants.

Immink et al. report that carbohydrates tended to be a more important source of energy for nonmigrants and return migrants, whereas protein and fat were more important sources of energy for forward migrants. Three socioeconomic variables—income, schooling, and mass media use—were imputed in a regression model and controlled for, to test for significant differences in the macronutrient composition of the dietary intake and their migration status. The results, shown in Figure 4.4, suggest that these variables were not related to the fat-energy and carbohydrate-energy ratios.

Controlling for these three socioeconomic variables, Immink et al. found that the difference in the macronutrient composition between the forward migrants and the two groups in Puerto Rico remained. Furthermore, for all groups the macronutrient composition was not significantly related to repeat migration status; and among return and forward migrants, the macronutrient composition of their diets was not correlated with the length of U.S. residence.

Migration Status and the Prevalence of Obesity   In the full sample of women, body mass index (BMI) was highly correlated with body weight (r =

FIGURE 4.4 Macronutrient composition of the diets of three migrant groups
Least square means; controlling for income, schooling and mass media use.

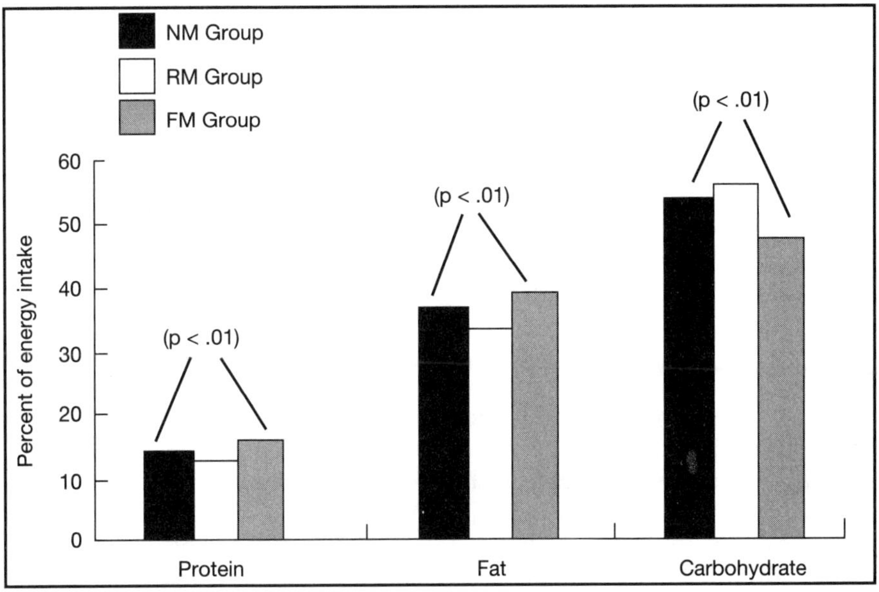

SOURCE: M.D.C. Immink, D. Sanjur, and M. Burgos, Nutritional consequences of U.S. migration patterns among Puerto Rican women. *Ecology of Food and Nutrition, 13* (1983), 139–148.

.91) and not correlated with height (4 = 0.09). The *body mass index* (weight/height^2) was calculated from the height and weight measurements taken from the mothers. This index is the most appropriate indicator of body fat content when skinfold measurements are not available. This is particularly true in population groups that tend to be obese.[48] Thus BMI may be considered a good indicator of body fat content. Obesity was defined as a BMI value greater than 27.[49] By this definition, 29.6% of the forward migrants were obese, as compared to 42.3% of the nonmigrants and 42.5% of the return migrants.

The BMI was negatively correlated with the homemakers' formal schooling after controlling for their age (-0.133; $p \geq .01$). The prevalence of obesity among homemakers with six or fewer years of schooling was 50.6%, versus 29.7% for those with schooling beyond primary education ($p \geq .01$). An inverse relationship between the prevalence of obesity in women and their socioeconomic status has been extensively reported in the literature. The prevalence rates of obesity also increased with length of U.S. residence, as shown in Table 4.8. The return migrants tended to have more body fat and were more likely to be obese the longer they had resided in the United States.

The results of the Immink et al. analysis suggest that U.S. migration patterns of Puerto Rican women are associated with "nutritional selectivity." Different kinds of migrants are exposed to different macroenvironments, and the migration process tends to select for socioeconomic characteristics.

TABLE 4.8 Prevalence of Obesity of Return/and Forward Migrants, by Length of U.S. Residence

| | Prevalence of Obesity (BMI > 27) Length of U.S. Residence (years) | | | |
Migrant-Group	≤5 (%)	>5–10 (%)	>10 (%)	Chi square
Return migrants	22.6	40.0	66.7	11.53
(N)	(31)	(15)	(27)	(p <.01)
Forward migrants	20.0	30.0	29.9	0.45
(N)	(10)	(20)	(157)	(p<.50)

SOURCE: M.D.C. Immink, D. Sanjur, and M. Burgos, Nutritional consequences of U.S. migration patterns among Puerto Rican women. *Ecology of Food and Nutrition, 13* (1983), 139–148.

However, two caveats are in order: First, the sample tended to include low-income women. Thus the results do not represent the complete U.S.–Puerto Rican migration pattern and its association with nutritional selectivity. Second, it is not clear whether the differences among the three groups in levels of formal schooling and per capita income reflect a selection process or merely differences in opportunities for mobility between the United States and Puerto Rico. Immink et al. explain that the answer to that question depends on knowing the schooling and income levels of the migrants before they departed from the United States or Puerto Rico.

Interestingly enough, return migrants seemed to revert rapidly to customary dietary patterns upon return to Puerto Rico. The only effect of having lived in the United States may have been increased intakes of calcium and vitamin C. Whether Puerto Rican migrants to the United States also rapidly change their dietary patterns in response to the macroenvironment is difficult to assess from this study, because most forward migrants were long-term U.S. residents.

Migration Status and Macronutrient Profile: A Comparison with the U.S. Dietary Goals

In 1977, the U.S. Senate Committee on Nutrition issued a set of dietary goals for the United States based on research regarding diet-disease relationships. The goals recommended that daily diets contain 12% kilocalories from protein, 30% from fat, and 58% from carbohydrates.

Figure 4.5 compares the U.S. Dietary Goals for 1977 with actual intakes by mothers in the South Bronx and in Puerto Rico in 1980. In the South Bronx the mean daily caloric intake was 1,985. Of these, the percentage of kilocalories from protein was 19% and from fat 35%. These were somewhat above the recommendations. On the other hand, in Puerto Rico, even though the total mean caloric intake of 1,588 was lower than in South Bronx, the distribution of the macronutrients was relatively similar. An examination of macronutrient distribution in the individual communities shows the following results:

FIGURE 4.5   U.S. Dietary Goals and Puerto Rican macronutrient intake

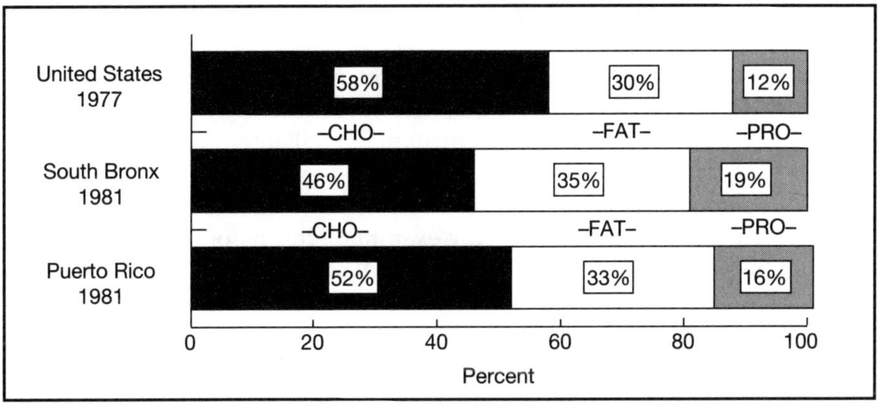

SOURCE: D. Sanjur, M.D.C. Immink, M. Colón, L. Bentz Rivera, L. B. Collachi, S. Alicea, and M. Burgos, *The effect of environmental changes on food consumption and nutrient intake among Puerto Rican families: South Bronx and Puerto Rico.* Research report, Division of Nutrition Science, Cornell University, Ithaca, NY, December 1981.

COMMUNITY	N	MEAN KILOCALORIES	PROTEIN (%)	FAT (%)	CARBOHY-DRATES (%)
South Bronx	200	1,985	19	35	46
Naranjito	109	1,851	15	33	52
Fajardo	62	1,545	16	34	50
Luquillo	60	1,521	16	29	55
Río Grande	95	1,294	15	35	59
Puerto Rico	326	1,588	16	33	52

These figures show that residents of Naranjito, Rio Grande, and Fajardo had quite similar relative intakes of protein and fat, and in Luquillo mean intakes of kilocalories and fat were much lower than in the South Bronx. On the other hand, carbohydrate intake was higher in all four Puerto Rican communities than it was in the South Bronx. A comparison of macronutrient intakes in Puerto Rico to those in the South Bronx shows that in Puerto Rico the percentages of protein (16% versus 19%) and fat (33% versus 35%) were lower, and the percentage of carbohydrates was higher (52% versus 46%). This higher consumption of carbohydrates was also reflected by the dietary pattern (Table 4.1) that exhibited a much higher consumption of sugar (38% more in the South Bronx), soft drinks (27% more than in the South Bronx), and starchy vegetables (13% more than in the South Bronx).

CONTEMPORARY HISPANIC DIETARY AND NUTRIENT INTAKE IN NEW YORK STATE

Data from a recent nutrition surveillance report, *New York State: Nutrition—State of the State Report,*[50] published by the Division of Nutritional Sciences at Cornell University in cooperation with the Nutrition Surveillance Program of the New York State Department of Health, can help put in perspective some of the historical trends in Puerto Rican food consumption discussed in this chapter. One caveat, however, must be made before examining this report: These data were collected from Hispanics in New York State. (According to the 1990 census, 12.4 percent of the entire population of New York State and 24.1 percent of the population of New York City is Hispanic.) If the assumption that the majority of Puerto Ricans in the United States live in New York City holds true, then it can also be assumed that the data reflect habits of a predominantly Puerto Rican population. However, Hispanics in New York State also include large numbers of Dominicans, Central Americans, Cubans, and other Latinos.

Food Consumption Patterns

Dietary choices influence health by providing the nutrients needed to maintain health and by limiting such nutrients as fat, saturated fat, cholesterol, and sodium that have been linked to increased risk of chronic disease. Because people eat foods, not nutrients, it is important that food constituents be known so that dietary counseling can be based on practical information.

In 1990, the USDA recommended that people consume at least three servings of vegetables, two servings of fruits, six servings of grain products, two servings of dairy products, and two servings of meat, legumes, and/or eggs per day. Table 4.9 shows the percentage of New York State adults with less than optimal consumption of foods from the five groups. These data indicate that Hispanics were least likely to report less than optimal intakes of vegetables, fruits, and meats, legumes, and/or eggs than were whites or African-Americans. The findings on Hispanic consumption of fruits and veg-

TABLE 4.9   New York State Survey Results

Food Groups	White (%)	African-American (%)	Hispanic (%)	Total (%)
≤ 3 Vegetables	75	78	69	75
≤ 2 Fruit	51	46	37	48
≤ 2 Dairy	71	81	69	73
≤ 6 Grain	84	77	79	80
≤ 2 Meat, legumes, eggs	45	37	22	41

SOURCE: New York State Department of Health, Bureau of Nutrition, *Dietary survey*, Albany, 1991.

etables, key sources of fiber and vitamins A and C, were quite encouraging, because these two food groups have not been an integral part of traditional Hispanic diets.

Vitamin and Mineral Intake

The optimal levels of essential nutrients for most healthy Americans are defined by the recommended dietary allowances (RDAs), which are set at levels high enough to account for individual variation in nutrient needs within the population. The percentages of men and women in New York State consuming less than the RDA for nine nutrients is shown in Table 4.10. In general, women were more likely than men to consume less than the RDA for energy and the eight nutrients. Similarly, larger percentages of adults between age 50 and 64 consumed less than recommended levels of nutrients than did adults younger than 50 years of age. Among the racial/ethnic groups, Hispanics were least likely to consume less than the RDA for most nutrients.

TABLE 4.10 Percentage of New York State Adults with Nutrient Intakes below the Recommended Dietary Allowances (RDAs).

	Race/Ethnicity			Age (Years)			
	White	African-American	Hispanic	18-34	35-49	50-64	Total
			Women				
Energy	75	72	53	63	71	88	72
Calcium	55	72	64	59	55	71	60
Iron	82	75	63	72	80	88	78
Thiamin	39	47	24	31	42	50	39
Riboflavin	26	39	26	23	28	41	29
Niacin	49	47	32	40	47	59	46
Phosphorus	24	41	25	28	25	33	28
Vitamin A	0	0	0	0	0	0	0
Vitamin C	10	9	3	9	11	5	9
			Men				
Energy	59	78	49	43	64	78	57
Calcium	43	62	50	45	47	52	47
Iron	16	16	12	10	18	26	16
Thiamin	42	43	24	28	51	54	40
Riboflavin	27	33	21	20	32	40	28
Niacin	36	37	24	24	42	49	35
Phosphorus	7	16	11	8	8	13	9
Vitamin A	0	0	0	0	0	0	0
Vitamin C	6	12	2	4	8	9	6

SOURCE: Division of Nutrition Sciences, Cornell University, *New York State: Nutrition—State of the State Report.* In cooperation with Nutrition Surveillance Program, New York State Department of Health, Ithaca, NY, 1992.

Table 4.11 Percentage of New York State Adults with Intakes of Fat, Saturated Fat and Cholesterol That Exceed Recommendations

	Men				Women			
	White	African-American	Hispanic	Total	White	African-American	Hispanic	Total
Fat (>30% of calories)	87	79	80	84	83	73	76	80
Saturated Fat (>10% of calories)	89	85	83	87	84	79	91	84
Cholesterol (>300 mg/day)	60	62	77	62	32	44	58	38

SOURCE: Division of Nutrition Sciences, Cornell University, *New York State: Nutrition—State of the State Report.* In Cooperation with Nutrition Surveillance Program, New York State Department of Health, Ithaca, NY, 1992.

Fat, Saturated Fat, Cholesterol, and Sodium Intake

The Dietary Guidelines for Americans recommend that people choose diets low in fat, saturated fat, and cholesterol and use salt and sodium in moderation. Specifically, no more than 30% of total calories should come from fat and no more than 10% from saturated fat;[51] daily consumption of cholesterol should not exceed 300 mg; and sodium intake should be limited to 2,400 mg/day.[52]

Table 4.11 shows that more than three-quarters of adults in New York State consumed greater than recommended amounts of fat and saturated fat, with very small differences across gender or racial/ethnic groups. Cholesterol intake was above the recommended limit for 62% of the men and 38% of the women. For both sexes, however, Hispanics were more likely than whites or African-Americans to consume more than 300 mg of cholesterol daily.

Food-related Practices

Certain food-related practices can help reduce intakes of fat and sodium. The Dietary Guidelines for Americans recommend using fats and oils sparingly in cooking, trimming fat from meat, removing skin from poultry, and using salt sparingly, if at all, in cooking and at the table. Interesting enough, although the majority of adults in New York State reported following dietary practices that helped limit their intake of fat and saturated fat, only 39% reported never adding salt to their food (Table 4.12). Hispanics (54%) were less likely than whites (75%) or African-Americans (74%) to avoid using fat in cooking.

Weight Loss Practices

Regular physical activity provides significant health benefits and contributes to maintenance of appropriate body weight, thus decreasing risk of devel-

TABLE 4.12 Percentage of New York State Adults' Dietary Practices That Reduce Fat and Sodium Intake

	Male	Female	White	African-American	Hispanic	Total
Cook with fat <1 time/day	72	72	75	74	65	72
Avoid:						
Chicken skin	52	59	60	43	58	56
Fat on meat	79	87	83	85	85	83
Salting food	35	41	38	43	36	38

SOURCE: Division of Nutrition Sciences, Cornell University, *New York State: Nutrition—State of the State Report*. In Cooperation with Nutrition Surveillance Program, New York State Department of Health, Ithaca, NY, 1992. Also New York State Department of Health, Bureau of Nutrition, *Dietary* Survey, Albany, NY 1991.

oping other chronic diseases. Information about the exercise practices of adults in New York State was classified as follows: sedentary (no regular physical activity); irregular (physical activity ≥ 3 times/week and/or ≥ 20 minutes/time); or regular (≤ 3 times/week or ≥ 20 minutes/time).[53] Surveys indicated that 70% of adults had sedentary or irregular patterns of physical activity. The New York State nutrition surveillance report found only small differences among the racial/ethnic groups, with 38, 32, and 30% of Hispanics reporting sedentary, irregular, and regular activity patterns, respectively. Based on this report, there appear to be some positive changes in the food behaviors of New York State Hispanics, but further improvement is needed in others.

SUMMARY

This chapter profiled Puerto Rican diets and nutrient intakes using several approaches. First, it highlighted several macroenvironmental factors that influence present-day Puerto Rican lifestyles and, consequently, health and nutrition patterns. Understanding the Puerto Rican culture is a major first step in attempting to work with them. A comparison of the Puerto Rican Food Guide with the USDA Food Guide Pyramid illustrated similarities and differences in the island's approach to nutrition education. A discussion of the Puerto Rican diet followed.

The chapter provided a historical perspective of food consumption trends in Puerto Rico and in the United States, especially in New York State, where most Puerto Ricans settle. Historical trends relative to food consumption patterns of any population group are important from an epidemiological point of view, especially the association between food intake and chronic diseases. Islandwide surveys spanning more than four decades were reviewed, as well as a large cross-sectional study conducted in four communities in Puerto Rico and in the South Bronx, New York City.

Changes in dietary practices also merited extensive discussion, as they are important in identifying factors that foster or hinder dietary changes. Dietary changes—in food groups, in typical meal patterns, and in reasons given by mothers for having changed their food intake patterns—were reviewed for Puerto Rico and New York City. Elements of continuity and change of Puerto Rican dietary patterns were identified. The chapter ended with a review of contemporary dietary and nutrient intake patterns for Hispanics living in New York State.

GLOSSARY OF PUERTO RICAN FOODS AND DISHES*

acerola	West Indian cherry
adobo	seasoning powder made with salt, garlic, and oregano
ajonjolí	sesame seeds
albóndigas	meatballs
alboronía	boiled *chayotes* cooked with eggs and sofrito
alcapurrias	tannier fritters stuffed with meat
almojábanas	rice and cheese meal crullers
amarillos	ripe plantains consumed as a cooked vegetable— boiled, fried, or baked
arroz con calamares	stewed rice with squid
arroz con gandules	stewed rice with pigeons peas
arroz con pollo	stewed rice with chicken
arroz con salchichas	stewed rice with Vienna sausages
arroz guisado	stewed rice colored with annato
arroz mamposteado	stewed rice with pink or kidney beans
asopao	stewed, soupy rice
bacalaítos	codfish fritters
bacalao	dried salted codfish
batata	sweet potato, yellow and white
batida	milk shake
berro	watercress
biftec	thin slices of beef, fried with oil, garlic, vinegar, and onions
bolitas de queso	cheese puffs
budín/pudín	bread pudding, usually with raisins

*SOURCE: 73 B. Cabanillas, and C. Ginorio, *Puerto Rican dishes* (Rio Piedras: Editorial de la Universidad de Puerto Rico, 1984. D. Sanjur, *Puerto Rican food habits* (Ithaca, NY: Cornell University, 1970). V. Dávila, *Puerto Rican cooking* (Secaucus, NJ; Castle Books, 1988.) M. Coll-Camalez, et al., *Siluetas que pueden cambiar,* 4th ed. (San Juan, PR, 1991). C. Bueso, personal communication, University of Puerto Rico, Rio Piedras, 1992.

buñuelos	crullers, often made with grated *viandas*
butifarra	pork sausage, grayish in color
carne al pincho	shish-kebab-style meat chunks
carne empanada	breaded beef
carne vieja	stewed, boiled shredded beef
casquitos de guayaba	guava shells in syrup
cazuela	sweet potato and pumpkin pudding
coditos	elbow macaroni
coquito	coconut, rum egg nog
culantro/recao/cilantro	long, broad, serrated leaf coriander
champola	fruit and milk drink
chicharrón	pork cracklings
chillo/pargo	red snapper
china	orange
chorizo	dry Spanish-style sausage
chuleta	pork chop
dulce de papaya	green papaya slices in syrup
empanadilla	large turnover
flan	custard made in caramel-lined mold
fritura	fritter
galletas de soda	soda crackers
gandinga	stew of liver, kidney, heart, and lungs of pork
gandules/gandures	pigeon peas
garbanzos	chick-peas
gaseosas/sodas	carbonated beverages
granos	legumes
guineítos verdes	green bananas
jíbaro envuelto	ripe ladyfinger bananas in a flour fritter
jueyes	crabs
leche de coco	coconut milk
lechón asado	pork roasted on an open fire
limón dulce	sweet lime
lomillo	loin of beef
longaniza	pork sausage, colored with *annato*
mabí	fermented beverage made with the bark of the mabí tree
majarete	rice meal pudding flavored with cinnamon and lemon rind
mallorca	spanish-style sweet roll
malta	nonalcoholic malt beverage
manteca/aceite con achiote	*annato* colored lard/oil used to season rice, stews, and other dishes

mantecaditos	cookies made with shortening and butter
mantecado	ice cream
mazamorra	grated green corn, coconut, milk, and sugar
melao	molasses
mofongo	fried green plantain slices mashed with pork rinds and garlic
mojo	sauce with olive oil, tomato sauce, garlic, onions, vinegar, and olives
mollejas guisadas	chicken gizzard stew
mondongo	tripe stew
morcilla	pork blood sausage
paella	spanish-style saffron-seasoned rice with various vegetables, meats, and/or seafood, chicken, or pork
panapén/pana	breadfruit, one of the *viandas*
parcha	passion fruit
pasta	fruit bar or preserve, made with guava, mango sweet-potato, coconut, or bitter orange
pastel	grated starchy vegetable stuffed with meat or chicken wrapped in banana leaves, tied and boiled
pastelillos	fried turnovers filled with meat, cheese, or guava paste
pastelón	meat or chicken pie made with potatoes or *viandas*
patitas de cerdo	stewed pigs' feet
pernil	baked fresh ham, seasoned with *adobo*
picadillo	stewed ground beef or pork
piñón	casserole made with layers of fried ripe plantain slices, ground meat, string beans, and beaten eggs
pionono	fried ripe plantain slices, rolled and stuffed with meat, covered with beaten eggs or flour batter
pique	hot sauce prepared with chili peppers
polvorones	lard cookies
ponche	egg nog
ponqué	pound cake
queso del país	Puerto Rican white cheese
quimbombó	okra
refresco	soft or fruit drink
revoltillo	scrambled eggs
salchicha	Vienna sausage
salcocho/sancocho	thick soup made with various vegetables and meats
salmorejo	crab meat stew
serenata	boiled codfish with potatoes, *viandas*, onions, olive oil, and vinegar, garnished with tomato, avocado, and boiled eggs
sidra	fermented apple cider

sofrito	mixture of chopped ham/bacon with onions, tomato, peppers, garlic, and *culantro*; basic Puerto Rican seasoning
surullitos	fried cornmeal sticks with cheese
tasajo	jerked beef stew
tembleque	coconut milk and cornstarch dessert
tostones	fried green plantain slices, flattened and fried again
yuca	cassava eaten boiled, fried, or grated and then roasted in banana leaves; used in various mixed dishes

NOTES

1. Sonia Badillo Ghali, Understanding Puerto Rican traditions. *Social Work* (January 1982). 361. 605 567

2. Clara Rodríguez, *Puerto Ricans—Born in the U.S.A.* (Boulder, CO: Westview Press, 1991).

3. Ibid.

4. Roger A. LaBrucherie, *Puerto Rico, Borinquen Querida—A loving portrait of an island* (Hong Kong: Imágenes Press, 1992).

5. J. M. Czaijkowski, . . . *Puerto Rican foods and traditions*, booklet, Cooperative Extension Service, University of Connecticut, Storrs, 1971.

6. Lizette Vicéns de Sánchez, Doña Elena twenty-seven years later. Ed.D. thesis, Teachers College, Columbia University, New York, 1986.

7. Puerto Rico Census Data Center, February 1993.

8. M. D. C. Immink, D. Sanjur, and M. Burgos, Nutritional consequences of U.S. migration patterns among Puerto Rican women. *Ecology of Food and Nutrition, 13* (1983), 139–148.

9. Nilda Tirado, The changing Puerto Rican diet: Implications for nutrition education, paper presented at the Ethnic Foods Symposium, New York Medical College, March 8, 1978.

10. J. J. Putnam and J. E. Allshouse, *Food consumption, prices, and expenditures, 1968–1989*, Statistical Bulletin no. 825 (Washington, DC: U.S. Department of Agriculture, 1991).

11. Division of Nutrition Sciences, Cornell University, *New York State: Nutrition—State of the State Report.* In cooperation with Nutrition Surveillance Program, New York State Department of Health, Ithaca, 1992.

12. Putnam and Allshouse, *Food Consumption.*

13. M. Green, G. Von Nostitiz, R. Simpson, and J. Grader, *The poor pay more . . . for less. Part I. Grocery shopping* (New York: Department of Consumer Affairs, 1991).

14. Division of Nutrition Sciences, Cornell University, *New York State: Nutrition.*

15. Tirado, *Changing Puerto Rican diet.*

16. Rodríguez, *Puerto Ricans.*

17. Tirado, *Changing Puerto Rican diet.*

18. L. J. Roberts and R. Stefani, *Patterns of Living of Puerto Rican families* (Rio Piedras: University of Puerto Rico Press, 1949); Nelson A. Fernández, Nutritional status of the Puerto Rican population: Master sample survey. *American Journal of Clinical Nutrition, 24* (1968), 952–965.

19. Berta Cabanillas de Rodríguez, *El Puertorriqueño y su alimentación a través de su historia* (San Juan: Instituto de Cultura Puertorriqueña, 1973).

20. Mirta Colón, Home food production and household income as predictors of nutritional status of Puerto Rican preschool children and their mothers. M. S. thesis, University of Puerto Rico Medical Campus, June 1981.

21. Laura Bentz Rivera, Patrones de consumo de alimentos e ingestión de nutrientes en Río Grande, Puerto Rico: Un enfoque sociocultural. M.S. thesis, University of Puerto Rico Medical Campus, June 1981.

22. D. Sanjur, E. Romero, and M. Kira, Milk consumption patterns of Puerto Rican preschool children in rural New York. *American Journal of Clinical Nutrition, 24* (1971), 1320.

23. Bentz Rivera, Patrones de consumo de alimentos.

24. Roberts and Stefani, *Patterns of living.*

25. Lydia J. Roberts, *The Doña Elena project: A better-living program in an isolated rural community* (Rio Piedras: Department of Home Economics, University of Puerto Rico, 1963).

26. Fernández, Nutritional status.

27. Puerto Rican Department of Health, *Estudio del estado nutricional de la población puertorriqueña,* Estado Libre Asociado de Puerto Rico, San Juan, 1983.

28. USDA, *Food Consumption and Dietary Levels of Households in Puerto Rico, Summer and Fall, 1977.* Nationwide Food Consumption Survey 1977–78, Preliminary Report no. 9, Washington, DC.

29. D. Sanjur, M. D. C. Immink, M. Burgos, and S. Alicea, Trends and differentials in dietary patterns and nutrient intake among Puerto Rican families. *Archivos Latinoamericanos de Nutrición, 36*(4) (December 1986), 625–641.

30. D. Sanjur, E. Romero, and G. Neville, *A community study of food habits and sociocultural factors of families participating in the East Harlem nutrition education program.* Research report, New York State College of Human Ecology, Cornell University, Ithaca, NY, 1972.

31. Sanjur, Romero, and Kira, Milk consumption patterns.

32. S. L. Parker and J. Bowering, Folacin in diets of Puerto Rican and black women in relation to food practices. *Journal of Nutrition Education, 8*(2) (April–June 1976).

33. Alan Harwood, The hot-cold theory of disease. *Journal of the American Medical Association, 216*(7) (May 1971).

34. Tirado, *Changing Puerto Rican diets.*

35. R. L. Duyff, D. Sanjur, and H. Y. Nelson, Food behavior and related factors of Puerto Rican teenagers. *Journal of Nutrition Education 7*(3) (July–September 1975).

36. Tirado, *Changing Puerto Rican diets.*

37. Sanjur, Romero, and Kira, Milk consumption patterns.

38. Immink, Sanjur, and Burgos, Nutritional Consequences.

39. M. B. Melville, Selective acculturation of female Mexican migrants. In M. B. Melville (ed.), *Twice a minority: Mexican-American women* (St. Louis, MO: C. V. Mosby, 1980), pp. 155–163; K. G. Dewey, M. A. Strode, and Y. Ruiz Fitch, Dietary change among migrant and nonmigrant Mexican-American families in northern California. *Ecology of Food and Nutrition, 14* (1984), 11–24. S. L. Black and D. Sanjur, Nutrition in Rio Piedras: A study of internal migration and maternal diets. *Ecology of Food and Nutrition, 10* (1980), 25–33.

40. Roberts and Stefani, *Patterns of living.*

41. Colón, Home food production; Immink, Sanjur, and Colón, Home gardens.

42. Roberts and Stefani, *Patterns of living.*

43. Ibid.

44. Colón, *Home food production.*

45. Sanjur, Romero, and Kira, Milk consumption patterns.

46. Immink, Sanjur, and Burgos, Nutritional consequences.

47. E. E. Sandis, Characteristics of Puerto Rican migrants to, and from, the United States. *International Migration Review,* 11:22–43, 1970.

48. M. B. Kohrs, L. L. Wang, D. Eklund, B. Paulsen and R. O'Neal, The association of obesity with socioeconomic factors in Missouri, *American Journal of Clinical Nutrition,* 32:2120–2128, 1979.

49. Ibid.

50. Division of Nutrition Sciences, Cornell University, *New York State Nutrition.*

51. United States Department of Agriculture, *Nutrition and your health: Dietary guidelines for Americans.* Home and Garden Bulletin No. 232, 3rd ed., revised 11/90, U.S. Government Printing Office, 1990.

52. National Research Council, National Academy of Science. *Diet and health: Implications for reducing chronic disease risk.* Washington, DC: National Academy Press, 1989.

53. Behavioral Risk Factor Surveillance System, unpublished data, New York State Department of Health, Albany, 1991.

5

Other Hispanic Diets and Nutrient Intake

Dominican Diets and Nutrient Intake
Dominican Dietary Patterns in New York City
Differential Dietary Patterns of Puerto Ricans and
Dominicans in New York City
Dietary Changes and Nutrient Profile
Infant Feeding Practices
Folk Beliefs and Infant Feeding
Diets in the Sierra Highlands of the Dominican Republic
Weaning Foods in Las Cuevas, Dominican Republic

Cuban Diets and Nutrient Intake
Maintaining Cuban Culture and Food Traditions
Nutritional Status of Cuban Refugees
The Health Status of Cubans in Cuba
HHANES Dietary Data on Cuban-Americans

Panamanian Diets and Nutrient Intake
Health and Nutritional Status
Food Consumption and Meal Patterns
Frequency of Consumption of Vitamin A–Rich Foods
Nutrient Intake

Salvadoran Diets and Nutrient Intake
Food Consumption: Rural/Urban Differences
Food Preparation Methods
Nutritional Status of Preschool
Children in La Paz
Vitamin A Deficiency Among Salvadoran Children
Breastfeeding Practices
Salvadorans in the United States

Glossary of Hispanic Foods

153

DOMINICAN DIETS AND NUTRIENT INTAKE

As discussed in Chapter 1 the largest influx of Dominicans to the United States, and specifically to New York City, occurred in the early 1980s. Estimates of the number of Dominicans living in New York City range from 300,000 to 500,000.[1]

Although Puerto Ricans and Dominicans come from Caribbean islands only 60 miles apart and thus share many commonalites, they differ in distinct and subtle ways. According to Tirado,[2] Puerto Ricans and Dominicans differ in their English-speaking skills. Generally, Puerto Ricans have a stronger command of English than do Dominicans. This is understandable because the majority of Puerto Ricans in the United States are second- or third-generation immigrants, whereas the majority of Dominicans are more recent immigrants. Also, early Puerto Rican immigrants in the 1950s came primarily from rural areas; most Dominicans have come from urban areas. Another fundamental difference between Puerto Ricans and Dominicans is that Puerto Ricans are U.S. citizens and Dominicans are not.

Tirado notes that because both groups have been exposed to mass media and American food products, these influences contributed to changes that have affected the traditional food patterns, perhaps in a negative way, which may ultimately result in similar chronic disease patterns seen in the larger population. Increased rates of high blood pressure, obesity and overweight, gastrointestinal disorders, and diabetes are observed in both Puerto Rican and Dominican groups, although (except for diabetes) not at a rate as alarming as in the general population. Interestingly enough, Tirado reports that in two school surveys a significant number of Dominican children were identified as obese and/or having high blood pressure. These findings point to a need for increased public health awareness of the traditional dietary pattern and implementation of changes in order to promote a healthy diet.

In subsequent sections we discuss in depth Tirado's studies of dietary and food selection patterns of Dominican women based on 76 dietary surveys (recalls and food frequencies) collected during home interviews in 1983 and 1987, as well as on numerous clinic contacts documented over many years.[3] The women in these studies were, on average, 23.7 years of age when they arrived in the United States and had lived here between 5 and 9 years. Forty-one percent had less than an eighth-grade education; 39% had attended high school. Furthermore, 72% reported being single heads of households, and 51% participated in the Special Supplemental Foods Program for Women, Infants, and Children (WIC) program.[4] Tiffany's work[5] on food preferences and dietary change of Dominican women in Upper Manhattan, New York City, and Mort's[6] and Smith et al.'s[7] studies in the Sierra highlands of the Dominican Republic are also examined.

Dominican Dietary Patterns in New York City

Following is Tirado's listing of the major food groups consumed by Dominican women in New York City:[8]

FOOD GROUPS	COMMENTS
Milk and Dairy Products	
Milk, whole fresh	80% have milk daily, mostly in coffee and *batidas* (shakes)
Cheese, cheddar/white	Cost of white cheese is high; women not
evaporated, condensed milk	adapted to using skim milk
and yogurt	
Cereal/Grains	
Rice, white long grain	83% have rice daily
Bread, white enriched	
Cereal/oatmeal, farina	
Pasta and specialty breads	
(rolls, Italian)	
Fruits and Vegetables	
Citrus juices	60% have juices daily
Fresh fruits/juices	
Green plantains	53% have plantains daily
White potatoes	
Yucca (starchy root)	
Ñame (starchy root)	
Calabaza (*Auyama*)	
Lettuce	
Tomatoes	
Cucumber	
Cabbage	
Carrots	
Broccoli, fresh	
Mixed vegetables	
Peppers, onions	
Meats/Meat Substitutes	
Beef or chicken	36% have beef or chicken daily
Fish, canned, fresh, dried	
Pork	
Salchichón (salami)	
Salted processed meats	
Oxtails	
Beans	80% have beans daily
Eggs	

Other

Sugar, coffee

Vegetable oil

Soda beverages

Desserts

Olive oil (widely used)

When Tirado and coworkers compared these dietary data with the U.S. Dietary Guidelines, they ascertained the distribution of calories by macronutrient sources as follows:

	Percent of Calories	
	In the Dominican Republic	In New York City
Protein	12	15
Fat	30	33
Carbohydrate	58	52

Meat and beans were the main sources of protein; milk and meat were the main sources of fat; rice, bread, cereals, and green plantains were the main sources of carbohydrates.

When the data were examined for nutrient intake per 1000 calories, the following were observed for 1983 and 1987:

	Nutrient Intakes per 1000 Calories	
	1983	1987
Protein	33.5 g	35.6 g
Calcium	383 g	410 g
Iron	7.2 mg	6.7 mg
Vitamin A	2680 IU	2870 IU
Vitamin C	77.2 mg	79.0 mg

Iron was derived mainly from meats, beans, and cereals; vitamin A from carrots, plantains, cheese, and milk; vitamin C from citrus fruits and juices; and calcium from milk. Based on these studies, Tirado concluded that:

Intakes appeared adequate for all nutrients except calcium and iron.

Intakes of vitamin A, vitamin C, and protein were 100% over the RDAs for 60% of the Dominicans studied. However, some individuals were low in these nutrients.

There is a need to focus on decreasing fat intake and reinforcing use of vegetables and fruits and other complex carbohydrates.

Caloric intake of women merits attention, as 25% had more than 2200 calories and another 20% consumed fewer than 1500.

There were no fundamental changes observed in the traditional dietary pattern among the women studied. However, there was a slight increase in the amount of meat eaten, as well as a tendency to consume a light meal at lunch.

Coming from a rural or urban area in the Dominican Republic did not have a major impact on nutrient intake. Food consumption was more dependent on economics and availability than on region of origin.

Tirado concluded that for Dominicans in New York City, nutrition education should emphasize lowering the consumption of total calories and the percentage of calories from fat. Similarly, education should emphasize increasing the consumption of foods high in iron and calcium. A shift from the widely used evaporated milk to low-fat milk might also be encouraged.

Differential Dietary Patterns of Puerto Ricans and Dominicans in New York City

In New York City both Puerto Ricans and Dominicans have had little problem in obtaining their traditional foods. Literally thousands of *bodegas* (small grocery stores), street vendors, and fruit and vegetable markets provide, albeit at a high cost, a wide variety of tropical foods. Because both the Puerto Rican and Dominican populations are very young, opportunities for health practitioners to influence major changes in the diet, whenever merited, do exist. Furthermore, because both populations participate in various nutrition education programs, it is important for health workers to become familiar with both similarities and subtle differences in their dietary patterns.

Tirado's comparative analysis of the ethnic dietary patterns of both groups is summarized below:[9]

1. *Rice and beans.* These are the traditional staple foods for both Dominicans and Puerto Ricans. In both countries people prefer short-grain shiny white rice that is usually well washed and then cooked with oil and salt. Rice can be combined with meat and vegetables; when eaten with beans, it is known as *moro* by the Dominicans. Large quantities of rice are eaten by both groups, commonly up to three large serving spoons per person.

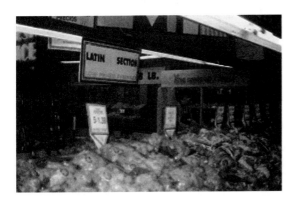

A Latin section in an American supermarket.

Red beans are the favorites, although white, pink, black, and pinto beans are also eaten. Unlike Puerto Ricans, Dominicans also use beans to make a beverage and to make a well-liked dessert called *habichuela con dulce*.

2. *Starchy roots.* Known as *viandas* in Puerto Rico and *víveres* in the Dominican Republic, starchy roots are an important part of the meal pattern of both populations. The counterpart of potatoes for the mainlanders, the principal roots include cassava, tanier, *malanga, ñame,* yams and green plantains, and bananas. Although these starchy vegetables contribute mainly energy from complex carbohydrates, they also provide varying amounts of other nutrients. For example, yam and yellow tanier provide vitamin A and others provide small amounts of B vitamins. There are, however, slight variations in the frequency and preference with which some of these are consumed. Puerto Ricans often eat green bananas and breadfruit, but Dominicans rarely eat these foods. Cassava, on the other hand, is especially important for Dominicans. It is usually eaten boiled, but also can be used in stews, as a dessert, or grated and dried to form *casabe* (flat dried bread). Plantains, whether green or yellow, are consumed by both groups, although they are especially important for Dominicans. *Mangú* (mashed boiled green plantain with onions and seasonings sausage) is a typical breakfast food. Plantians are also eaten fried as *tostones,* or they can be cooked on top of the stove with sugar or honey. The almost daily consumption of plantains provides Dominicans with a fairly good source of vitamin A.

3. *Convenience foods.* Tirado notes that major food companies have made available a number of traditional Hispanic foods, including stewed beans with sauce, *sofrito* (mixed condiments), and fritters ready for frying, that enable a homemaker to serve traditional foods without spending hours in the kitchen. Similarly, changing lifestyles have enabled Hispanic working women to choose frozen pizzas, precooked cereals, frozen TV dinners, prepared seasoning mixes, frozen cassava, prepared oatmeal beverages (consisting mostly of sugar), cake mixes, prepackaged Chinese and Mexican dishes, as well as hundreds of canned or frozen vegetables, fruits, and desserts. Tirado considers these products as early warning signals that it will not be long before Dominican homemakers will be changing their family's traditional dietary patterns. Many of these convenience foods are higher in salt, preservatives, and sugars and may be lower in nutrients than similar foods prepared from starch. Dominican women may need help in understanding the potential problems that can result from excessive use of convenience foods.

Dietary Changes and Nutrient Profile

Tiffany studied 180 low-income immigrant women from the Dominican Republic who were living in the Washington Heights area of New York City and were participating in the Expanded Food and Nutrition Education

Program (EFNEP).[10] To find out whether their diets changed, Tiffany administered a family record questionnaire and a 24-hour recall within a woman's first three visits after entering EFNEP. A follow-up questionnaire and another 24-hour recall were repeated after six months in the program. Tiffany examined dietary changes reported by these women since coming to the United States, along with the women's migration history, food preferences, food preparation and purchasing practices, and eating-out and snacking patterns.

In general, the meal patterns for these women appeared to have changed somewhat. In the Dominican Republic they reported preparing "more substantial meals" three times a day, especially at noon, whereas in New York City, women reported that they cooked less and also ate less often. However, the women felt "they were eating better here because there is more variety, abundance, and opportunity to get food." Much of the opportunity, Tiffany notes, may be related to economics as well as to the availability of food. Women often stated that "they have more money here and the foods are more economical and easier to get." One woman explained a common situation: "In my country when I was young I ate chicken only on Sunday and meats only on special occasions. All I ate was plantains, rice and beans, and dried codfish on Friday. Here I eat more variety."

Interestingly, when mothers were asked if their diets had changed during the last year, 94% claimed that they had. The following percentages of women reported consuming the listed foods more frequently than they had before:

Meats	35%
Milk	35
Vegetables	24
Fruits	13
Rice	11
Chicken	10

Although, very few women reported decreased food consumption, 5% reported eating less "beef" and 3% less plantains, rice, and/or fats. The main reasons for decreases were related to "less fresh products and/or poorer flavor in the products" available in the United States.

Tiffany found a significant improvement in the variety and quality of the diets consumed and a significant improvement in intakes of all 11 nutrients between the first and second 24-hour recalls. For example, during the first 24-hour recall, only 32% and 35% consumed at least two-thirds of the recommended amounts of calcium and iron, respectively. After six months, 73% and 57% consumed two-thirds or more of the recommended amounts of calcium and iron, respectively. Tables 5.1 and 5.2 summarize Tiffany's findings.

Tiffany hypothesizes that the following reasons may explain the dramatic dietary changes observed:

TABLE 5.1   Dietary Changes Among Dominican Women In New York City

First Dietary Recall (N = 188)	Percent	Second Dietary Recall (N = 178)	Percent
Food Consumed by at Least 50% of the Sample			
Oil	92	Oil	96
Rice	75	Milk	88
Ingredients for *sofrito*	69	Rice	82
Milk	67	Sugar	78
Sugar	64	Ingredients for *sofrito*	78
Coffee	55	Coffee	74
		White bread	59
		Green plantain	55
		Eggs	53
		Orange juice	52
Food Consumed by at Least 30% of the Sample			
Green Plantain	46	Beans	48
Beans	43	Chicken	36
White Bread	38	Beef	35
Chicken	37	Other cooked vegetables	32
Eggs	37	Margarine, butter	30
Orange Juice	36		
Beef	35		
Food Consumed by at Least 10% of the Sample			
Raw vegetables	23	American cheese	28
Lettuce	22	Lettuce	26
Other cooked vegetables	19	Potato	21
Carbonated beverages	19	Pork	21
Margarine, butter	17	Ripe plantain	19
Pork	16	High vitamin A vegetables	17
Potato	13	Citrus fruits	15
American cheese	11	Banana	15
Malta[a]	11	Apple	13
		Mayonnaise	13
		Sausage	12
		Cassava	12
		Pigeon peas	11
		Spaghetti	10

[a]Carbonated beverage made from barley, malt, and sugar, often drunk with sweetened condensed milk.

SOURCE: Adapted from Jean M. Tiffany, Dietary patterns and nutritional status of immigrant women from the Dominican Republic living in New York. Master's thesis, Cornell University, Ithaca, NY, May 1984.

1. Women had adjusted to the United States and to New York City and were able to buy more adequate foods.

2. Nutrition aides collecting the dietary data were better trained to probe for accurate estimates of intakes.

3. Homemakers were complying with the perceived expectations of the program interviewers.

TABLE 5.2 Total Nutrient Intake and Comparison with the Recommended Dietary Allowances (1980)

Nutrient	First Recall (N = 188)			Second Recall (N = 188)		
	Mean ± S.D.	Median	Percent of RDA	Mean ± S.D.	Median	Percent of RDA
Calories	1406 ± 472	1364	—	1855 ± 455	1847	—
Protein, g	46.6 ± 19.1	45.9	104	63.1 ± 18.5	61.0	139
Fat, g	57.4 ± 24.4	57.2	—	76.3 ± 26.4	75.9	—
Carbohydrate, g	182 ± 66	179	—	238 ± 61	235	—
Calcium, mg	461 ± 255	427	53	730 ± 295	698	87
Iron, mg	10.1 ± 4.6	9.5	53	13.2 ± 4.1	12.7	71
Vitamin A, IU	4065 ± 6626	2474	102	8146 ± 10,385	5098	211
Thiamin, mg	.835 ± .412	0.7	70	1.2 ± 0.3	1.1	110
Riboflavin, mg	1.2 ± 0.8	1.0	83	1.9 ± 1.1	1.6	133
Niacin, mg	13.7 ± 10.7	10.6	82	23.4 ± 17.8	14.9	115
Vitamin C, mg	105 ± 80	84.2	140	151 ± 82	139	232

SOURCE: Jean M. Tiffany, Dietary patterns and nutritional status of immigrant women from the Dominican Republic living in New York. Master's thesis, Cornell University, Ithaca, NY, May 1984.

4. Homemakers were indeed eating better after six months in New York City.

A closer look at Table 5.2 shows that at the first food recall, the nutrient intake for five nutrients did not meet the recommended dietary allowance (RDA) set by the National Research Council (1980). Median intakes of calcium and iron were only equal to 53% of the 1980 RDAs. On the other hand, intakes exceeded the RDAs for protein at 104%, vitamin A at 102% and vitamin C at 140%. At the second dietary recall, only median intakes of calcium (87% of RDA) and iron (71% of RDA) were below the recommended levels. Intakes of all other nutrients surpassed the recommendations.

Interestingly enough, in a national survey by Sebrell[11] taken a number of years ago among 5500 people in the Dominican Republic, intakes of both vitamin A and riboflavin were exceptionally low for the majority of the population studied. The nutritional intakes of pregnant and lactating women were particularly poor. These women did not increase their food consumption to meet the elevated physiological nutrient needs of pregnancy because their diets were so marginal to begin with. In short, this survey described a population in a precarious nutritional situation, with a strikingly low consumption of green leafy vegetables "except among wealthy urban families, and even there the quantities were small."

A comparison of Sebrell's work with the findings of Musgrove[12] indicates that nutrition seems to have improved over the last two decades. On a nationwide basis, average kilocalorie and protein intakes have improved by roughly one-third. In Musgrove's study rice, plantains, and oil were the main sources of calories; animal products (milk, chicken, eggs) and rice and beans were the major sources of protein.

Infant Feeding Practices

Studies conducted in the Dominican Republic over the last 20 years and cited by Tirado[13] indicate that although the number of women who breast-feed has decreased, it is still practiced by a substantial percentage of low-income women and by almost half of middle- and upper-income women. A study by Rondón et al. further substantiated these findings.[14] These investigators note that many Dominican mothers, even those of urban and upper socioeconomic strata, breast-feed. However, many of them breast-feed for short periods of time and then introduce formula if funds are available or change to whole cow's milk. The mean duration of breast feeding is about six months, although some women breast-feed for prolonged periods, sometimes as long as three years. Tirado indicates that health professionals working in the Dominican Republic have noticed a definite decrease in breast feeding, especially in urban areas. In the United States, very few studies have documented breast-feeding trends among Dominican mothers.

Myers' study of pregnant Dominican women in a Presbyterian Hospital clinic in New York City showed that although many expressed interest in breast feeding, less than half of them actually breast-fed their babies.[15] Similarly, Tirado reports that many Dominican participants in the EFNEP program expressed a strong interest in breast feeding. Tirado notes that when nutrition aides provided continued and frequent support to new mothers, they were more likely to continue breast feeding than mothers who were visited less often. The program found that mothers who breast-feed continue for up to three months. After that, friends and others discourage continuation because they call breast feeding "old-fashioned."

Reasons given by mothers for discontinuing breast feeding before one month include "painful nipples, lack of milk, not customary in the United States, embarrassment, mother was too upset, too uncomfortable or inconvenient, or husband did not like it."[16] Conversely, among the reasons mothers choose to breast-feed, "baby's health and baby's enjoyment" were most often mentioned. It appears that additional support and encouragement can help new Dominican mothers to initiate and continue breast feeding.

When mothers switch from the breast to the bottle, it is usually after the child is 3 months old and is generally in response to a child's illness. Cow's milk seems to be the preferred milk. However, Tirado expresses concern over the practice of giving children older than 6 months of age fruit juice or punch in place of milk.

Folk Beliefs and Infant Feeding

Dominican mothers, like others in rural developing areas, have a legion of folk beliefs about which foods to avoid or consume during lactation. High-protein foods to avoid during breast feeding include fresh fish, liver, eggs, dried fish, and pork. Foods believed to increase mother's milk supply include milk, orange juice, chocolate milk, noodle soup, black beer, and dried codfish. (It is worth noting the internal inconsistencies in these folk beliefs; an almost equal number of women in the EFNEP program reported that lactating women should avoid eating dry fish.[17])

There is some question about how strongly Dominican mothers are committed to these beliefs. Mothers reported that "they have been told these things but they really did not know how true these were." However, mothers have told nutrition aides that "one should drink more malt beer and lemon leaf tea to increase milk, while one should avoid eating pork and fish." Although Puerto Rican mothers give their babies tea before they switch from breast to bottle feeding, it is common for Dominican mothers to give their babies a purgative tea before introducing a new milk. Allergies or gastrointestinal disturbances in infants are often blamed on formula, especially if the formula contains iron. Illness is often treated by withholding formula and giving tea for several days until the child's health improves. In regard to these practices, Tirado has observed:

> During the short period of time that we have been working with the Dominican population, we have seen several cases of severe dehydration and increased

severity of child's illness due to lack of medical attention for gastrointestinal disturbances often not related to infant formula. These are often considered child neglect problems by personnel at area hospitals, when in reality they are more often due to lack of economic resources, and the adherence to an accepted behavior pattern in times of illness. Use of home remedies especially as related to infant feeding needs to be discussed in counseling mothers, especially those who are from rural areas, or who are older than 35 years of age.[18]

In contrast to Puerto Ricans, Dominicans tend to introduce solid foods somewhat later and to rely less on commercially prepared baby foods. Tirado notes that mothers have commented that commercially prepared foods are of "inferior nutritional quality," and that only mothers who are lazy use them. Tirado's listing of the foods most frequently introduced to infants by Dominican mothers is shown here:

Milk	78%
Orange juice	78
Rice water	73
Tea, herbal, lime, oregano	60
Rice	43
Mashed *viandas*	40
Puréed beans	37
Noodle soup	23
Eggs	20
Meat	17
Cornstarch cereal	17
Oatmeal	17
Coca-Cola	12

Diets in the Sierra Highlands of the Dominican Republic

The information in this section comes from two cross-sectional studies conducted 10 years apart. Mort, in 1990, studied 79 homemakers who were participating in a rural development agroforestry project in the Sierra Highlands of the Dominican Republic,[19] Mort evaluated their food intake by using two independent dietary methods, 24-hour recall and food frequency. She found that women's diets were similar to diets of people in many developing countries, proportionally low in nutrients and high in energy. Staple foods consisted mainly of rice, beans, and starchy vegetables, mostly plantain and yucca. Table 5.3 lists the foods most frequently eaten.

Rice, red beans, sugar, coffee, spices, and condiments were consumed daily by at least 60% of the sample. Mort defined these foods as daily staples that were mainly purchased at *colmados* (small grocery stores). Rice and beans, the most frequently consumed staples, provided energy, protein, and many vitamins and minerals. More than 81% of the women reported eating both of these foods daily.

TABLE 5.3 **Foods Consumed by at Least 60% of the Sample in the Dominican Republic (N = 79[a])**

Frequency	Food Group	Food Item	Percent	N
Every day:	Cereal products	Rice	92.4	73
	Legumes	Red beans	81.0	64
	Fats	Oil	97.5	77
	Sugars and sweets	Sugar	98.7	78
	Miscellaneous	Coffee	69.6	55
	Spices and condiments	Salt	100.0	79
		Spices	98.6	71
		Bouillon cubes	92.4	73
		Onion	97.4	77
		Tomato paste	88.6	70
3–4 times weekly	Fruits	Limes	70.4	50
	Starchy vegetables	Plantain	70.9	56
1–2 times weekly	Fruits	Mango	65.8	52
	Cereal products	Spaghetti	70.9	56
		Bread/cracker	64.6	51
	Meat/poultry/fish	Eggs	59.5	47
	Dairy products	Raw milk	31.6	29
		Powdered milk	39.2	31
	Sugars and Sweets	Chocolate powder	63.3	50
	Starchy vegetables	Yucca	65.8	52
1–3 times monthly	Meat/poultry/fish	Chicken	78.5	62
		Pork	74.7	59
	Starchy vegetables	Pumpkin	60.8	48
		White sweet potato[b]	67.1	53
	Vegetables	Green pepper	73.4	58
	Dairy products	Cheese	63.3	50
	Cereal products	Corn flour	73.4	58

[a]Cases where sample size differs are noted in the N column.

[b]White sweet potato, or *batata*, is a white- or yellow-fleshed vegetable with a slightly sweet chestnutlike flavor. It is high in energy and rich in vitamin A and has some protein and vitamin C and small amounts of some B vitamins.

SOURCE: Margaret M. Mort, Effects of women's characteristics, household characteristics, and food acquisition practices on the dietary practices and nutritional status of rural Dominican women. Master's thesis, Cornell University, Ithaca, NY, January 1990.

Oil, mainly of vegetable origin, was the major fat source in the diet and was used widely to prepare rice, beans, soups, and stewed meats and to fry such foods as plantains, eggs, and meats. The only alternative fat was pig lard, which was used by a few women. Spices and condiments commonly used included salt, bouillon cubes, coriander, *bija* (*annato* seed coloring), pepper, oregano, garlic, cloves, cinnamon, tomato paste, and onions. Salt was used in almost all recipes, and the other spices and condiments were used to prepare such staple foods as beans, soups, stewed meats, and spaghetti.

Raw sugar was the major sweetening agent, and it was used daily by everyone in Mort's study. *Azúcar crema* (raw sugar) has been centrifuged but not refined and so is light brown in color. It retains more vitamins and minerals from the sugarcane than *azúcar refinada* (white sugar).[20]

Mort reported two interesting general findings about the sample studied. One was that most households reported having a *huerta casera* (home garden) and a *conuco* (larger agricultural plot). Because these families were participating in a rural development project, food produced in these gardens made a significant contribution to the overall household food supply. The second was that friends, neighbors, and relatives commonly shared food.

Reciprocal food exchanges were also reported in a national food consumption survey,[21] where the monetary value of foods given and those received by households were virtually equal within every income group. However, the nutritional impact of food gifts was strongest among the poorest households, where food gifts contributed roughly one-fifth of the total calories consumed by the household.

As a comparison with Mort's findings, Table 5.4 shows food data collected in the same region ten years earlier (1980) by Smith et al.[22] Although there have been some slight changes in the diet, the data show that traditional diets have persisted. Table 5.5 shows one of the most significant findings from Mort's data. One single food item, in this case, mango, can make a significant impact on the diet. Mango, a free and abundant fruit in tropical areas, is high in energy from carbohydrates, particularly rich in vitamins C and A, and is also a source of iron and thiamin and riboflavin. This finding highlights the impact of seasonality on food intake.

Weaning Foods in Las Cuevas, Dominican Republic

Bruce and Lieberman surveyed 280 children 6 to 54 months of age in Las Cuevas, a southwestern region of the Dominican Republic.[23] The researchers found that breast feeding is common practice in the Dominican Republic. In this study 60% of the mothers breast-fed their children for 6 to 24 months; the mean age for weaning was 12 months. Twenty-five percent of the babies received cow's milk and 10% received formula; the combination of feeding both was not explored. The average age for introducing solid foods was 6 to 7 months. In some cases children were not introduced to solid foods until they were 12 months old. The most severe cases of malnutrition were found among children who were not given solid foods until 16 to 24 months of age and who had continued breast feeding, often in competition with a younger sibling. The most common weaning foods were modifications of adult foods. Rice, puréed tubers and beans, along with plantains, *guineo*, and coffee, were the most common. Sources of protein such as cow's milk, eggs, stewed meats, and breast milk complemented the infant's diet.

In summary, the results of the Bruce-Lieberman study indicated that preschool children experienced the greatest growth deficits in the second year of life, and that these deficits were caused by chronic under-nutrition rather than by acute food shortages or recent episodes of disease.

TABLE 5.4 Food Reported Consumed During the Previous Day in the Plan Sierra Project, April–May 1980

	Morning			Midday			Evening		
Food	Percent	(N)	Food	Percent	(N)	Food	Percent	(N)
Milk	36.6	(108)	Rice	83.7	(247)	Plantain	43.4	(128)
Bread	33.2	(98)	Kidney beans	72.9	(215)	Eggs	38.6	(114)
Eggs	29.5	(87)	Meat	34.6	(102)	Spaghetti	34.6	(102)
Plantain	28.8	(85)	Spaghetti	27.8	(82)	Yucca	31.9	(94)
Oats	21.3	(63)	Salad[a]	23.0	(68)	Soup[c]	30.5	(90)
Yucca	19.0	(56)	Moro[b]	17.6	(52)	Bread	20.3	(60)
Sweet potato	18.3	(54)	Salted cod	10.5	(31)	Sweet potato	16.9	(50)
Spaghetti	10.5	(31)	Soup[c]	10.2	(30)	Oats	14.2	(42)
Sausage	9.8	(29)	Pigeon peas	9.5	(28)	Milk	14.2	(42)
						Meat	14.2	(42)
						Tubers	12.2	(36)
						Chocolate	10.2	(30)

[a]Usually contains shredded cabbage or lettuce, plus sliced tomatoes.

[b]Rice and bean mixture.

[c]Usually contains plantain, various tubers, or squash, plus small amount of meat or sausage.

SOURCE: M. F. Smith, B. Santos, and M. Fernández, Nutrition and public health in the Dominican Republic. *Archivos de Latinoamericana Nutrición*, 23(4) (December 1982).

TABLE 5.5 Effect of Seasonal Consumption of Mangos on the Nutrient Intake of Dominican Women and Comparisons with the Recommended Dietary Allowance (RDA)

Nutrient	Without Mango (N = 36)			With Mango (N = 43)		
	Mean ± SD	Range	Percent of RDA	Mean ± SD	Range	Percent of RDA
Kilocalories	1644 ± 657	630–3458	76.4	2314 ± 1035[b]	410–5209	103.3
Protein, g	36 ± 16	12–73	84.5	45 ± 19[a]	5–84	99.8
Fat, g	46 ± 28	9–133	—	48 ± 29	3–126	—
Carbohydrate, g	271 ± 103	102–508	—	426 ± 102[c]	87–991	—
Iron, mg	8.5 ± 3.7	3–16.9	77.7	16.2 ± 7.5[c]	5.2–39.3	124.6
Calcium, mg	473 ± 296	91–1220	89.3	622 ± 391	74–1860	102.3
Vitamin A, IU	906 ± 1006	12–4721	12.9	6710 ± 4260[c]	1555–20,154	90.8
Vitamin C, mg	71 ± 55	1–262	233.1	528 ± 330[c]	155–1462	1519.1
Thiamin, mg	0.71 ± 0.44	0.23–2.16	81.8	1.23 ± 0.58[c]	0.34–2.76	135.3
Riboflavin, mg	0.52 ± 0.44	0.08–2.07	44.0	1.03 ± 0.48[c]	0.33–2.42	83.1
Niacin, mg	4.8 ± 3.1	0.7–13	32.7	8.6 ± 4.2[c]	2.4–20.8	56.6

[a]$p < .05$ [b]$p < .001$ [c]$p < .0001$

SOURCE: Margaret M. Mort, Effects of women's characteristics, household characteristics, and food acquisition practices on the dietary practices and nutritional status of rural Dominican women. Master's thesis, Cornell University, Ithaca, NY, January 1990.

CUBAN DIETS AND NUTRIENT INTAKE

During the summer of 1980, thousands of Cuban refugees entered the United States.[24] Though there is a reasonable amount of information about immigrants' acculturation and sociodemographic and economic patterns, there is little information about dietary intake and nutritional status. Research has been done on such specific issues as liver-storage iron in normal populations in Cuba,[25] daily intake of nitrates and nitrites of children in Cuba,[26] and impact of kin, friend, and neighbor networks on infant feeding in Florida.[27] Cross-sectional studies of diets, meal patterns, and changes in nutritional status after migration to the United States are almost nonexistent. The lack of nutrition information about Cuban-Americans could be due to the fact that, as shown in Chapter 1, Cubans have the highest socioeconomic standing among U.S. Hispanics. Consequently, they are not as likely to participate in federally funded nutrition programs, where dietary data are systematically collected.

Our discussion on Cubans' dietary intake briefly touches on two studies that give glimpses of the dietary and nutritional situation of Cubans in Cuba, as well as some of the dietary data collected using a 24-hour recall as part of the Hispanic Health and Nutrition Examination Survey (HHANES). The methodology employed in this large-scale survey of the U.S. Hispanic population is described in Chapter 7. Additional comparative data on Cuban-Americans, Mexican-Americans, and Puerto Ricans are presented in Chapter 8.

Maintaining Cuban Culture and Food Traditions

According to Mohl,[28] the Cubans have maintained their culture in America extremely well, and Roman Catholicism has remained an important part of Cuban-American culture. With several other Catholic immigrant groups, Cubans pray to saints and the Virgin Mary. Afro-Indian religious beliefs grafted onto Catholicism in Cuba persist among Cubans in Miami. A similar pattern can be found in adherence to *santería*, a cult religion of Afro-Cuban origin that is sometimes described as a Cuban form of voodoo. With its elaborate system of ceremony and ritual, and magic and medicine, *santería* has become more popular in recent years, perhaps because it serves as a link to the Cuban past.[29]

Mohl reports that although some Cuban family patterns have changed in America, Cubans have held tenaciously to their traditional food habits. By the 1980s, the Miami area boasted some 700 Cuban groceries, or *bodegas*, and more than 400 Cuban restaurants, an institutional pattern that has helped ensure preservation of traditional Cuban food habits.

Nutritional Status of Cuban Refugees

In 1980, as part of a U.S. Public Health Service survey, Gordon studied the nutritional status of newly arrived Cuban refugees.[30] The survey sample consisted of 138 Cubans who were newly arrived in Florida; data included

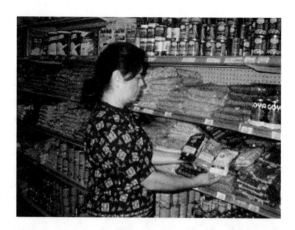

Hispanics are a major consumer group and are heavily targeted by food manufacturers.

medical, socioeconomic, and dietary histories, physical examinations, anthropometric measurements, and biochemical analyses. The results revealed that 25% of the children suffered from malnutrition, mostly of the first degree. Obesity was found in 17% of the women. Fifteen percent of adults and 12% of the children had anemia.

The frequency of food consumption, as reported and discussed by Gordon, is presented in Table 5.6. Milk was consumed daily by 29% of the adult refugees. Most of the milk consumed was condensed; no one reported using dry milk or skim milk. One out of three refugees never consumed milk, and consumption of ice cream and cheese was infrequent.

The products that at least half of the refugees reported eating every day were eggs (89%), bread (89%), rice (71%), *garbanzo* (chick-pea) (68%), sugar (62%), lard and oil (52%), and crackers (51%). Seafood, fruit juices, canned fruit, and corn were the least often eaten; 90% ate these foods rarely or never. Cheese, beef, veal, pork, fresh fruits, squash, green leafy vegetables, and cereals were also rarely consumed; 70 to 89% ate these products less often than once a week. Eggs were the main source of protein in the daily diet (89%), followed by fish (30%).

Intake of any good source of vitamin C was infrequent. According to Gordon, 37% of adults in Cuba took multivitamins. Most of these supplements were provided by relatives living in the United States. In Cuba, vitamin and mineral supplements were widely available only for children younger than 7 years of age and for pregnant women.

Interestingly Gordon notes that the dietary survey suggests that refugees had a low intake of dietary iron. The iron enrichment policies of Cuba are not well documented, and Gordon notes that despite claims by Navarro that parasitism has been eradicated from Cuba,[31] reports in the Cuban medical literature have documented that 60% of the rural population has intestinal parasites.[32] Among parasitic infections *Necator* infestation is most common among adults in Cuba, and this type of parasite is associated with iron deficiency anemia.

TABLE 5.6 **Frequency of Consumption of Selected Foods by Adult Cuban Refugees**

Food	Percentage of Consumption (N = 48)		
	Daily	Occasionally[a]	Never[b]
Milk	29	42	29
Ice cream	6	46	48
Cheese	0	29	71
Egg	89	8	3
Fish	30	37	33
Seafood	0	3	97
Poultry	7	33	60
Beef	1	28	71
Pork	0	11	89
Veal	1	28	71
Garbanzos	68	27	5
Black beans	0	66	34
Lard and oil	52	45	2
Butter and margarine	32	37	31
Fruit juices	0	1	99
Fresh fruits	0	19	81
Canned fruits	0	1	99
Green peas	0	9	91
Corn	0	0	100
Squash	0	15	85
Boniato (sweet potato)	0	27	73
Carrot	0	15	85
Malanga	1	23	76
Potato	15	58	27
Green plantain	1	23	76
Green leafy vegetables	0	21	79
Cereals	9	15	76
Rice	71	27	2
Pasta	42	39	19
Bread	89	9	2
Crackers	51	41	8
Cake	0	33	66
Pizza	15	50	35
Sugar	62	38	0
Coffee	36	56	8
Carbonated beverages	4	39	57

[a]Consumption of food item at least once a week and three times or less a week.
[b]Consumption of food item less than once a week.

SOURCE: A. H. Gordon, Jr., Nutritional status of Cuban refugees: A field study on the health and nutrition of refugees processed at Opa Locka, Florida. *American Journal of Clinical Nutrition*, 35 (March 1982), 582–59.

The Health Status of Cubans in Cuba

Terris provides some interesting biostatistics regarding the health status of Cubans in Cuba and makes some recommendations regarding epidemiological investigations and public health policy.[33] Cuba in 1985 had a population of about 10 million, with approximately three-quarters living in urban areas. The age distribution of Cuba's population differs from the average distribution in Latin America. In Cuba there is a greater proportion of older adults, as shown here:

	United States	Cuba	Latin America
Under 15 years	22.5%	31.3%	39.4%
15–64 years	66.2	61.4	56.4
Over 65 years	11.3	7.3	4.3

According to Terris, diarrheal disease causes an enormous drain on Cuban health services. In 1984, 877,000 cases of acute diarrhea occurred in Cuba (MINSAP, *Balance Anual 1984*, p. 26). According to Francisco Rojas Ochoa, approximately 60,000 people were hospitalized for acute diarrhea in Cuba in 1978.[34] Acute diarrhea results in the unnecessary use of health personnel and facilities and the waste of human and material resources. A major cause of diarrhea is inadequate sanitation: In 1982, only 61.2% of the population had access to potable water and 31.0% had access to sanitary waste disposal.

Based on the data compiled by Terris, there were 2,929 available calories per capita per day in 1983 in Cuba and 77 available grams of protein. Thus, according to information from the Institute of Nutrition in Cuba, "it would be desirable to import sunflower oil, construct adequate refining facilities within the next few years, and provide polyunsaturated oils and margarine at low prices."[35] Additional recommendations on food and nutrition policy were

> Cuba should market low-fat milk at low prices.
>
> Cuba should produce more lean beef and pork.
>
> Cuba should produce more fish and chicken.
>
> Nutrition education programs should focus on decreasing consumption of saturated fat.
>
> The price mechanism should be used to favor the consumption of foods containing little or no saturated fat.
>
> Saturated fats should be replaced in all commercial food processing, cooking, and baking.
>
> Facilities for measuring serum cholesterol levels should be expanded immediately.
>
> Epidemiologic studies should be undertaken to determine the prevalence of high serum cholesterol, hypertension, cigarette smoking, and lack of physical exercise in the population.

Hispanic HANES Dietary Data on Cuban-Americans

The Hispanic Health and Nutrition Examination Survey (HHANES) collected information on 1001 Cuban-Americans, including 297 children aged 1 to 17 years, 444 adult women; and 360 adult men aged 18 to 74 years.[36]

TABLE 5.7   Mean Daily Frequency of Consumption of Food Groups for Cuban-Americans

A. Twenty-four Hour Recall for Children

	Age Group (total N = 297)			
Food Group	1–2 yrs. (N = 39)	3–5 yrs. (N = 40)	6–11 yrs. (N = 101)	12–17 yrs. (N = 117)
Milk	3.91	3.73	3.13	2.25
Meat	2.63	2.43	2.47	2.31
Bread	2.51	2.48	2.38	1.79
Vegetable	0.85	0.64	0.50	0.48
Fruit	1.51	1.41	0.91	0.85
Fat	0.76	1.01	1.21	0.99
Sugar	3.02	2.92	2.63	2.96

B. Twenty-four Hour Recall for Women

	Age Group (total N = 444)			
Food Group	1–2 yrs. (N = 58)	3–5 yrs. (N = 116)	6–11 yrs. (N = 142)	12–17 yrs. (N = 128)
Milk	1.65	1.49	1.67	2.03
Meat	2.50	1.97	1.80	1.47
Bread	1.85	1.76	1.84	1.77
Vegetable	0.64	0.65	0.72	0.62
Fruit	0.78	0.88	1.01	1.05
Fat	1.13	1.28	0.96	0.87
Sugar	2.47	2.34	2.89	2.03

C. Twenty-four Hour Recall for Adult Men

	Age Group (Total N = 360)			
Food Group	1–2 yrs. (N = 50)	3–5 yrs. (N = 86)	6–11 yrs. (N = 126)	12–17 yrs. (N = 98)
Milk	2.04	1.75	1.41	1.76
Meat	2.88	2.25	1.91	1.73
Bread	1.72	1.74	1.69	1.79
Vegetable	0.62	0.68	0.63	0.58
Fruit	0.68	0.87	0.77	0.78
Fat	1.39	1.30	1.14	0.89
Sugar	3.12	2.69	2.68	2.18

SOURCE: U.S. Department of Health and Human Services, Public Health Services, *Hispanic HANES—Dietary practices, food frequency and total nutrient intakes, ages 6 months–74 years*, tape no. 6525, Hyattsville, MD, 1991.

Mean Daily Frequency of Servings of Food Groups   Table 5.7 shows the average daily consumption of servings of foods from various food groups by Cuban-Americans as elicited by 24-hour food recall. (For a comparison of the mean daily consumption of foods in various food groups by Mexican-Americans, Puerto Ricans, and Cubans, based on the USDA Food Pyramid, see Chapter 8.) Children were most likely to consume foods from the milk, sugar,

FIGURE 5.1   Macronutrient distribution as percentage of kilocalories among Cuban children (N = 297)

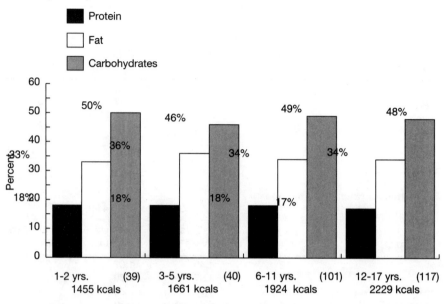

SOURCE: U.S. Department of Health and Human Services, Public Health Service, HHANES, unpublished dietary data, 24-hour recall.

bread, and meat groups. Conversely, children were less likely to consume vegetables and fruits. Meat and sugar were the food groups most frequently consumed by adult women in both the youngest (18–24 years) and oldest (55–74 years) age categories. Across all ages, the vegetable group, followed by the fruit group, showed the lowest daily consumption. For Cuban-American adult men, consumption of foods in the sugar group ranked the highest across all ages, followed by meat in the youngest age group and milk in the oldest age group.

   Macronutrient Contribution as Percentage of Energy   Figures 5.1, 5.2, and 5.3 show the energy consumption and the percentage distribution of the macronutrients derived from energy for the Cuban-American population surveyed by HHANES. Cuban-Americans in these age groups consumed less energy from fat and more from protein and carbohydrate than did the U.S. population as a whole.[37] The children's dietary pattern, apart from revealing the expected trend that as they grow older they eat more (1455 kcal versus 2429 kcal), does not show any major differences in the macronutrient contribution as a percentage of energy consumption. Furthermore, the consistency of the percentage contributions is quite remarkable.

   Among women, the younger age groups consumed substantially more energy from fat than did the older age groups. The proportion of energy from fat for the younger women resembled the proportion for the U.S. population in general. This finding may suggest that younger Cuban women are more

FIGURE 5.2   Macronutrient distribution as percentage of kilocalories among Cuban women (N = 444)

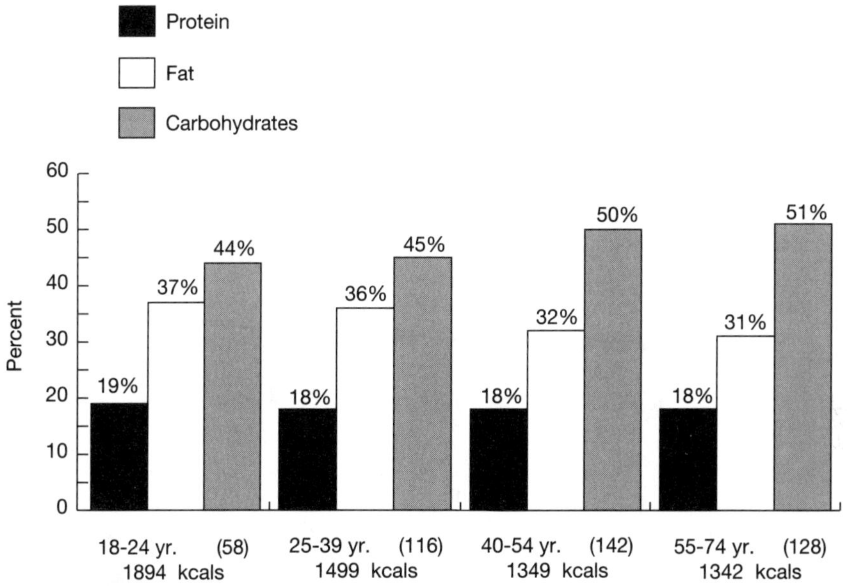

SOURCE: U.S. Department of Health and Human Services, Public Health Service, HANES, unpublished dietary data, 24-hour recall.

likely to follow U.S. dietary patterns than traditional Cuban patterns. Although less well defined among men, a similar trend appeared.

PANAMANIAN DIETS AND NUTRIENT INTAKE

The Isthmus of Panama in Central America has a total land area of about 77,082 square kilometers, with a Pacific coastline extending to 1188 kilometers and a Caribbean coastline of 624 kilometers.[38] Humidity in Panama is high, averaging 80% throughout the country. The rainy season lasts nine months, with January to March being the period of lightest rainfall (the dry season). In 1991, the population of Panama was estimated to be 2.5 million, with 52% urbanized. Interestingly, the province of Darién, which accounts for 33% of the national territory, only had 2% of the population. The age profile shows that 37.5% of the population is under 14 years, 58% between 15 and 64 years, and 4.5% over 65 years.[39]

Panama has a historical dependence on world commerce for prosperity. The construction of the Panama Canal in 1914 brought rapid economic growth to the country. In 1991, according to a recent UNICEF report,[40] the GNP per capita was U.S. $1830. Agricultural products account for 36.7% of exports, with bananas, seafood, sugar, and coffee being exports of the highest value.

FIGURE 5.3   Macronutrient distribution as percentage of kilocalories among Cuban men (N = 360)

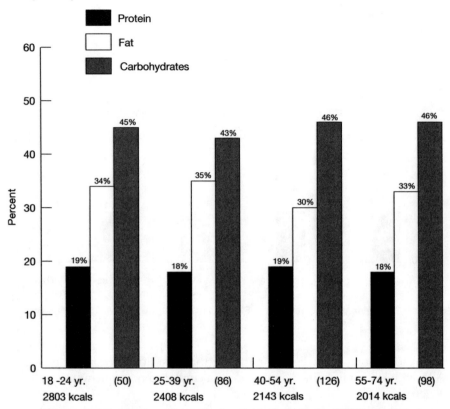

SOURCE: U.S. Department of Health and Human Services, Public Health Service, HANES, unpublished dietary data, 24-hour recall.

Cocoa, beef, fruit, and vegetables are also exported. Industries did not develop because an abundance of goods are imported from North America.

Health and Nutritional Status

Public investment in health in Panama has historically been a high official priority and is one of the highest among developing countries. This expenditure has resulted in substantial improvement in health indicators since 1970. For example, the infant mortality rate dropped from 40.5 per 1000 in 1970 to 21.5 in 1981[41] to 21.0 in 1991.[42] For the country as a whole, health indicators show that in relation to other Latin American countries, quality of life is generally high in Panama. For example, 100% of the urban and 66% of the rural population have access to safe water; 95% of the urban and 64% of the rural population have access to health services; and 82% of 1-year-old children were fully immunized for DPT.[43] Life expectancy is 68 years for men and 73 years for women in Panama.

Although statistics show Panama to be more highly developed with better overall health and nutrition indicators than most other developing countries, malnutrition remains a problem. According to Parillón et al., malnutrition in Panama is linked to low incomes that limit food acquisition.[44] In 1982, a national survey carried out to determine the nutritional status of children attending first grade found that 22% of the children showed severe or chronic growth retardation. The 1993 UNICEF report indicates a much lower figure of only 16%. The same earlier study also found that the nutritional status of children in Panama was associated with the occupation of the head of the household. Almost 70% of the malnourished children lived in households whose head was dependent on the agricultural sector for incomes and employment.

Besides low income, large family size, unemployment, poor sanitation, and lack of potable water, particularly in rural areas, are factors associated with malnutrition in Panama. Data from 1984 indicate that 5.5% of all deaths were caused by infectious diseases and 8.5% by parasitic diseases.[45] Specific nutrient deficiencies were also found in Panama, with inadequate intakes of iron and riboflavin affecting, respectively, 60% and 18% of the population. It was estimated that availability of calcium and vitamin A was limited. However, mean percent adequacy, in relation to recommended levels, was greater than 100% for protein, iron, thiamine, niacin, and vitamin C.[46]

Researchers in three provinces in Panama (Chiriquí, Panamá, and Coclé) have studied the relationships among intestinal parasitic infections, nutritional anthropometry, and dietary intake.[47] In addition, these cross-sectional studies have examined socioeconomic and maternal characteristics that could predict nutritional status and *Ascaris* infection among preschool and school children. In general, the prevalence of *Ascaris lumbricoides* was found to be 27%, *Trichuris trichiura* 34%, and hookworm about 14%. Ascariasis was related to lower socioeconomic status. Children with *Ascaris* infection lived in houses with larger family size, crowded conditions, lower housing index, poor sanitary facilities, inadequate water supply, and inadequate cooking facilities. Dietary data indicated that noninfected children had significantly higher mean intakes of energy and nutrients. Tucker and Sanjur's study also found that maternal employment in Panama had a positive effect on child nutrition.

Food Consumption and Meal Patterns

Using a 24-hour recall method, Tucker analyzed the foods consumed by more than 25% of 207 children and 208 mothers in Chiriquí province (Table 5.8). The most important foods were rice, oil, and sugar, followed by bread, which seemed to be replacing the more traditional tortillas. The major protein sources were evaporated milk, beef, and eggs. With the exception of oranges, fruits and vegetables were notably missing from the list. The importance of soups or broth in the children's diet is worth noting. The mothers generally followed a similar consumption pattern, except that fewer mothers consumed milk, eggs, and oranges and more consumed coffee.[48]

TABLE 5.8   Foods Consumed by More than 25% of Panamanian Mothers and Children.

	Children (N = 209)		Mothers (N = 208)	
Food	No.	%	No.	%
Rice	204	99	202	97
Oil	204	99	206	99
Sugar	192	93	184	89
Bread	129	62	108	52
Evaporated milk	119	58	90	43
Beef	102	49	108	52
Egg	95	46	66	32
Soup/broth	94	45	76	37
Plantain	85	41	96	46
Guiso[a]	72	35	69	33
Powdered milk	71	34	33	16[b]
Kidney beans	70	34	64	31
Whole milk	66	32	61	29
Butter/margarine	65	31	56	27
Chicken	61	30	72	35
Oranges/juice	55	27	43	21[b]
Coffee	(49)	(24)	161	77

[a]*Guiso* is a sauce used on meat and chicken, usually made with tomato sauce, onion, green pepper, celery, and garlic.

[b]Consumed by less than 25% of the sample.

SOURCE: K. L. Tucker, Maternal time use, differentiation, and child nutrition. Ph.D. thesis, Cornell Univeristy, Ithaca, NY, 1986.

Table 5.9 shows meal patterns of a group of 150 Panamanian mothers and children in Coclé province as analyzed by Furumoto. In most cases breakfast for the children consisted of bread with margarine, *crema,* fried eggs, and *chicha de naranja* (fresh orange juice diluted with water and sugar). For midmorning snack, sweet bread, *hojaldra* (fried dough), and cheese puffs were typically eaten during school recess.

At lunch, soup was a basic item. *Sopas* (soups) have a pivotal place in the Panamanian diet, and they consist of meat bones boiled with *verduras* (starchy roots) and vegetables. The most common roots are *yuca, ñame,* and *otoe;* the most common vegetables are squash, potato, and *chayote.* Another typical ingredient in soup is *plátano verde* (green plantain). The spices used most often in soups are garlic, onion, sweet pepper, and *culantro* (fresh coriander). Soups are also prepared with fish, chicken, beans, or with noodles and a boiled egg.

For the evening meal rice was the main dish, eaten with boiled beans or lentils and fried ripe plantain. Fried beef or chicken were animal sources of protein. Evening snacks were often fruit juice or milk with bread.

The diets of the mothers generally followed the same pattern as those of the children. Breakfast was most often bread with margarine and coffee with sugar. Soup was the typical lunch. Rice and beans were the core foods of the dinner meal. Legumes (beans and lentils), an important source of veg-

Table 5.9 Meal Patterns of Panamanian Mothers and Children (N = 150)

Meal	Mothers		Children	
	Basic Items	Variations	Basic Items	Variations from Pattern
Breakfast	Coffee with sugar Bread with margarine	Evaporated milk Cheese Fried egg	Crema[a] Bread with margarine Coffee with evaporated milk	Bread with cheese Milk with sugar Fried frankfurter Chicha de naranja
Morning Snack	Cookie Banana	Chicha de naranja[b]	Sweet bread Orange or banana Hojaldra (fried dough)	Soda Cheese puffs Chicha de naranja Popsicle
Lunch	Soup, with beef bones or fish, yuca, otoe, ñame[c]	Rice Plantain Squash Fried beef or fish Chicha de naranja	Beef or fish soup, with otoe, yuca and ñame	Rice Fried beef or fish Plantain and squash Chicha de naranja
Dinner	Rice Lentils Fried beef Fried ripe plantain	Beans Vegetable salad Fried fish	Rice Lentils Beef Vegetable salad Fried ripe plantain	Fried chicken Beans
Evening snack	Bread Tea with sugar Soda	Cheese Evaporated milk	Milk Sweet bread Orange	Soda Bread with margarine

[a]A gruel made with evaporated milk, sugar, and cereal (usually oatmeal or rice).
[b]A fruit drink made of orange juice, water, and sugar.
[c]Otoe is tannier; yuca is cassava; and ñame is yam.
SOURCE: Adapted from R. M. Furumoto, Ascaris infection and nutritional status of school children from Coclé province, Panama: Master's thesis, Cornell University, Ithaca, NY, 1990.

etable protein in addition to rice, were eaten at dinner with fried beef and *plátano maduro* (fried ripe plantain). The mothers' snacks were mainly fruit or tea with a cookie or bread.[49]

Frequency of Consumption of Vitamin A–Rich Foods

Studies on *Ascaris* infection and vitamin A status have shown a negative association between the two. The Panama studies referred to earlier compared the vitamin A status and consumption of vitamin A–rich foods by *Ascaris*-infected children with the status and consumption by noninfected children. Table 5.10 lists 20 food sources of vitamin A and beta-carotene in the diets of the population under study. Vegetable oil, the most commonly used fat, was reportedly consumed daily by 94% of the children. Vegetable oils were consumed in fried foods such as meats and eggs at breakfast and fried ripe plantain at dinner. Rice was often stir-fried in vegetable oil and then boiled. Coconut oil was used to prepare rice, known as *arroz con coco*. *Chicharrones* (fried pork skins) were also often consumed.

Among the fruits and vegetables, sweet peppers were reportedly consumed on a daily basis, often in soups and sauces, followed by carrots and squash, also boiled in soups. According to Furumoto, few of the children had ever eaten leafy green vegetables such as watercress, spinach, mustard leaves, beet leaves, and cassava leaves. This supports data from previous dietary studies showing that green leafy vegetables were very limited in the diets of Panamanian children.

Among the vitamin A–rich fruits, the most frequently consumed was mango, consumed daily when in season. Papaya, guava, and prunes were the next most frequently consumed, and their daily consumption varied from 36% to 57%. Although these fruits were consumed only when in season, they have different seasons. Therefore a fruit source of vitamin A (and vitamin C) is available throughout the year.

Data on the frequency of consumption of organ meats and eggs are shown in Table 5.10. Beef liver is very popular among Panamanians and is reportedly consumed at least once a week by 24% of the children. Eggs were eaten almost daily and were a basic breakfast food for children.

Nutrient Intake

Barbeau analyzed the energy and nutrient intakes of mothers and children in Chiriquí province using a 24-hour recall method, and her findings are shown in Table 5.11. Mothers had a mean energy intake of 1709 kcal, consisting of 48 g of protein, 63 g of fat, and 238 g of carbohydrates. The mean daily intakes were 8 mg of iron, 60 mg of vitamin C, and 545 RE (Retinol Equivalents) of vitamin A. Children had a mean energy intake of 1580 kcals, consisting of 45 g of protein, 52 g of fat, and 234 g of carbohydrates. Mean daily intakes were 665 mg of calcium, 7 mg of iron, 61 mg of vitamin C, and 523 RE of vitamin A. According to Barbeau, there was a wide range of intakes for all nutrients

Table 5.10   Panamanian Children's Consumption of Vitamin A–Rich Foods (N = 150)

	Daily (%)	Weekly (%)
Fats and Oils		
Vegetable oil	94	5
Coconut oil	7	18
Pork lard	1	3
Chicken fat	1	4
Butter	14	5
Margarine	59	13
Fried pork skin	0	7
Fruits and Vegetables		
Sweet pepper	67	17
Watercress	0	7
Carrot	17	50
Squash	12	36
Prunes	34	10
Guava	36	9
Mamey	6	6
Mango	71	4
Melon	16	16
Papaya	57	16
Coconut	12	11
Organ Meats and Eggs		
Beef liver	0	24
Kidney	0	6
Eggs	44	49

SOURCE: Adapted from R. M. Furumoto, *Ascaris* infection and nutritional status of school children from Coclé province, Panama. Master's thesis, Cornell University, Ithaca, NY, 1990.

analyzed. For vitamin A especially, the standard deviation was greater than the mean values for the children's intake.

The adequacy of the dietary intakes of both mothers and children was compared with the Food and Agricultural Organization's nutritional requirement[50] and the U.S. recommended dietary allowances (RDAs).[51] The percentages of mothers meeting three levels of dietary adequacy are shown in Table 5.12. About 3% and 2% of the mothers had energy intakes below one-third of that recommended by the FAO and the U.S. RDA, respectively. More than 88% (FAO) and 71% (RDA) had protein intakes greater than two-thirds of the respective recommended levels. Inadequate intake was more common for micronutrients than for macronutrients. For example, nearly 50% and 35% of the mothers had intakes below one-third of the NAS and RDA recommendations for calcium, respectively. In the case of iron, 46% (RDA) and 67% (FAO) of the mothers had intakes less than one-third of the recommendations. Mothers were most deficient in vitamin A; 64% (RDA) and 59.6% (FAO) had intakes under one-third of the recommendations.

TABLE 5.11   Mean Nutrient Intake of Panamanian Mothers and Children

	Mean	SD
Mothers		
Kilocalories	1709	661
Protein, g	47	24
Fat, g	63	33
Carbohydrates, g	238	283
Calcium, mg	372	283
Iron, mg	8	4
Vitamin C, mg	60	70
Vitamin A, RE	545	207
Children		
Kilocalories	1508	588
Protein, g	45	21
Fat, g	52	25
Carbohydrates, g	234	96
Calcium, mg	665	546
Iron, mg	7	5
Vitamin C, mg	61	72
Vitamin A, RE	523	1011

SOURCE: Adapted from I. S. Barbeau, Child nutrition in Panama: An investigation of sex bias and maternal allocation of food and other resources. Ph.D. thesis, Cornell University, Ithaca, NY, 1987.

TABLE 5.12   Dietary Adequacy of Panamanian Mothers Compared to Levels Recommended by the Food and Agriculture Organization (FAO) and National Academy of Sciences (U.S. RDAs)

	FAO Recommendation			RDA Recommendation		
	0–33%	34–65%	66%	0–33%	34–65%	66%
Kilocalories	2.9	45.7	51.4	1.9	35.6	62.5
Protein	1.4	10.1	88.5	6.3	22.5	71.2
Calcium						
Minimum	25.0	29.3	45.7			
				49.6	30.7	20.7
Maximum	34.6	28.4	37.0			
Iron						
Minimum	21.6	46.2	32.2			
				45.7	42.3	12.0
Maximum	67.8	29.8	2.4			
Vitamin C	21.2	11.5	67.3	35.1	21.2	43.7
Vitamin A	59.6	24.5	15.9	63.9	22.2	13.9

NOTE: Minimum value applies when more than 5% of calories in the diet came from animal fats and maximum value applies when animal foods represent less than 10% of calories.

SOURCE: Adapted from I. S. Barbeau, Child nutrition in Panama: An investigation of sex bias and maternal allocation of food and other resources. Ph.D. thesis, Cornell University, Ithaca, NY, 1987.

SALVADORAN DIETS AND NUTRIENT INTAKE

El Salvador is one of the smallest and most densely populated countries in Central America. It comprises approximately 21,041 square kilometers, and the population was about 5 million people according to the 1988 census. The country is divided into 14 *departamentos* (provinces) and 263 municipalities, with 57% of the population living in rural areas. El Salvador has a tropical climate, with a rainy season from May to October and a dry season from November to April. As a result of political conflicts since 1980, as well as an earthquake in 1986, there has been a great displacement of the population within the country (from rural to urban areas, in particular to the capital, San Salvador) and emigration to other countries. This has caused profound economic and social changes in urban areas.[52]

Agriculture is the most important sector of the economy, bringing in about 70% of the foreign currency and accounting for 50% of the internal consumption. Exports of coffee, sugar, and cotton, as well as cereals and beans, have decreased since 1960. The internal deficits in food production have been alleviated in great part by food donations.

In the last decade El Salvador experienced the worst economic, political, and social crises in its history. The deteriorating health and nutritional situation has had the greatest impact among poor families, a segment that in 1985 made up approximately 66% of the total population. The nutritional situation continues to be a serious problem, as reflected in an infant mortality rate of 55 per 1000 births in 1985. A high prevalence of infectious diseases is also a serious health issue. Malnutrition due to lack of protein, calories, iron, and vitamin A is a major problem for Salvadorans today, particularly for children under age 5.

Food Consumption: Rural/Urban Differences

Dietary information about the nutrient intake of Salvadoran children and families is quite limited. A 1990 assessment by ESANES-88[53] notes that the basic diet of the Salvadoran people is composed mainly of corn (tortillas) and beans as staple foods (Table 5.13). However, there are significant regional differences in food consumption. The basic diet varies according to socioeconomic status and geographic location. The rural diet is quite monotonous, with corn, beans, and sugar being the main items; less often consumed are rice, eggs, bread, and sometimes small quantities of meat (pork, beef, or chicken). Milk and dairy products are often unaffordable.

The urban diet includes a slightly greater variety of foods. Beans, eggs, coffee, and sugar are eaten at breakfast; rice, tortillas, and beans at lunch; and beans, tortillas, eggs, coffee, and cheese at dinner. Residents in the capital city have the most varied diet because more foods are available, and they can afford a variety of dairy products. Also, urban and other metropolitan residents have more access to meat (pork, beef, or chicken) and *pupusas* (Salvadoran

TABLE 5.13 Distribution of Families in El Salvador According to Their Levels of Consumption of Foods of Animal Origin and of Basic Grains and Derivatives.

Foods	Sector					
	Metropolitan		Urban		Rural	
	Percent	(N)	Percent	(N)	Percent	(N)
Fresh milk	32.9	(47)	36.0	(85)	42.9	(181)
Powdered milk[a]	60.8	(87)	44.1	(104)	33.9	(143)
Cheese[a]	87.4	(125)	84.3	(199)	74.9	(316)
Beef[a]	61.5	(88)	47.9	(113)	30.8	(130)
Pork	23.8	(34)	26.3	(62)	23.7	(100)
Chicken[a]	73.4	(105)	51.3	(121)	53.1	(224)
Fish	49.0	(70)	39.0	(92)	38.2	(161)
Eggs[a]	96.5	(138)	94.1	(222)	88.6	(374)
Beans[a]	88.8	(127)	95.8	(226)	91.2	(385)
Rice[a]	96.5	(138)	90.7	(214)	85.3	(360)
Maiz[a]	100	(143)	100	(236)	99.8	(421)
French bread[a]	93.7	(134)	90.3	(213)	76.8	(324)
Pastries	90.2	(129)	88.1	(208)	83.7	(353)
Pasta[a]	64.3	(92)	50.0	(118)	43.1	(182)

[a]Significant differences found among sectors.

SOURCE: ESANES-88, Asociación Demográfica Salvadoreña, Ministerio de Salud Pública y Asistencia Social, Instituto de Nutrición de Centroamérica y Panamá, El Salvador, 1990.

tortillas filled with meat, cheese, or beans and sold in the *pupuserías,* popular restaurants in urban and metropolitan areas).

Other differences between rural and urban/metropolitan diets are the consumption of corn tortillas and the sources of food. Rural women make corn tortillas for family consumption and to sell in the urban/metropolitan areas. Consequently, rural people eat fresh corn tortillas at all three meals, whereas urban/metropolitan people eat fresh tortillas at breakfast and left-over tortillas or bread at lunch and dinner. Similarly, some rural residents produce at least part of their milk, eggs, poultry, fish, corn, beans, and coffee, whereas urban/metropolitan residents buy all of their foods. In addition, foodstands with a North American influence are beginning to appear in metropolitan areas, thus initiating Salvadorans into "fast-food culture."

Food Preparation Methods

Cooking conditions vary tremendously between rural and urban/metropolitan areas. In rural areas water is less accessible, and there is little or no electricity. Therefore electrical stoves are not used in rural sectors. Wood fires with *comales,* large round flat pans, are used instead of ovens. The cooking areas are often unsanitary because they are on a dirt floor or out in the open, exposed to flies and other contamination. In the urban/metropolitan areas, people have more access to electricity and potable indoor water systems. Therefore most people have an electric or gas stove. Generally, cooking areas are situated on brick floors and sheltered by walls, minimizing the number of flies and other contamination.

Nutritional Status of Preschool Children in La Paz

Wolfe and Trowbridge conducted a dietary survey among 194 children, 1 to 4 years old, as part of an assessment of the nutritional status of preschool children in El Salvador.[54] Intake of calories, protein, and retinol equivalents were estimated using a 24-hour recall technique. The average daily energy intake of 866 calories was only 60% of the level recommended in 1973 by the Institute of Nutrition of Central America and Panama (INCAP) for this age group, and 76% of the recommended level based on body weight. The average daily protein intake of 31.3 grams was 110% of the recommended level for the age group and 136% of the recommended level based on body weight. The estimated daily intake of retinol equivalent was 36% of the recommended allowance.

In their study, Wolfe and Trowbridge took special care to ensure the quality of the dietary data by conducting the dietary interviews in the children's homes and by employing a nutritionist who was fluent in Spanish. A child's mother or the person responsible for food preparation was asked to recall the types and amounts of food eaten by the child in the previous 24 hours. Food models, various sized cups, and spoons of known volume served as visual aids to improve quantitative estimates. In the case of tortillas, where large weight variations were observed among households, researchers weighed sample tortillas on portable scales. At the close of an interview the investigator cross-checked the dietary information by reviewing the child's share of the food prepared for the entire family during the 24-hour period. Last, all field methods were pretested with a comparable population outside the study area.

Table 5.14 shows the percent contribution of food groups to intake by age of the children. Cereal products were the major source of calories for all ages, as well as the major protein source for children age 1 to 4. Milk products contributed substantially to the calorie and protein intakes of 1 year olds but made lesser contributions in the older age groups. Sugar contributed most significantly to the calorie intake of the 1 year olds. Beans were an important source of both calories and protein, mainly for older children. Milk products and eggs were the main sources of retinol for all age groups. The intake of retinol was 36% of the recommended level, showing that vitamin A was the most limiting nutrient.

Both Wolfe and Trowbridge and ESANES-88 agree that past malnutrition is most prevalent in Salvadoran preschool children, although general and acute malnutrition are also significant health issues.

Vitamin A Deficiency among Salvadoran Children

A significant nutritional concern in El Salvador is vitamin A deficiency. Estimates of low retinol intake corresponded with low serum vitamin levels

TABLE 5.14 Percent Contribution of Food Groups to Intake by Age, La Paz, El Salvador

Food Group	Calories (age in years)				Protein (age in years)				Retinol (age in years)			
	1	2	3	4	1	2	3	4	1	2	3	4
Milk products	23	11	8	9	39	18	15	18	61	55	53	54
Eggs	4	4	4	4	8	9	7	7	15	30	29	24
Meat, poultry, fish	2	3	3	5	5	8	7	10	—	—	—	—
Beans	4	12	4	12	9	21	24	20	—	—	—	—
Fruits and vegetables	1	1	1	1	1	1	—	1	3	6	6	6
Cereals	40	50	53	54	30	34	37	36	—	—	—	—
Fats and oils	1	1	1	1	—	—	—	—	—	—	—	—
Sugar	16	9	8	6	—	—	—	—	—	—	—	—
Miscellaneous	9	9	8	9	8	9	10	8	21	8	12	14

SOURCE: P. Wolfe and F. L. Trowbridge, Dietary intakes of preschool children in La Paz, El Salvador, Central America. *Archivos Latinoamericanos de Nutrición, 30* (1980), 53–97.

as measured by an INCAP survey conducted in 1965.[55] More than 40% of El Salvadoran children 0 to 4 years of age had serum levels of vitamin A below 20 μg/100 ml—the highest deficiency level found in Central America. Although field studies have failed to document widespread clinically apparent vitamin A eye disease,[56] ample evidence indicates general low intakes and possible subclinical deficiencies. As such, vitamin A deficiency is a continuing concern in El Salvador.

Breast-feeding Practices

The results of a study that investigated breast feeding of children younger than 24 months of age showed that 43% of the children were breast-fed for six months or less and 30% for less than one year.[57] Children who were breast-fed usually also received other foods and water.

In El Salvador, even in rural areas, infants as young as 1 month of age are given water and cow's milk. Weaning practices start, on the average, at about 3 months, with cereals and *guineo* (banana) as the first foods. Vegetables, including potatoes, and eggs are given at 4 months. By the age of 6 months, Salvadoran children are eating most adult foods, including meat, tortilla, beans, rice, and banana. Extended breast feeding is more common in rural than in urban/metropolitan areas.

Salvadorans in the United States

Due to civil conflicts in El Salvador, many people, especially those from rural areas, emigrated from El Salvador to other countries. A great number moved to the United States as political refugees or illegal aliens. In the United States there are approximately 1 million Salvadorans, mainly in Los Angeles, Washington, D.C., Houston, and San Francisco. A study sponsored by the University of Central America found that three-quarters of the Salvadorans arrived in the United States after the civil conflict of 1979.[58] However, almost half immigrated after 1982 and thus cannot qualify for amnesty.

For Salvadorans living in the United States, the different customs and lifestyles have affected their food habits and food consumption patterns. A food-frequency questionnaire attempting to assess changes in meal patterns and dietary practices of newly arrived Salvadorans was administered in the summer of 1992 by Tagle and Marchante in New York City.[59] They conducted 30 home interviews among a random sample of people of various ages, and their findings are shown in Table 5.15. Their data show that tortillas and beans continued to be the core diet of Salvadorans in their new environment, followed by soup, coffee, eggs, and cheese. Traditional foods such as *chayote*, plantains, *pasteles, empanadas,* and *atol* also showed up in the diet, albeit less frequently. Items such as green salads and fresh fruits were also reported as consumed, perhaps indicating a newly acquired American influence in their dietary patterns.

TABLE 5.15   Foods Commonly Consumed by Salvadorans in New York City (N = 30)

Morning Food	Percent	Noon Food	Percent
Beans	73	Tortilla	73
Coffee	60	Rice	63
Eggs	50	Fruit drink	43
Bread	43	Beans	37
Tortilla	35	Chicken	30
Hard cheese	30	Soup[a]	27
Milk	27	Green salad	20
Pastries	23	Meat (pork, beef)	17
Plantain	10	chayote[b]	
Heavy cream	10	Fresh fruit	4

Snacks (midafternoon food)	Percent	Evening Food	Percent
Pastries	43	Beans	66
Fruit	33	Tortilla	50
Candy	19	Eggs	40
Coffee	19	Coffee	40
Fruit drinks	14	Cheese	30
Soda	14	Plantain	23
Bread	10	Rice	13
Pasteles[c]	5	Fruit drink	10
Green salad	5	Soda	10
Flan (custard)	5	Bread	7
Atol[d]	5	Milk	6
Empanadas	5	Heavy cream	6
Bread with rice/beans	5	Soup	6
Enchilada	5	Casamiento[e]	4

NOTE: Immigrant fear of deportation, lack of eligibility to participate in federally funded nutrition programs, and researchers difficulty in gaining access to the Salvadoran population settled in urban areas are some of the major barriers to studying dietary patterns among this group. Given the small sample size, the data in the table represent only a small sample of a particular group of Salvadorans residing in New York City and do not necessarily represent the dietary intake of all Salvadoran immigrants to the United States.

[a]Soup includes a variety of meat/chicken, and vegetables.

[b]*Chayote* is usually consumed stuffed with cheese.

[c]Beef patties mixed with tomatoes, potatoes, onions, and spices.

[d]*Atol* is a thick hot drink made from fresh immature corn dough.

[e]*Casamiento* is a mixture of refried rice and beans.

SOURCE: A. Tagle and I. E. Marchante, A review of the nutritional status of El Salvador and Nicaragua. Unpublished research monograph, Cornell University, Ithaca, NY, Summer 1992.

Tagle and Marchante concluded that food habits and diets of Salvadoran families were affected in varying degrees by immigration to the United States. Some Salvadorans stated that their meal patterns had become more like those in North America, mainly due to job pressures and fast-paced lifestyles. Others stated that they no longer ate a large lunch as they were accustomed to in El Salvador; dinner had now become their main meal. In addition, the types of foods that they cooked were determined by the availability and cost of traditional foods in the area.

SUMMARY

This chapter has attempted to provide nutritionists and health practitioners with information about the culture and eating habits of four Hispanic groups from the Caribbean and Central America. More knowledge about their ways of eating may lead to better and more relevant nutrition counseling.

The diets of Dominicans in New York City and in two areas of the Dominican Republic were examined, mainly to illustrate changing patterns and continuity. This was followed by a brief discussion of Cuban diets, with examples taken from a study of Cuban refugees in Florida, food policy issues in Cuba, and recent dietary data from Hispanic HANES. Panama and El Salvador were used to illustrate Central American countries with two distinctly different dietary patterns, Panama representing a "rice-eating culture" and El Salvador a "maize-eating culture."

GLOSSARY OF DOMINICAN FOODS AND MIXED DISHES*

adobo	dry mixture of salt, garlic, oregano, black pepper, and monosodium glutamate
arepas de yuca/catibia	mixture of grated cassava, eggs, butter or margarine, milk, and a touch of anisette; shaped like a small tortilla and deep-fried
asopao	soup made with dried beef or sausages and chicken, with condiments and rice; or a soupy rice with chicken
azúcar crema	raw sugar, light brown in color
batata	sweet potato
batidas	milk shakes made of tropical fruits with sugar
berenjena	eggplant
bija/achiote	coloring from *annato* seeds extracted with hot oil
carnes guisadas	stewed meats (goat, pig, chicken) briefly sautéed, and then cooked in a tomato sauce with added condiments and *sofrito*
casabe	dessert made of *yuca amarga* (bitter cassava), grated and dried to form a flat dried bread
cerdo	pork
chicharrones	small pieces of chicken, cut and marinated, then breaded in flour and deep-fried
galletas de soda	soda crackers
habichuelas con dulce	dessert made with beans, raisins, cinnamon, coconut milk, cloves, sweet potatoes, and sugar
leche condensada	condensed milk
limón agrio	lime

*Sandra Santos helped in the development of this glossary.

locrío	popular mixed dish prepared like *moros y cristianos*, made of meat instead of beans
maltas	carbonated beverage made from barley, malt, and sugar; often drunk with sweetened condensed milk
mangú	green plantain purée, with some oil and salt added
morir soñando	drink made with milk, orange juice, sugar, and ice (other fruit juices, such as grapefruit or lime, could also be used); common snack in the afternoon or evening
moros y cristianos	boiled dish of rice and beans, with oil, onions, pepper, garlic, tomato sauce, and vinegar
pica pica	sardines
plátano verde	green plantain
recao	fresh mixture of parsley, green pepper, rosemary, coriander, and other herbs used to flavor beans and meats
sofrito	principal mixed condiment used to flavor stewed beans; main ingredients include oil, diced tomatoes, garlic, and *recao*
salcocho or sancocho	soup made with dried beef or sausage and chicken (preferably old hens), condiments and various starchy *víveres*
tayota	chayote (white pear-shaped vegetable)
tostones	deep-fried plantains
víveres	starchy vegetables, also known as *viandas* in Puerto Rico
yuca	one of, if not the, favorite and most versatile starchy vegetables in the Dominican Republic

GLOSSARY OF CUBAN FOODS AND MIXED DISHES*

ajiaco	thick soup made with various vegetables and meats
aporreado de tasajo	jerked beef meats with starchy vegetable
arroz con almejas	rice with clams
arroz con calamares	rice with squid
arroz con leche	rice pudding
arroz con pollo	rice with chicken
bistec de puerco	thin pork loin steak, fried
boliche	beef (round eye) filled with ham and carrots
boniato frito	fried sweet potato
calamares en su tinta	squid in their ink
caldo de pescado	fish broth
camarones enchilados	shrimp creole
cangrejitos de jamón	ham pastries

*Dr. Lisa Peréz helped in the development of this glossary.

carne "ripiada"	shredded beef with potatoes and tomato sauce
casabe	flat dried bread made of cassava
cocido español	spanish stew
congrí	rice with black or kidney beans
"cubano"	Cuban sandwich made of ham, roast pork, and cheese
escabeche	pickled king fish
escudella catalana	Catalan stew
flan de leche	cream caramel
frijoles negros	stewed black beans
frijoles negros refritos	black bean hash
fufú de plátano	mashed green plantains with garlic and pork cracklings
jalea de guayaba con queso	thick guava jelly with white cheese
judías con puerco	pigs' trotters with chick-peas
lengua guisada	stewed tongue
mantecadas	cupcakes
mariquitas	green plantain chips
merenguito	meringue
mojo agrio	dressing for vegetables made of garlic, lime, salt, and olive oil
moros y cristianos	rice with black beans
muñeta	stewed chick-peas
pan con timba	bread with thick guava jelly
pastica	cheese paste
picadillo	beef hash
plátanos en tentación	whole ripe plantain with syrup
plátanos maduros fritos	fried ripe plantain
rabo alcaparrado	oxtails with capers
revoltillo	scrambled eggs
ropa vieja	stringed beef
sesos	brains
sopa de plátano	plantain soup
tortilla de huevo	omelette
yuca con mojo	boiled cassava in garlic dressing

GLOSSARY OF PANAMANIAN FOODS AND MIXED DISHES

alfajores	corn dough fritters with white cheese
agualpán o fruta pan	bread fruit
arroz con coco	rice with pigeon peas and coconut milk
arroz con pollo	chicken with rice

bienmesabe	dessert made with evaporated milk, cornstarch, and coconut milk
bollo de maíz nuevo	immature grated corn rolled into a corn husk and then boiled
caimito	star apple
caña de azúcar	sugarcane
carimañolas	cassava fritters with ground meat filling
carne de iguana	*iguana* meat
ceviche	raw fish marinated in lime juice and hot pepper
chicha	beverage made with various fresh fruits, sweetened with sugar or molasses
chicha fuerte de maíz	alcoholic beverage made from fermented corn
chicharrones	fried pork skin, eaten at breakfast
chicheme	sweetened beverage made of mature corn
cocada	popular dessert, consisting of grated coconut meat and molasses ("panela")
crema de cebada	sweetened barley, plantain, or corn
crema de plátano o crema de maíz	meal gruel consumed at breakfast
duros	popsicles made of fruit drinks
empanada	corn dough with ground meat filling
gallo pinto	soupy rice with beans and various kinds of meats and starchy roots
gelatina	gelatin dessert, often given to children
guacho	soupy rice often made with beans
guanábana	soursop
guandú	pigeon peas
hojaldra	fried flat bread made from wheat flour
huevito faldiquero	milk candy
malteada	sweetened malt beverage
mamón	genip
marañón	cashew fruit
merengue	baked egg whites with sugar
mollejitas cocidas	stewed gizzards
mondongo	stewed tripe
morcilla	blood sausage
ñame	yam
nance	yellow rounded fruit, somewhat acidic in taste, well-liked by Panamanians; when in season, it is often used to make *chichas* or *pesada de nance* (custard); high in ascorbic acid
otoe	starchy root
pan de huevo	wheat flour bread to which eggs have been added; *Rosca de pan de huevo* is very popular at Christmas or Mother's Day

patacones	fried green plantains
patitas de puerco	stewed pig's feet
pescado seco/ahumado	dry or smoked fish
pifá	peach palm fruit
pipa	fresh coconut
plátanos en tentación	ripe plantains cooked in syrup
queso blanco	white cheese
rapadura	molasses
ropa vieja	shredded meat prepared with spices and hard boiled eggs
sancocho de gallina	soup made with an old hen and white yam
sopa de pescado	fish soup with starchy roots added
tajadas de plátano maduro	fried ripe plantains
tajadas de plátano verde	fried green plantains
tamales	corn dough with chicken meat and spices
tasajo	beef jerky
torrejitas de maíz nuevo	fresh corn fritters
tortilla asada de maíz	tortilla baked over open fire
tortilla frita de maíz	fried tortilla
ubre de vaca	cow's udder
yuca frita	fried cassava

GLOSSARY OF SALVADORAN FOODS AND MIXED DISHES

arroz con ostiones y verduras	fried rice with oysters and vegetables, such as potatoes, carrots, *chayote,* and onions
arroz en leche	rice pudding
arroz frito	fried white rice with condiments such as green peppers, tomato, onions, and salt, a favorite preparation for rice
atol de elote	gruel of immature fresh corn with added milk and cinnamon
carne adobada	seasoned meat (pork), often marinated the night before in mustard and mayonnaise, garlic, vinegar, tomatoes, and red pepper
carne asada	barbecued meat, usually marinated or seasoned overnight with garlic, mustard, pepper, and tomatoes; usually accompanied by *chirmol* (a sauce of fresh, diced tomatoes, onion, and seasonings)
carne o pollo guisado	stewed meat or stewed chicken
cebada	sweet drink made of imitation barley flavoring and cinnamon, bread crumbs, water, sugar, and pink artificial coloring
chilate	a thick sour drink made of toasted corn, water, cinnamon, pepper, and *ananias* (anise); often accompanied by *torrejas* or very ripe plantains in honey

conserva de coco	fresh coconut preserve
dulce de ayote	sweet pumpkin made with brown raw sugar
empanadas	small oval patties, made of sweet ripe plantains, filled with milk custard
fresco de ensalada	drink made from various fresh fruits like cashew, pears, and apples
fresco de tamarindo	drink made of tamarind pulp, with sugar and water
horchata	drink made from ground pumpkin seeds, rice, cinnamon, nuts, and sugar
iguana en alguashte	iguana meat roasted with *alguashte* (sauce made of ground pumpkin seed, onion, garlic, bread, flour, paprika, tomato, and salt)
pasteles de masa	maize dough, stuffed with beef or pork or only vegetbles
pescado forrado	fried salted fish, made especially during Holy Week (Good Friday); fish is usually left in water overnight to remove salt, then prepared with spices, eggs, potatoes, and chick-peas
pupusas	round tortillas stuffed with either hard cheese (*pupusas de queso*) or beans (*pupusas de frijol*) or fried pork skin (*pupusas de chicharrón*); very popular foods, eaten mainly at night at foodstands called *pupuserías.*
quesadilla de queso	sweet bread made of rice flour, cheese, sugar, heavy cream, and lard or margarine
riguas	fresh young corn dough, cooked in banana leaves, and served with cottage cheese and heavy cream
shuco	a thick drink made of toasted corn and black beans, water, salt, and *alguashte* (pumpkin seed powder)
sopa de cabeza de pescado	fish-head soup prepared with tomatoes, onion, pepper, and garlic
sopa de frijoles negros o rojos	black/red bean soup prepared with *chayote* and often meat and corn dough patties; a major source of iron
sopa de gallina india	chicken soup, prepared with potatoes, carrots, tomatoes red pepper, mint, and coriander
sopa de patas	cows-hoof soup mixed with intestines and various vegetables, including green plantain, tomato, corn, and cassava
tamales de carne o pollo	fresh maize dough, shaped into rectangles, wrapped in banana leaves; filled with beef or chicken, potatoes, tomatoes, and spices
tamales dulces	fresh maize dough made with sugar, lard, cinnamon sticks, prunes, and raisins; no meat is added
tamales de elote	fresh maize dough sweetened with sugar, cooked in corn husks, usually accompanied by heavy cream
torrejas	sweet bread made with eggs, melted sugar, cinnamon sticks, and lard or oil, typically consumed at Lent

| tortillas | yellow corn ground to dough, the main form of maize consumption, they accompany most meals consumed by Salvadoran people |
| tortitas de carne de res | fried ground meat patties, mixed with vegetables, cumin, and eggs |

NOTES

1. Nilda Tirado, Dietary and food selection patterns of Dominican women living in the upper Manhattan area. Paper presented at the Conference on Hispanic Health Care Approaches in New York: A Focus on Dominicans, Columbia Presbyterian Medical Center, New York City, October 15, 1987.

2. Nilda Tirado, Puerto Rican and Dominican ethnic food habits. Paper presented at the Food and Nutrition Council Symposium, Teachers College, Columbia University, New York City, May 10, 1983.

3. Nilda Tirado, Multicultural perspectives on infant feeding—The Dominican and Puerto Rican experience. Paper presented at New York University Medical Center, New York City, October 29, 1982; C. A. Barbano, V. Acosta, H. D. Reyes, and N. Tirado, Culturally appropriate nutrition education information for Dominicans. Paper presented at the Conference on Hispanic Health Care Approaches in New York: A Focus on Dominicans. Columbia University, New York City, October 15–16, 1987.

4. Tirado, Dietary and food selection patterns.

5. Jean M. Tiffany, Dietary patterns and nutritional status of immigrant women from the Dominican Republic living in New York City. Master's thesis, Cornell University, Ithaca, NY, May 1984.

6. Margaret M. Mort, Effects of women's characteristics, household characteristics, and food acquisition practices on the dietary practices and nutritional status of rural Dominican women. Master's thesis, Cornell University, Ithaca, NY, January 1990.

7. M. F. Smith, B. Santos, and M. Fernández, Nutrition and public health in the Dominican Republic. *Archivos Latinoamericanos de Nutrición, 23*(4) (December 1982).

8. Tirado, Dietary and food selection patterns.

9. Tirado, Puerto Rican and Dominican ethnic food habits.

10. Tiffany, Dietary patterns.

11. W. H. Sebrell, Nutritional status of middle and low income groups in the Dominican Republic. *Archivos Latinoamericanos de Nutrición, 23*, número especial (July 1972).

12. P. Musgrove, Household food consumption in the Dominican Republic: Effects of income, price and family size. *Economic Development and Cultural Change, 34*(1) (1985), 833.

13. Tirado, Multicultural perspectives.

14. Haydee Rondón de Nova, J. M. Vázquez, and V. Suero, *Situación actual de la lactancia meaterna en Santo Domingo de la República Dominicana*, Secretaría de Salud Pública, Division de Nutrición, Santo Domingo, 1980.

15. B. Myers, Breast or bottle—An analysis of the choices made by Dominican women in New York City. Thesis, Institute of Human Nutrition, Columbia University, New York, 1981.

16. Tirado, Multicultural perspectives; Myers, Breast or bottle.

17. Tirado, Multicultural perspectives.

18. Tirado, Multicultural perspectives.

19. Mort, Effects of women's characteristics.

20. Musgrove, Household food consumption.

21. Ibid.

22. Smith et al., Nutrition and public health.

23. L. Bruce and L. S. Lieberman, Nutritional anthropometry and dietary intake of children from the Las Cuevas region of the Dominican Republic. *Archivos Latinoamericanos de Nutrición, 26*(2) (June 1987), 250.

24. Center for Disease Control, Health status of Cuban refugees. *Morbidity and Mortality Weekly Report, 29* (1980), 217.

25. H. Gautier, R. Puente, B. Vidal, E. Pérez, and H. Vidal, Liver storage iron in normal population of Cuba. *American Journal of*

Clinical Nutrition, 88 (January 1980), 133–136.

26. M. O. García Roché, A. Bécquer, and N. Moraleza, Estimation of the daily intake of nitrates and nitrites which children six to eleven years old, who attend primary schools in the city of Havana, may consume. Cuban National Hygiene Institute, *Die Nahrung, 29*(2) (1985), 191–195.

27. Carol A. Bryant, The impact of kin, friend, and neighbor networks on infant feeding practices: Cuban, Puerto Rican and anglo families in Florida. *Social Science and Medicine, 16* (1988), 193–195.

28. R. A. Mohl, An ethnic boiling pot: Cubans and Haitians in Miami. *Journal of Ethnic Studies, 13*(2) (1985).

29. Juan J. Sosa, La santería: A way of looking at reality. Master's thesis, Florida Atlantic University, 1981.

30. A. M. Gordon, Jr., Nutritional status of Cuban refugees: A field study on the health and nutrition of refugees processed at Opa Locka, Florida. *American Journal of Clinical Nutrition, 35* (March 1982), 582–590.

31. V. Navarro, Health, health services, and health planning in Cuba. *International Journal of Health Services, 2* (1972), 397–432.

32. R. Rodríguez, Parasitismo en el área rural de Bernardo. *Revista Cubana de Medicina,* (1967), 497–498.

33. M. Terris, The health status of Cuba: Recommendations for epidemiologic investigation and public health policy. *Journal of Public Health Policy, 10*(1) (1989), 78–87. This article drew heavily on data published by the Pan American Health Organization: *Annual Report of the Director, 1984,* and *Health Conditions in the Americas, 1981–1984*. Two other sources are quoted: Ministry of Public Health (MINSAP), *Balance Annual 1984,* and L. A. Bernal and J. L. Figueroa, *La lucha por la salud en Cuba* (Mexico City: Siglo XXI, 1985).

34. Francisco Rojas Ochoa, in Bernal and Figueroa, *La Lucha,* pp. 301–303.

35. Terris, Health status of Cuba.

36. U.S. Department of Health and Human Services, Public Health Service, Hispanic HANES—Dietary practices, food frequency and total nutrient intakes, ages 6 months–74 years, tape no. 6525, Hyattsville, MD, 1991. The contribution of Dr. Rey Martorell and Dr. Laura Kahn in sharing their HHANES unpublished 24-hour recall dietary data is hereby acknowledged.

37. National Research Council, *Diet and health: Implications for reducing chronic disease risk* (Washington, DC: National Academy Press, 1989).

38. Dirección de Estadística y Censo, *Panamá en cifras: Años 1981–1985,* Panama, 1986.

39. R. M. Furumoto, *Ascaris* infection and nutritional status of school children from Coclé Province, Panamá. Master's thesis, Cornell University, Ithaca, NY, 1990.

40. UNICEF, *The state of the world's children, 1993* (Oxford: Oxford University Press, 1993).

41. V. Valverde, H. Delgado, A. Noguera, and R. Flores, Malnutrition in tropical America. *Current Topics in Nutrition and Diseases, 10* (1983), 3–15.

42. UNICEF.

43. Furumoto, *Ascaris* infection.

44. C. Parillón, V. Valverde, and H. L. Delgado, Political and administrative distribution of nutritional status in Panama according to the height census of first grade school children. *Ecology of Food and Nutrition, 19* (1987), 333–343.

45. D. J. Bogue, *Population and socioeconomic development in Central America and selected countries of Latin America and the Caribbean* (Chicago: Social Development Center, 1985).

46. V. Valverde, H. L. Delgado, and A. Noguera, Nutrition in Central America and Panama: Comparative data and interpretations. *Food and Nutrition Bulletin, 9*(3) (1987), 3–14.

47. E. Carrera, M. C. Nesheim, and D. W. T. Crompton, Lactose maldigestion in *Ascaris*-infected preschool children. *American Journal of Clinical Nutrition, 39* (1984), 255–264. I. S. Barbeau, *Child nutrition in Panama: An investigation of sex bias and maternal allocation of food and other resources.* Ph.D. thesis, Cornell University, Ithaca, NY, 1987; C. V. Holland, D. L. Taren, D. W. Crompton, M. C. Nesheim, D. Sanjur, I. Barbeau, K. Tucker, J. Tiffany, and G. Rivera, Intestinal helminthiases in relation to the socioeconomic environment of Panamanian children. *Social Science and Medicine* 26 (1988), 209–213; K. Tucker and D. Sanjur, Maternal employment and child nutrition in Panama. *Social Science and Medicine 26* (1988), 605–612: D. L. Taren, Effects of *Ascaris lumbricoides* on the nutritional status of

children in Panama. Ph.D. thesis, Cornell University, Ithaca, NY, 1986; K. L. Tucker, Maternal time use, differentiation, and child nutrition. Ph.D. thesis, Cornell University, Ithaca, NY, 1986; A. C. García, Socioeconomic and maternal determinants of nutritional status and ascaris infection among school children in Coclé, Republic of Panama. Ph.D. thesis, Cornell University, Ithaca, NY, 1989.

48. Tucker, Maternal time use.

49. Furonoto, *Ascaris* infection.

50. R. Passmore, *Handbook on nutritional requirements.* Food and Agricultural Organization FAO Nutritional Studies no. 28, Rome, 1974.

51. Food and Nutrition Board, National Academy of Sciences, National Research Council, *Recommended dietary allowances,* rev., Washington, DC, 1980.

52. A. Tagle and I. E. Marchante, A review of the nutritional status of El Salvador and Nicaragua. Unpublished research monograph, Cornell University, Ithaca, NY, Summer 1992.

53. ESANES-88, *Evaluación de la situación alimentaria nutricional en El Salvador.* Aso-

ciación Demográfica Salvadoreña, Ministerio de Salud Pública y Asistencia Social, Instituto de Nutrición de Centroamérica y Panamá. El Salvador, 1990.

54. Wolfe, P. and F. L. Trowbridge, Dietary intakes of preschool children in La Paz, El Salvador, Central America. *Archivos Latinoamericanos de Nutrición, 30* (1980), 53–97.

55. *Nutritional Evaluation of the Population of Central America and Panama. Regional Summary.* Institute of Nutrition of Central America and Panama (INCAP) and Nutrition Program, Center for Disease Control, USHEW, Washington, DC, 1972.

56. A. Sommer, A preliminary report of vitamin A prophylaxis assessment program in El Salvador. In *Vitamin A deficiency and blindness prevention* (New York: American Foundation for Overseas Blind, 1974).

57. ESANES-88.

58. T. Barry, *El Salvador: A country guide* (Albuquerque, NM: Interhemispheric Resource Center, 1991).

59. Tagle and Marchante, A review of nutritional status.

6

Diet-Related Diseases
and Other Health Issues

Health Care Utilization
Poverty Levels and Medicaid Coverage

Life Expectancy and Causes of Mortality
Excess Deaths among Hispanic Groups
Deaths Due to Heart Disease and Stroke
Deaths Due to Cancer
Deaths Due to Diabetes

Cancer Incidence

Cardiovascular Disease
Tobacco Use
Impact of Acculturation and Assimilation
Effects of Obesity

Noninsulin-Dependent Diabetes Mellitus
Effects of Body Fat Distribution
Association with Amerindian Ancestry
Severity of NIDDM among Mexican-Americans

Gallbladder Disease

Dental Disease

Overview

Dr. Cutberto Garza, Cornell University, is guest author of this chapter.

Indices of the general health status of Hispanic-Americans are mixed and difficult to interpret for four principal reasons: (1) the Hispanic population is highly heterogeneous; (2) immigration patterns make it a particularly dynamic subset of the general population; (3) survey designs used to obtain data often are not sufficiently rigorous to ensure external validity; and (4) the classification of Hispanics and Hispanic subgroups is inconsistent or is inconsistently applied. Nonetheless, in 1980, 87% of Hispanic-Americans self-assessed their health as good or excellent compared with 87% of non-Hispanic whites and 82% of African-Americans. The incidence (per 100 persons per year) of acute medical conditions for the same general period was higher only for Puerto Ricans (321.8) compared with non-Hispanic whites (224.6). Comparable rates for Mexican-Americans, Cuban-Americans, and other Hispanics were 188.9, 172.5, and 223.3, respectively. The percentages of Hispanic-Americans, however, whose daily activities were limited by chronic health conditions during the same period were generally higher than those of non-Hispanic whites (10.3%), 15.5% of Puerto Ricans, 11.4% of Mexican-Americans, 10.9% of Cuban-Americans and 10.0% of other Hispanics.[1]

A report on health variables among Hispanics and non-Hispanic children with chronic health conditions (where 80% of Hispanics identified themselves as Puerto Ricans) living in a city in the Northeast concluded that despite sociodemographic disparities among groups, traditional measures of morbidity were similar among Hispanics and non-Hispanics.[2] Qualitatively, similar conclusions were reached in a study of indigent adolescents participating in the San Diego Job Corps in California—that is, no differences in the incidence of chronic illness were noted among indigent Mexican-Americans, whites, and black adolescents.[3] In sharp contrast, in an "exploratory" survey conducted in Wisconsin, the incidence of chronic disease conditions was reported to be several times greater in children of migrant farm workers, of whom more than 90% were Hispanic.[4]

HEALTH CARE UTILIZATION

Two issues continue to dominate Latino criticism of health care delivery systems in the United States: Latino families' lack of access to medical services and health promotion efforts and the ineffectiveness of monocultural/English models used by health care professionals.

Health insurance coverage, which in turn influences health care utilization, is a major health concern among Hispanics (see Table 6.1). A paper by Trevino and Ray reports findings relative to this topic.[5] Data on 13,000 Mexican-Americans, Puerto Ricans, and Cuban-Americans between 6 months and 74 years of age obtained between 1982 and 1984 in the Hispanic Health and Nutrition Examination Survey (HHANES) and data from the 1989 Current Population Survey (CPS) conducted by the Bureau of Census were studied. To date, HHANES is the most culturally and linguistically sensitive large-

TABLE 6.1   Major Health Concerns of Latino Communities

Children and Adolescents

1. Malnutrition, inadequate protein consumption and vitamin deficiencies
2. Upper respiratory diseases
3. Lead poisoning
4. Child abuse
5. Household accidents
6. Substance abuse
7. High rates of teenage pregnancy
8. Parasitic infection among children

Service Delivery Responses

1. Negative reactions and blaming of parental values and health care efforts
2. Ignorance and biases about ethnic diets
3. Lack of dental, visual and hearing screening, diagnosis and treatment
4. Inaccurate psychological testing and diagnosis of mental retardation or learning disabilities
5. Culturally inappropriate educational programs and materials in schools and health promotion efforts
6. Lack of counseling and inappropriate educational and vocational tracking in schools

Adults

1. Nutritional inadequancies due to low income and lack of information
2. Cardiovascular disease and hypertension
3. Diabetes
4. Lack of obstetrical/gynecological care
5. Contraception needs: education, choices, and assurances of voluntary consent
6. High stress
7. Spouse and family abuse
8. Substance abuse
9. Workplace hazards
10. Death and injuries due to social violence
11. Need for preventive health education, detection of cancers, consequences of chemical substance use during pregnancy, family communications skills
12. Pesticide exposure (migrants)
13. Liver disease
14. HIV infection

Service Delivery Responses

1. Failure to acknowledge socioeconomic causes of prevalent Latino health condition—attribution of cultural explanations
2. Culturally inappropriate health prevention and treatment interventions
3. Inaccurate psychological assessment and treatment of mental illness
4. Failure to accept professional responsibility to address environmental and public health issues affecting Latinos
5. Biases about dietary evaluation

SOURCES: Planned Parenthood Federation of America, *Latino families in the United States: A resource book for family life education* (New York 1983), and U.S. Department of Health and Human Services, Public Health Service, *Healthy people 2000,* Publication no. 01-50213 (Washington, DC, 1991).

scale survey conducted of the U.S. Hispanic population, with a net coverage of about 80%. Persons were interviewed in the language of their choice. Interestingly, 62% of Mexican-Americans chose to be interviewed in English, compared with 45% of the Puerto Ricans and 19% of the Cuban-Americans. However, because the sampling frame was regional rather than national, and because HHANES did not sample non-Hispanics, cross-ethnic comparisons cannot be made. HHANES is also becoming outdated since it was conducted over ten years ago. The 1989 CPS, on the other hand, was a national survey that sampled white and black non-Hispanics as well as Hispanics, thus allowing for comparisons between these groups. However, CPS did not use a Spanish-language questionnaire and used bilingual interviewers to a very limited degree, and had other characteristics that may limit the validity and reliability of findings for Hispanics. CPS contained 13,996 observations on Hispanics of all ages, including 8157 Mexican-Americans, 1760 Puerto Ricans, 890 Cubans, and 3189 other Hispanics.

More than a third of the Mexican-American population, one-fifth of the Puerto Rican population, and one-fourth of the Cuban-American population were uninsured for medical expenditures, compared with one-fifth of the black non-Hispanic and one-tenth of the white non-Hispanic populations. Furthermore, compared with Hispanics with private health insurance, uninsured Hispanics were less likely to have a regular source of health care, to have visited a physician in the past year, to have had a routine physical examination, and to rate their health status as excellent or very good.[6]

One very interesting point made by the investigators is that Hispanic groups, when studied by national origin, differed with respect to their use of medical services. Mexican-Americans had the lowest overall utilization of physician services (3.7) and Cuban-Americans had the highest (6.2) during the course of one year. Mexican-Americans were found to have the least health insurance coverage, to be the least likely to have regular health care, and to be the least satisfied with the care they received. These variations in health care utilization, Trevino and Ray note, may be due in part to differences in health insurance coverage among these groups. Of special concern are children of migrant farm workers. Less than 50% of migrant children under the age of 16 receive recommended preventive medical care.[7]

Higher rates of noncoverage of health insurance among Hispanics were found in the 1982–84 HHANES compared with the 1989 CPS. Trevino and Ray attributed the observed differences to a better understanding of the questions rather than to true changes over time, because Hispanics were interviewed in the language of their choice in HHANES. Regardless, it would appear that the Hispanic population studied was at significant risk for catastrophic out-of-pocket expenditures for medical care and for failing to receive medical care when needed.

Poverty Levels and Medicaid Coverage

Among the uninsured, Trevino and Ray found that 53% of Mexican-Americans, 60% of Cuban-Americans, and 46% of Puerto Ricans were employed; however, 53% of Mexican-Americans, 40% of Cuban-Americans, and 47% of Puerto Ricans were living at the poverty level. Thus these investigators suggest that among employed Hispanics, the low rates of insurance coverage may have been the result of their low income levels and employment by firms that do not provide health insurance benefits.

A final important point made by Trevino and Ray was that Medicaid does not appear to provide proportionately comparable coverage to all Hispanic groups. For example, Puerto Ricans are five and a half times more likely to receive Medicaid coverage than Mexican- or Cuban-Americans. The researchers offered two possible explanations for this. First, because there are proportionately twice as many female-headed households among Puerto Ricans as among the other two groups, Puerto Ricans may be more likely to qualify for Medicaid coverage under Aid to Families with Dependent Children. Second, Puerto Ricans are more likely to reside in states that provide greater optional coverage under Medicaid (e.g., New York); Mexican- and Cuban-Americans are more likely to reside in states with more restrictive Medicaid programs (e.g., Texas and Florida).

LIFE EXPECTANCY AND CAUSES OF MORTALITY

Life expectancy at birth for Hispanics in the American Southwest appears to be very close to that for non-Hispanic whites (68.7 years for men; 76.0 for women). In California, life expectancy in 1969 to 1971 of Hispanic-American men and women was 68.3 and 75.2 years, respectively. Mexican-born and Cuban-born males less than 45 years of age, however, had a higher risk of death from any cause, 1.4 and 1.2, respectively, compared with non-Hispanic white men. Homicide, however, accounted for much of the increased risk.[8] The 1985 report of the Task Force on Black and Minority Health identified cancer, cardiovascular disease (CVD), chemical dependency (measured by deaths due to cirrhosis, most often caused by alcoholism), diabetes, homicide and accidents, and infant deaths as responsible for more than 80 percent of the age-adjusted excess mortality observed among minority groups in the United States.[9] Excess mortality was defined as the difference between the number of deaths that occurred among minority groups and the number expected from age- and gender-specific death rates of the non-Hispanic white population. Although it is obvious that dietary excesses, deficiencies, and imbalances do not fully explain the excess mortality experienced by minority groups in the United States, the association of dietary risk factors with certain cancers, CVD, complications due to alcoholism, diabetes, and neonatal and infant deaths suggests that diet plays a significant role.[10]

Key demographic variables (economic status, age distribution, educational attainment), environmental factors (urban and rural environmental hazards), occupational exposures (hazards related to white- and blue-collar jobs), and sociocultural mechanisms for coping with stress (personality traits, activity patterns, use of preventive, diagnostic, and therapeutic health services) also are expected to modulate diet and non-diet-related causes of morbidity and mortality. Unfortunately, excess mortality due to specific causes (cancer, cardiovascular disease) cannot always be estimated for Hispanic-Americans, and seldom are estimates available for more than two or three Hispanic-American subgroups. Few states include a Hispanic identifier on death certificates, and when identifiers are available, criteria for their application are neither uniform nor applied consistently. Furthermore, the categorization is often not sufficiently precise to identify Hispanic subgroups.[11]

Similar concerns apply to estimates of dietary factors related to ethnicity and associated with increased risk of chronic diseases and of morbidity related to diet. These shortcomings should be recognized in the material reviewed in this chapter. Although recent surveys that have targeted Hispanic groups or oversampled Hispanic groups are expected to improve the data base significantly, summaries of much of those data are not available.

Excess Deaths among Hispanic Groups

Excess deaths were estimated for three Hispanic populations by the 1985 Task Force on Black and Minority Health: those with Spanish surnames in Texas for the period between 1970 and 1980 and Cuban-born and Mexican-born populations living in the United States between 1979 and 1981.[12] For the Hispanic subgroups, the magnitude of excess deaths was smaller than expected from data available for another major minority group, African-Americans. Deaths between 1970 and 1980 for the Texas population with Spanish surnames exceeded the expected number by only 14%. For Cuban-born and Mexican-born individuals dying between 1979 and 1981, the number of deaths exceeded the expected levels by only 2.2% and 7.2%, respectively. In 1980 age-adjusted death rates among African-American males and females were 50% greater than among white males and females. Changing demographic characteristics of Texas populations during the index periods and the problems described in the preceding section preclude any inferences regarding possible trends.

Table 6.2 summarizes data for the period between 1979 and 1981. Homicides accounted for all of the excess deaths among Cuban-born males, and unintentional injury accounted for all of the excess deaths among females. Cirrhosis, unintentional injuries, and homicide accounted for all of the excess deaths among Mexican-born males, and diabetes and homicide accounted for excess deaths among the females. Excess alcohol consumption probably contributed significantly to deaths due to cirrhosis and possible unintentional injuries.

TABLE 6.2 Hispanics (Foreign-Born) Average Annual Number of Deaths by Disease Category, United States, 1979–1981.

	CVD[a]	Cancer	Cirrhosis	Infant Mortality	Diabetes	Unintentional Injuries	Homicide	Other	Sub-Total[c]	Total Deaths
Mexican-born Hispanics, age 0–64										
Males Observed	585	334	136	3	32	1322	848	554	(3814)	3814
Expected[b]	947	622	106	39	34	769	147	727	(3391)	3391
Excess	−362	−288	30	−36	−2	553	701	−173	(423)	1284
Percentage of total Excess[d]	0	0	2	0	0	43	55	0		100
Females Observed	292	367	39	2	40	184	53	309	(1286)	1286
Expected[b]	331	512	45	28	28	186	33	357	(1520)	1520
Excess	−39	−145	−6	−26	12	−2	20	−48	(−234)	32
Percentage of total Excess[d]	0	0	0	0	38	0	63	0		100
Cuban-born Hispanics, age 0–64										
Males Observed	351	243	32	0	12	143	179	204	(1164)	1164
Expected[b]	540	337	53	1	17	172	31	268	(1419)	1419
Excess	−189	−94	−21	−1	−5	−29	148	−64	(−255)	148
Percentage of total Excess[d]	0	0	0	0	0	0	100	0		100
Females Observed	114	215	14	0	9	39	25	102	(518)	518
Expected[b]	208	307	26	1	16	56	9	158	(781)	781
Excess	−94	−92	−12	−1	−7	−17	16	−56	(−263)	16
Percentage of total Excess[d]	0	0	0	0	0	0	100	0		100

[a]Cardiovascular disease (CVD) combines heart disease and stroke.
[b]The expected number is calculated from the rate observed in the white population.
[c]Sub-total is the sum of negative and positive excess deaths. Total deaths sums positive excess deaths only.
[d]Percentages based on total deaths.

Source: Duke University analysis commissioned by the Task Force on Black and Minority Health, 1984–1985.

Data that describe the age of onset of alcohol use among Hispanic youth and the pattern of use among Hispanics of specific ages and subgroups are poor.[13] The percentage of Hispanic-American males (24%) who report heavy drinking was higher than that of non-Hispanic whites (21%), but Hispanic-American women were more likely to report abstaining from alcohol (33% versus 18%) and less likely to report heavy drinking (3% versus 4%) than were non-Hispanic white women.[14]

The lower than expected number of deaths due to heart disease and stroke (listed as CVD in Table 6.2) and cancer and the lower than expected rates of infant mortality among Mexican-Americans compensate for the extraordinarily high rates of death due to homicide among Mexican- and Cuban-Americans (almost 600% of the expected rate for men) and unintentional injury among Mexican-American men (approximately 175% of the expected number).

Except for Puerto Ricans, Hispanic-Americans and non-Hispanic whites have similar proportions of low-birth-weight (LBW) infants. Overall, the low-birth-weight rate among Hispanics was 7.1% and 7.0% among non-Hispanic whites; the rate among Mexican-Americans was 5.7%. For women born in Mexico, the rate was 5.0% in 1987; for those born in the United States, 6.7%. For Cuban-Americans the rate was 5.9% and Puerto Ricans, 9.3%.[15] In all groups, LBW rates were higher for mothers with limited educational attainment. These data were derived from the 1987 National Vital Statistics System and the Hispanic Health and Nutrition Examination Survey (1982–84). Figure 6.1 summarizes the rates of LBW among various minority groups and non-Hispanic whites according to trimester of prenatal care. Table 6.3 summarizes childbirth patterns of Hispanic-American and non-Hispanic white women who gave birth in 1982.

Despite the relatively favorable distribution of birth weights among Mexican-Americans, neonatal mortality rates are high in some studies.[16] For Cuban-Americans, mortality rates are consistent with their favorable birth-weight profiles and rates of prematurity. Mortality rates of Puerto Rican infants reflect unfavorable birth-weight profiles and rates of prematurity among that subgroup. Among Hispanic teenage groups, the rate of prematurity among Puerto Ricans in the mainland was 14.6%, among Mexican-Americans, 13.5%, and among Cuban-Americans, 12.6%. These rates are higher than observed among non-Hispanic whites, 11.4%.

While the heterogeneity of Hispanic-Americans is nowhere more overt than in fertility statistics, it is important to note that fertility rates of young Hispanic-American girls and women between the ages of 13 and 19 is much higher (4.41%) than among their non-Hispanic white counterparts (1.68%).[17] As for smoking, only 10% of Mexican-American women smoke during pregnancy; approximately 25% of non-Hispanic white women smoke at that time.[18]

The risk factors associated with poor perinatal outcomes suggest that the high percentage of LBW infants among Puerto Ricans is due to socioeco-

Figure 6.1   Percentage of LBW (<2500 g) infants born to Hispanics according to trimester of prenatal care, 1987

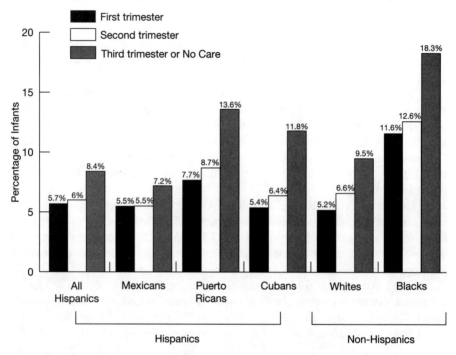

SOURCE: F.S. Mendoza et al., Selected measures of health status for Mexican-American, mainland Puerto Rican, and Cuban-American Children. *JAMA, 265* (1991), 227–232.

nomic factors. In contrast, the low rates among women of Mexican descent suggest that successful coping mechanisms can be implemented to overcome some of the risk associated with poor socioeconomic status.

The Task Force on Black and Minority Health identified the following risk factors:

Low income and inadequate insurance coverage

Preexisting disease conditions

Poor nutrition

Inadequate housing and crowded living conditions

Limited maternal education

Stressful work environments

Disrupted families and lack of social supports

Problems of transportation and child care that impede use of services associated with improved health outcomes

Table 6.3   Childbearing Patterns of Hispanic and Non-Hispanic White Women, 1982.

Age of Mother	Hispanic[a]	Non-Hispanic Whites
Under 15	1,288	4,153
15–19	60,369	357,948
20–24	115,275	958,509
25–29	90,393	961,053
30–34	47,999	503,847
35–39	18,056	136,664
40–44	3,809	19,027
45–49	201	853
Percent of births to mothers under age 20		
	18.3	12.3
Percent of births to mothers over age 35		
	6.5	5.3
Marital status: out-of-wedlock births		
Number	86,488	355,180
Percent	25.6	12.1
Parity		
Percent first births	37.8	43.3
Percent high parity (4+)	16.4	8.6

[a]Refers to births to residents of 23 states reporting Hispanic origins of the mother on birth certificates. These states accounted for an estimated 95% of all births of Hispanic origin in the United States in 1982.
SOURCE: National Center for Health Statistics. Adapted from Table 15, M.M. Heckler, *Report of the Secretary's Task Force on Black & Minority Health*, Washington, DC: U.S. Department of Health and Human Services, August 1985), p. 176.

In contrast to the low infant mortality noted for most Mexican-American children, results of a retrospective survey suggest that childhood mortality among migrant farm workers is 1.6 times higher than among the general population of children.[19]

Infant Mortality and Low Birth Weight   Infant mortality rates are a composite of *neonatal mortality* (deaths that occur within the first 28 days of postnatal life) and *postneonatal mortality* (deaths that occur between 28 days of postnatal life and the first year of age). Low birth weight is defined as 2500 g. Infants with low birth weight may be born prematurely and be of an appropriate birth weight for age (AGA) or may be small for gestational age (SGA).

Deaths Due to Heart Disease and Stroke

The reported number of deaths due to heart disease and stroke were 55% to 65% of expected levels for Cuban-born men and women and Mexican-born men, respectively. Reported deaths for Mexican-born women, however, were relatively higher, 88% of the expected number. The difference between Mexican-born men and women may be explained partially by the greater relative increase in risk to fatal ischemic heart disease imposed by diabetes in women than in men (see the section on non-insulin-dependent diabetes). The relative risks of ischemic heart disease in diabetics versus nondiabetics were 1.8 and 3.3 in a predominantly white affluent population of men and women, respectively, after adjusting for age, systolic blood pressure, cholesterol, body mass index, and cigarette smoking.[20] A similar difference may exist among diabetic men and women of Mexican descent. Importantly, however, this does not mean that diabetic women are at greater risk of fatal ischemic heart disease than are diabetic men, but rather, the difference in risk between nondiabetics of both genders is larger than that between diabetic men and women.

Although mortality statistics for CVD may look encouraging, data for Mexican-Americans in Texas suggest that the trend in cardiovascular mortality between 1970 and 1980 was not as favorable for Mexican-American men as for non-Hispanic white counterparts. Rosenthal et al. reported declines of 27% among non-Hispanic white men in mortality from acute myocardial infarction during that period, but only about half that relative decline, 14%, among Mexican-American men.[21] Mortality from all ischemic heart disease fell 21% in non-Hispanic white men and only 13% in Mexican-American men. Conversely, Hispanic women experienced greater declines in mortality due to myocardial infarction and all ischemic heart disease than did non-Hispanic white women.

Deaths Due to Cancer

The pattern of deaths due to cancer differed from that seen for heart disease and stroke. The reported number of deaths were 70% to 72% of expected levels for Cuban-born men and women and Mexican-born women. Reported deaths for Mexican-born men, however, were low, 54% of the expected number. Unfortunately, comparable data for native-born Hispanic-Americans are not available for reasons already cited.

Deaths Due to Diabetes

The pattern of deaths due to diabetes is also different. Mexican-born men and Cuban-born men and women have lower than expected deaths due to diabetes. The range is from 56% (for Cuban-born females) of the level observed in non-Hispanic white women to 94% (Mexican-born males) of the level observed in non-Hispanic white women and men. Deaths due to diabetes among Mexican-born women, however, are 143% of the expected number.

In addition to the already mentioned factors that complicate the interpretation of data, migration patterns must also be considered. The number of reported deaths may be falsely low if a significant number of Mexican-Americans return "home" to die. Gender differences among Mexican-born men and women in the relative risk of death due to heart disease and stroke may be due to a greater likelihood of early diagnosis among men than women. An earlier diagnosis would provide additional time for men to return "home." Alternatively, women may be less likely to return "home" with the onset of a life-threatening illness, risk factors associated with life-threatening chronic disease may be lower among a significant proportion of Hispanic Americans, or risks to specific diseases may be ameliorated by unidentified genetic and/or behavioral factors.

Migration patterns, however, are unlikely to explain the mortality patterns of Cuban-Americans, for Cubans are unlikely to return "home" upon the onset of a life-threatening illness. Gender differences of deaths due to diabetes among the Mexican-born also are not as easily explained by migration patterns, unless, as considered earlier, men are likelier to return "home" than are women. Alternatively, interactions between the environment and gender-specific genotypes may account for these disparities. A specific example cited earlier is the increased risk in diabetic women for fatal coronary heart disease. Each of these explanations is highly speculative and impossible to evaluate without better morbidity and population tracking data.

CANCER INCIDENCE

Age-adjusted cancer incidence is lower for Hispanic-Americans than it is for non-Hispanic whites (see Table 6.4). This estimate, however, may not be very reliable because at the time when the report of the Task Force on Black and Minority Health was issued, only approximately 12% of Hispanic-Americans were covered by the Surveillance, Epidemiology, and End Results (SEER) Program of the National Cancer Institute, a national cancer monitoring program. The incidence of cancer among Hispanic-Americans, however, is not lower

Table 6.4   Cancer Incidence Rates: Average Annual Age-adjusted (1970 U.S. Standard) Cancer Incidence Rates by Primary Site and Racial/Ethnic Group

Selected Primary Site	Hispanics	Non-Hispanic Whites	Percent Expected
All sites	246.2	335.0	69
Esophagus	1.6	3.0	53
Stomach	–	–	–
Colorectal	25.2	49.6	51
Colon	15.8	34.6	46
Rectum	9.4	15.0	63
Pancreas	10.8	8.9	121
Larynx	2.6	4.6	56
Lung			
Male	34.3	81.0	42
Female	13.0	28.2	46
Breast	54.1	85.6	63
Cervix	17.7	8.8	201
Prostate gland	76.5	75.1	102
Multiple myeloma	2.5	3.4	74

SOURCE: Adapted from Table 12, in M. M. Heckler, *Report of the Secretary's Task Force on Black and Minority Health* (Washington, DC: U.S. Department of Health and Human Services, August 1985), p. 91.

for all sites. The incidence of cancer (rates per 100,000 population) of the stomach (15.7 versus 8.0), prostate (76.5 versus 75.1), pancreas (10.8 versus 8.9), and cervix uteri (17.7 versus 8.8) is higher among Hispanic-Americans than among non-Hispanic whites. Cancer of the stomach is of particular concern because the rate is nearly twice that of non-Hispanic whites. Of those sites, cancer of the stomach has been related most often to a number of dietary factors, for example, the use of smoked and spicy foods. Generally five-year cancer survival rates are similar for Hispanics (47%) and non-Hispanic whites (50%).[22]

The reasons for the lower general cancer incidence among Hispanic-Americans and those for the site-specific differences between Hispanic-American and non-Hispanic whites have not been identified. The major risk factors for cancer are "unspecified" genetic predispositions and a number of behavioral, sociocultural, and environmental factors. Doll and Peto estimated that tobacco use, the combined use of tobacco and alcohol, diet, and occupational factors accounted for 72% of the mortality due to cancer and 69% of the incidence of cancer.[23]

Low socioeconomic status has been associated with an increased risk for cancer of the lung, breast, and cervix. Yet the incidence of breast cancer among Hispanic women is 63% of that reported for non-Hispanic whites. The incidence rate of breast cancer among Hispanic women (7.9) less than 40 years of age is approximately 90% of that found in non-Hispanic whites (8.2) but only 61% of that found in women over 40 years (134.9 versus 221.1).

When one considers the poor socioeconomic status of most Hispanic-Americans, the low incidence of breast cancer is especially noteworthy. The high fat content of many traditional Hispanic diets is also is not consistent with the lower reported incidence. Furthermore, Hispanics lag behind the general population in their awareness of major risk factors for cancer, they generally are unable to identify more than three warning signs of cancer, and are less aware of tests that detect cancer.[24]

Colon cancer also has been related to diet. The age-adjusted incidence rate of colon cancer among Hispanics (15.8) is 45% of the incidence rate reported for non-Hispanic whites (34.6%). The reasons for this difference are not known, nor is it clear that acculturation contributes to the risks for this disease.

CARDIOVASCULAR DISEASE

The rate of CVD among Hispanics appears to be lower than that among non-Hispanic whites. The incidence of CVD, however, is not well quantitated. Although risk factors (hypertension, elevated blood cholesterol, cigarette smoking, diabetes, and obesity) have been studied in non-Hispanic whites, the identification of risk factors among Hispanic-Americans and Hispanic subgroups has received much less attention. The low socioeconomic characteristics, the rural-to-urban migration, and the relatively higher prevalence of obesity, hypertension, and noninsulin-dependent diabetes among most Hispanic-Americans suggest that rates of CVD should be higher than are reported for the group.

Blood lipid profiles do not explain the apparent low levels of CVD relative to those reported for non-Hispanic whites. Fasting levels of cholesterol, triglycerides, high density lipoprotein (HDL) cholesterol and its subfractions (HDL$_2$ and HDL$_3$), α- and β-lipoprotein cholesterol, low density lipoprotein (LDL) cholesterol, and apolipoproteins A-I, A-II, B, C-II, C-III, and E were measured in Mexican-Americans living in Texas.[25] The lipoprotein distribution was similar to that of the general population except for higher triglycerides and lower HDL cholesterol among females. Where comparative data were available, apolipoprotein levels were similar or lower in the Mexican-American group that was studied. The high triglyceride and low HDL levels are not surprising given the high prevalence of obesity among Mexican-Americans. The lipoprotein profile of Mexican-Americans is similar to that observed in the Pima Indians, in whom unexpectedly low levels of cardiovascular disease are also reported despite high frequencies of diabetes and obesity.

Tobacco Use

The use of tobacco may help explain these findings. Although rates of smoking are higher among Hispanic-Americans than among non-Hispanic whites, the rate of heavy smokers appears lower among Hispanics.[26] Additional factors that complicate the assessment of tobacco use and CVD among Hispanics is the age distribution of the Hispanic population in the United States. Age-specific smoking habits among Hispanic subgroups are not well described.

Impact of Acculturation and Assimilation

Studies have been undertaken among Mexican-Americans to assess acculturation and assimilation into the American mainstream and socioeconomic status (SES) with preventive knowledge and behaviors related to CVD. These studies have found that measures of assimilation and SES are associated independently with knowledge and behaviors related to disease prevention. Measures of assimilation were associated more strongly with both preventive knowledge and behaviors. Regardless of the level of assimilation or SES, however, Mexican-Americans scored low on preventive knowledge and behavior.[27]

More recently, Ford and Jones[28] reported similar findings from analyses of the 1985 Health Promotion and Disease Prevention supplement[29] and the National Health Interview Survey.[30] Non-Hispanic white men and women scored higher on a cardiovascular disease knowledge index than either Hispanics or blacks after adjusting for age and education. Within each ethnic group, women had greater age- and education-adjusted knowledge of individual CVD risk factors. CVD knowledge increased with age and peaked in the fourth or fifth decade. Ethnicity in those studies was determined from self-reports. Of the various modulating factors that were assessed—age, education, income, marital status, access to medical care, and geographic region—education was the strongest predictor of cardiovascular disease knowledge.

Effects of Obesity

The observations are generally in agreement with changes in obesity-related cardiovascular risk factors.[31] For Mexican-American women, age-adjusted values of body mass index, the sum of subscapular and triceps skinfolds, and serum triglycerides were reported to decrease across populations living in the barrio, transition neighborhoods (50% Mexican-American and 50% non-Hispanic white), and the suburbs; HDL cholesterol was reported to increase across that spectrum. No trends were noted for age-adjusted total or LDL cholesterol. Similar trends were noted for non-Hispanic white women but not in Mexican-American men. Surprisingly, however, age-adjusted total (+20%) and LDL cholesterol (+20%) levels were higher in the suburbs than in transitional neighborhoods only for non-Hispanic whites; values for Mexican-American men were similar in both neighborhoods.

The high rates of obesity and body fat distribution among Hispanic-American women are of special concern because of the increased risk of coronary heart disease associated with obesity and a high waist-to-hip circumference. In a prospective study of 115,886 American women 30 to 55 years of age, increases in current Quetelet index (kilograms per square meter) from <21 to >29 were associated with steady increases in the relative risk to coronary heart disease (adjusted for age and cigarette smoking) from 1.0 to 3.3. The risk was attenuated after adjustments were made for hypertension, diabetes, and hypercholesterolemia. The current Quetelet index was more important as an explanatory determinant of risk than was weight at age 18.[32]

In a Swedish study of 1,462 women and 792 men, a fourfold higher risk of coronary heart disease was found for men during 12 years of follow-up.[33] Gender differences in serum cholesterol, smoking, and body mass index explained a marginal portion of the disparity in risk; however, when analyses controlled for waist-to-hip ratios, the disparity in risk of coronary heart disease between men and women became insignificant.

NONINSULIN-DEPENDENT DIABETES MELLITUS

Noninsulin-dependent diabetes mellitus (NIDDM) of adult onset is approximately three times more prevalent among Hispanic-Americans than among non-Hispanic whites. The severity of the problem, however, appears to vary enormously among localities and Hispanic subgroups. For example, in Texas for the period 1970 to 1981, county-wide death rates attributable to diabetes ranged from 2.5 to 52 per 1000 total deaths; the highest rates were observed in counties whose populations were >75% Hispanic.[34] In other areas of the Southwest, a 2.1-fold excess of confirmed NIDDM was reported for Hispanic males and a 4.8-fold excess for Hispanic females.[35] Among Hispanic-Americans the prevalence of this disease is highest among the least acculturated into the American mainstream (as determined by socioeconomic status) and appears to be positively related to the degree of genetic admixture with Amerindian populations.

Stern and colleagues studied three neighborhoods in San Antonio, Texas[36] and found the prevalence of NIDDM among Mexican-Americans living in the barrio was 16 percent; it was 10% among Mexican Americans living in transition neighborhoods (50% Mexican-American and 50% non-Hispanic white), and 5% in the suburbs. Hispanic men and women living in the barrio were two and four times, respectively, as likely to have the disease than their counterparts in the suburbs. Although NIDDM was slightly more prevalent among women in the barrio than among men, the converse was true in the suburbs.

Declines in NIDDM across socioeconomic groups represented by the barrio, transitional neighborhoods, and the suburbs were not unique to Mexican-Americans.[37] Non-Hispanic whites studied in transitional neighborhoods and the suburbs also showed declines in the prevalence of NIDDM. The prevalence of NIDDM among non-Hispanic white males in the suburbs was approximately 50 percent of that seen in transitional neighborhoods. The declines among women were much greater among non-Hispanic whites than Mexican-Americans. The prevalence of NIDDM among non-Hispanic white women living in the suburbs was only 30 percent of that for their counterparts in transitional neighborhoods.

Effects of Body Fat Distribution

Studies by Haffner et al. suggest that both Mexican-American men and women have more body fat than do their non-Hispanic white counterparts, and that waist-to-hip ratios are also higher among Mexican-Americans.[38] A predominance of body fat in the trunk or upper body predisposes individuals to diabetes. In studies of Mexican-Americans conducted by Mueller at al., the ratio of upper to lower body fat increased significantly with aging.[39] In males, this pattern appeared to emerge in adolescence and to continue through 40 to 50 years of age. In females, the pattern appears to start later, at about age 20.

Association with Amerindian Ancestry

Amerindian ancestry may help explain the high prevalence of NIDDM among Mexican-Americans. Genetic predisposition of Amerindians of the Southwest to NIDDM has been well documented. One explanation offered for such predisposition is the presence of a "thrifty" genotype that confers an enhanced efficiency to store excess energy. The advantages of this ability in populations at risk for severe food shortages are evident. Under conditions of a consistently plentiful food supply, the same genotype appears to result in obesity and NIDDM.[40]

In a heavily Mexican-American populated county in south Texas (Starr County; 97% Mexican-American), Hanis et al. used various genetic markers to estimate that approximately 35% of the gene pool among Mexican-Americans is of Amerindian origin and the remaining 70% European.[41] Gardner et al. made similar estimates and calculated that approximately 40% of the gene pool of Mexican-Americans in a barrio of the Southwest was of Amerindian origin; the corresponding percentages for Mexican-Americans in transitional neighborhoods and the suburbs were about 25% and 15%, respectively.[42] These genetic differences across socioeconomic groups were similar among men and women.

The potential contributions of genetic traits and learned behaviors to an increased predisposition to NIDDM among Amerindians are not known. Unfortunately, within neighborhoods, ethnic differences in the prevalence of NIDDM do not help distinguish effects of cultural and genetic influences.

Severity of NIDDM among Mexican-Americans

For reasons that are not fully understood, NIDDM among Mexican-Americans appears to be metabolically more severe than among non-Hispanic whites (see Table 6.5), and even before NIDDM fully evolves, Mexican-Americans demonstrate higher levels of hyperinsulinemia than can be explained by total adiposity or regional fat distribution patterns.[43]

For example, diabetes-related end stage renal disease is approximately six times more common and retinopathy appears to be two to three times more

TABLE 6.5   Distribution of Fasting and Two-Hour Plasma Glucose Concentrations
in Mexican-American and Non-Hispanic White Diabetics

	Mexican-Americans	Non-Hispanic Whites
Fasting plasma glucose (mg/dl)		
< 150	40	44
140–199	30	26
> 200	29	10
Two-hour plasma glucose (mg/le)		
< 200	5	6
200–299	47	70
> 300	49	23

SOURCE: Adapted from M. P. Stern, The epidemiology of diabetes in Mexican Americans. In R. Urby and J.H. Flores (eds.), *Proceedings of Hispanic Health Status Symposium.* (San Antonio, TX: Health Policy Development, Inc., 1988), pp. 17–23.

common among Mexican-Americans.[44] It is not known if these signs of increased severity reflect a poor utilization of medical services, poor compliance in the management of the disease, and/or genetically based differences that are expressed as more metabolically severe disease.

GALLBLADDER DISEASE

Diabetes, obesity, the excess intake of dietary fat, low-fiber diets, and a positive family history are risk factors in gallbladder disease. In industrialized countries, cholesterol is the principal component of most gallstones.[45] The formation of stones in the gallbladder is likely due to increased cholesterol synthesis by the liver and/or increased secretion in bile in combination with relative decreases in bile acid synthesis. The result is a supersaturated bile from which cholesterol crystals aggregate to form stones.

Hanis et al. estimated the frequency of gallbladder disease by either a self-reported history of the disease or a history of cholecystectomy in Mexican-Americans in Starr County, Texas. They found the prevalence to be 13% and 26% in males and females over the age of 35, respectively, a rate approximately threefold higher than reported in Framingham, Massachusetts.[46] In that study, the odds of a Mexican-American with diabetes having gallbladder disease were 2.4 times that of a nondiabetic.

Using data from the 1982–1984 Hispanic Health and Nutrition Examination Survey, researchers calculated the age-adjusted prevalence of gallstone disease (i.e., the presence of gallstones diagnosed by ultrasonography or history of a cholecystectomy) for Mexican-Americans (7.2% for men, 23.3% for women), Cuban-Americans (4.2% for men, 15.4% for women), and Puerto Ricans (4.0% for men and 13.5% for women) from 20 to 74 years of age.[47] Rates of cholecystectomies were similar in studies of Mexican-Americans residing in New Mexico and Texas.[48]

The higher prevalence of gallbladder disease among Mexican-Americans is ascribed to a genetic admixture with American Indians in the Southwest. Indeed, Pima Indian men and women have rates of gallbladder disease twice that of Mexican-Americans.

Other risk factors that contribute to the high rate of gallbladder disease among Mexican-Americans are the high rates of obesity and the unfavorable distribution of body fat.[49] Although there is no consensus on the best measure of regional fat distribution, ratios of subscapular to triceps skinfold thickness (a measure of central adiposity) and body mass index (estimated as the ratio of total body weight to height squared to reflect total adiposity) were found to be positively and independently associated with gallbladder disease in Mexican-American women but not in men; for men, only body mass index was found to be associated with the disease. However, the small number of men included in the reference study limits the ability to detect potential associations between fat distribution and disease.

DENTAL DISEASE

Dental disease among Hispanics is difficult to evaluate. Much of the available data are derived from convenience samples, and interpretation of the data is complicated by the lack or introduction of fluoridation. Hispanic-Americans generally have substantially poorer oral health and are less likely to receive treatment for dental disease than are non-Hispanic whites. The underlying reasons for the poorer dental health may relate to the failure of public health efforts to improve the knowledge base required to maintain good oral health, the lack of economic resources to implement what is known, and the lack of access to preventive and curative treatment.[50]

OVERVIEW

Several factors limit the inferences that can be drawn from relationships among diet, health, and sociocultural factors for Hispanics: the Hispanic population's heterogeneity, its dynamic characteristic imposed by migration patterns, and the varying quality in data sources. Conclusions, therefore, must remain tentative and be interpreted within the limits of an unsatisfactory context. Nonetheless, in the interest of discussion, several points can be made.

Available data present a community that self-assesses its health as good, despite an uneven but generally unacceptable access to health care. The community is dissatisfied with the care that it receives. Hispanics tend to lag behind the general population in awareness of major risk factors for cancer and in knowledge and behaviors related to cardiovascular disease prevention. Furthermore, educational attainment for this group remains unsatisfactory, rates of poverty are among the highest for identifiable subgroups in the United States, and teenage fertility rates are three times higher than those for non-Hispanic whites.

From that synopsis it is reasonable to expect a picture of health outcomes that is quite disparate from that portrayed by available data. If one accepts the estimate of life expectancy for Hispanics in the Southwest as representative of that for the general American Hispanic population, it is 99% of the life expectancy at birth of non-Hispanic whites. By a significant margin, the majority of excess deaths in Hispanic groups for whom data are available are due to preventable causes generally unrelated to physical health, that is, homicides and unintentional injury. Although it is true that unintentional injuries may be related to excess alcohol ingestion, there are other culturally based behaviors and beliefs or job-related risks that also may be suggested as potentially significant causes. Even more remarkable, however, is that the lower than expected deaths due to heart disease, stroke, and cancer and lower than expected infant mortality are sufficient to compensate almost completely for the extraordinarily high mortality due to homicide and unintentional injury. The major exception to this general picture is excess deaths due to diabetes among Hispanic women.

Potential modulators responsible for the disparity between observed and expected mortality due to diet-related chronic diseases fall into four broad categories: diet, health-related behaviors (e.g., smoking), environment, and genetics. The potentially adverse or positive influences of the interplay among variables in those four categories are obvious. For example, the genetically linked increased rates of obesity and diabetes among Amerindians become evident only with "modernization." And the lower than expected rate of cardiovascular mortality among Mexican-Americans cannot be explained by the usual risk factors identified by studies of non-Hispanic whites. Recognizing the importance of that interplay provides limited information regarding which specific variables are the most powerful modulators or how they interact. It appears that integration into the American mainstream ameliorates differences in health indices between Hispanics and non-Hispanic whites. Coincident with that integration are changes in health-related behaviors, diet, and environment. Furthermore, it is likely that gradual increases in integration are accompanied by progressively less Amerindian genetic admixtures. Therefore even opportunistic observational studies of this type are of limited use.

The most striking challenge is the identification and preservation of factors that promote health before they are lost in the assimilation of Hispanic-Americans. An improved understanding of these factors is of potential consequence to both the American Hispanic community and other groups. Their possible value in compensating for clear disadvantages is obvious. For example, the expected negative relationship between socioeconomic status and infant mortality is not evident when one compares American Hispanics and non-Hispanic whites; nor, however, is it evident in comparisons between selected American Hispanic groups (e.g., Mexican-Americans and Puerto Ricans). In an era when containment of health costs demands taking greater responsibility for one's own well-being, factors that account for "positive deviance" among any of the four categories take on added importance; however, those amenable to intervention (diet, health-related behaviors, and the environment) are of greater interest to the individual.

SUMMARY

Population heterogeneity, migration patterns, and flaws in study designs make the assessment of health status of the Hispanic-American population a difficult task. Morbidity and mortality are strongly affected by employment status, health-care access and insurance coverage, educational level, economic status, as well as genetic and environmental factors in the different Hispanic subgroups.

Mortality rates for cardiovascular disease, cancer, and diabetes are lower among Cuban-born males and females; for other Hispanic subgroups the data is less clear. The incidence of all-site cancer seems to be lower in Hispanics than in non-Hispanic whites. Site-specific cancer incidence rates are lower for cancers of the colon, rectum, breast, and larynx, but higher for stomach, pancreas, and cervix.

Documented risk factors play an important role in the incidence of some of the diseases affecting the Hispanic population. Tobacco use, alcohol consumption, and obesity have been reported to be high among the Hispanic population, although these factors differ by gender. Together with acculturation patterns and Amerindian ancestry, these may be important variables to explain the high prevalence of non-insulin dependent diabetes among this group. Clearly, further research relative to these factors will provide better data to evaluate diet-related diseases and other health issues among Hispanics.

NOTES

1. Office of Disease Prevention and Health Promotion, *Disease Prevention/Health Promotion, The Facts.* (Palo Alto, CA: Bull Publ. Co., 1988), pp. 213–227.

2. R. E. K. Stein and D. J. Jessop, Measuring health variables among Hispanic and non-Hispanic children with chronic conditions. *Public Health Reports, 104* (1989), 377–384.

3. S. B. Fitzpatrick, C. Fujii, G. P. Shragg, L. Rice, M. Morgan and M. E. Felice, Do health care needs of indigent Mexican-American, black, and white adolescents differ? *Journal of Adolescent Health Care, 11,* (1990), 128–132.

4. D. P. Slesinger, B. A. Christenson, and E. Cautley, Health and mortality of migrant farm children. *Social Science and Medicine, 23* (1986), 65–74.

5. F. M. Trevino, and L. Ray, Health insurance coverage and utilization of health services by Mexican Americans in Texas and the Southwest. In R. Urby and J. H. Flores (eds.), *Proceedings of the Hispanic Health Status Symposium* (San Antonio, TX: Health Policy Development, Inc., 1988), pp. 163–180.

6. M. M. Heckler , *Report of the Secretary's Task Force on Black and Minority Health. Vol. I: Executive Summary* (Washington, DC: U.S. Government Printing Office, 1985).

7. Trevino and Ray, Health insurance coverage.

8. Office of Disease Prevention and Health Promotion, *Disease prevention.*

9. Heckler, *Report of the Secretary's Task Force.*

10. U.S. Department of Health and Human Services, *The Surgeon General's report on nutrition and health* (Washington, DC: U.S. Government Printing Office, 1989).

11. Heckler, *Report of the Secretary's Task Force.*

12. Ibid.

13. S. R. Andrews, Research and evaluation of alcohol and drug use among Mexican American children and adolescents. In R. Urby and J. H. Flores (eds.), *Proceedings of the Hispanic Health Status Symposium* (San Antonio, TX: Health Policy Development, Inc., 1988), pp. 98–106.

14. Office of Disease Prevention and Health Promotion, *Disease prevention.*

15. F. S. Mendoza, S. J. Ventura, R. Burciaga Valdez, R. O. Castillo, L. E. Saldivar, K. Baisden, R. Martorell, Selected measures of health status for Mexican-American, mainland Puerto, Rican, and Cuban-American children. *JAMA, 265* (1991), 227–282.

16. Heckler, *Report of the Secretary's Task Force.*

17. M. H. Cantu-Moore, and T. Fields, Family planning and adolescent pregnancies: Issues for health promotion and prevention among Hispanics. In R. Urby and J. H. Flores (eds.), *Proceedings of the Hispanic Health Status Symposium* (San Antonio, TX: Health Policy Development, Inc., 1988), pp. 138–151.

18. Mendoza et al., Selected measures of health status.

19. Slesinger et al., Health and mortality.

20. E. L. Barret-Connor, B. Cohn, D. L., Wingard, and S. L. Edelstein, Why is dia-

betes mellitus a stronger risk factor for fatal ischemic heart disease in women than in men? *JAMA, 265* (1991), 627–631.

21. M. Rosenthal, H. Hazuda, and M. Stern, Trend in ischemic heart disease mortality among Mexican Americans in Texas. *American Journal of Epidemiology, 122* (1985), 532.

22. Office of Disease Prevention and Health Promotion, *Disease prevention.*

23. R. Doll, and R. Peto, *The causes of cancer* (New York: Oxford University Press, 1981).

24. J. A. Lopez. Cancer among Hispanics: An anatomy of a threat. In R. Urby and J. H. Flores (eds.), *Proceedings of Hispanic Health Status Symposium* (San Antonio, TX: *Health Policy Development, Inc.,* 1988), pp. 31–41.

25. C. L. Hanis, D. Hewett-Emmett, T. C. Douglas, and W. J. Schull. Lipoprotein and apolipoprotein levels among Mexican-Americans in Starr County, Texas. *Arteriosclerosis and Thrombosis, 11* (1991), 123–129.

26. H. P. Hazuda, Role of acculturation in disease prevention behavior: Implications for health policy. In R. Urby and J. H. Flores (eds.), *Proceedings of Hispanic Health Status Symposium* (San Antonio, TX: Health Policy Development, Inc., 1988), pp. 107–109.

27. Ibid.

28. E. S. Ford, and D. H. Jones, Cardiovascular health knowledge in the United States: Findings from the National Health Interview Survey, 1985. *Preventive Medicine, 20* (1991), 725–736.

29. C. A. Schoenborn, *Health promotion and disease prevention: United States, 1985.* DHHS Publ. no. (PHS) 88–1591, Vital and Health Statistics Ser. 10, no. 163 (Washington, DC: National Center for Health Statistics, 1988).

30. National Center for Health Statistics, *The National Health Interview Survey Design, 1973–1984, and Procedures, 1975–1983* DHHS Publ. No. (PHS) 85–1320, Vital and Health Statistics Ser. 1, no. 18 (Washington, DC, 1985).

31. M. P. Stern, M. Rosenthal, S. M. Haffner, H. P. Hazuda, and L. J. Franco, Sex difference in the effect of sociocultural status on diabetes and cardiovascular risk factors: The San Antonio Heart Study. *American Journal of Epidemiology, 120* (1984), 834–851.

32. J. E. Manson, G. A. Colditz, M. J. Stampfer, et al., A prospective study of obesity and risk of coronary heart disease in women. *New England Journal of Medicine, 322* (1990), 882–889.

33. B. Larsson, C. Bengtsson, P. Björntorp, et al., Is abdominal body fat distribution a major explanation for the sex difference in the incidence of myocardial infarction? *American Journal of Epidemiology, 135* (1992), 266–273.

34. C. L. Hanis, R. E. Ferrell, S. A. Barton, L. Aguilar, et al., Diabetes among Mexican Americans in Starr County, Texas. *American Journal of Epidemiology, 118* (1983), 659–672.

35. R. F. Hamman, J. A. Marshall, J. Baxter, L. B. Kahn, E. J. Mayer, M. Orleans, J. R. Murphy, and D. C. Lezotte, Methods and prevalence of non-insulin-dependent diabetes mellitus in a biethnic Colorado population. *American Journal of Epidemiology, 129* (1989), 295–311.

36. Stern et al., Sex difference.

37. Ibid.

38. S. M. Haffner, M. P. Stern, H. P. Hazuda, J. A. Pugh, and J. Paterson, Hyperinsulinemia in a high risk population for non-insulin dependent diabetes mellitus. *New England Journal of Medicine, 315* (1986), 220–224.

39. W. H. Mueller, S. K. Joos, C. L. Hanis, A. N. Zavaleta, et al., The diabetes alert study: Growth, fatness and fat patterning, adolescence through adulthood in Mexican Americans. *American Journal of Physical Anthropology, 64* (1984), 389–399.

40. J. V. Neel, Diabetes mellitus: A ``thrifty'' genotype rendered detrimental by ``progress''? *American Journal of Human Genetics, 14* (1962), 353–362.

41. C. L. Hanis, R. Chakraborty, R. E. Ferrell, and W. J. Schull, Individual admixture estimates: Disease associations and individual risk of diabetes and gallbladder disease among Mexican-Americans in Starr County, Texas. *American Journal of Physical Anthropology, 70* (1986), 433–441.

42. L. I. Gardner, M. P. Stern, S. M. Haffner, S. P. Gaskill, H. P. Hazuda, J. H. Relethford, and C. W. Eifler, Prevalence of diabetes in Mexican Americans: Relationship to percent of gene pool derived from native American sources. *Diabetes, 33* (1984), 86–92.

43. Haffner et al., Hyperinsulinemia.

44. M. P. Stern, The epidemiology of diabetes in Mexican Americans. In R. Urby and

J. H. Flores (eds.), *Proceedings of Hispanic Health Status Symposium* (San Antonio, TX: Health Policy Development, Inc., 1988), pp. 17–23.

45. U.S. Department of Health and Human Services, *Surgeon General's report.*

46. D. L. Hanis, R. H. Ferrell, B. R. Tullock, and W. J. Schull, Gallbladder disease epidemiology in Mexican Americans in Starr County, Texas. *American Journal of Epidemiology, 122,* (1985), 820–829.

47. K. R. Maurer, J. E. Everhart, T. M. Ezzati, et al., Prevalence of gallstone disease in Hispanic populations in the United States. *Gastroenterology, 96* (1989), 487–492.

48. J. M. Samet, D. B. Coultas, C. A. Howard, et al., Diabetes, gallbladder disease, obesity, and hypertension among Hispanics in New Mexico. *American Journal of Epidemiology, 128* (1988), 1302–1311.

49. S. M. Haffner, A. K. Diehl, M. P. Stern and H. P. Hazuda. Central adiposity and gallbladder disease in Mexican Americans. *American Journal of Epidemiology, 129* (1989), 587–595.

50. J. P. Brown, Dental health status and treatment needs among Mexican Americans. In R. Urby and J. H. Flores (eds.), *Proceedings of Hispanic Health Status Symposium* (San Antonio, TX: Health Policy Development, Inc., 1988), pp. 74–84.

7

Overweight and Obesity
In the United States
Hispanics

Professors Laura Kettel Khan, Cornell University, and Reynaldo Martorell,
Emory University, are guest authors of this chapter.

Clinical observations have long suggested a connection between obesity, particularly in its extreme forms, and a variety of chronic diseases. The strongest evidence that obesity has an adverse effect on physical health comes from population-based prevalence and cohort studies, findings that have been complemented by those from weight reduction trials. Studies have documented that obesity results in physiological stress manifested in increased rates of cardiovascular disease,[1] hypertension,[2] diabetes mellitus,[3] gallbladder disease,[4] cancers,[5] impaired respiratory function,[6] hematologic and immunologic consequences,[7] bone, joint, and skin disorders,[8] complications of pregnancy,[9] and endocrine disorders.[10]

Target population groups in the United States at risk for obesity and its health consequences are Hispanics, American Indians, and Afro-Americans (females).[11] The variability in estimates of obesity in minority populations reflects the many factors influencing the development and persistence of obesity, including physical activity, diet, income, education, ethnicity, and genetic susceptibility. This multitude of factors clearly indicates that obesity is a heterogeneous condition and that oversimplification in the characterization of individual factors that influence obesity may increase inconsistencies in research studies of obesity.

The increasing number of Hispanics in the United States, particularly in the Southwest, has been a dominant trend for many years. Hispanics generally exhibit increased levels of overweight and obesity and increased levels of obesity-linked disease than do American whites,[12] which points up the need to describe accurately the anthropometric characteristics of this population nationally. Studies conducted on regional populations of Hispanics have found that sociocultural and socioeconomic factors linked to diet may strongly influence health outcomes.[13] In addition, Native American ancestry, particularly for Mexican-Americans, may contribute to an increased risk of noninsulin-dependent diabetes mellitus (NIDDM) in obese Hispanics.[14] These findings indicate the need to enhance our knowledge about the levels of overweight and obesity in the American Hispanic population.

This chapter focuses on U.S. Hispanics, particularly Mexican-Americans, Cuban-Americans, and Puerto Ricans. Its objectives are to describe sources of data available for Hispanics; to describe the main features of the Hispanic "short and plump" physique; to discuss the determinants of the Hispanic physique; and to assess the public health implications of information available. The primary data source for this overview is the Hispanic Health and Nutrition Examination Survey (HHANES) conducted between 1982 and 1984, which was the first large-scale assessment of the health and nutritional status of the American Hispanic population.[15] This endeavor was supported by HATCH funds, grant #NY(C)-399457.

SOURCES OF DATA FOR HISPANICS

Most data on the growth, maturation, and body composition of Hispanic children, youths, and adults, primarily Mexican-Americans, were derived from samples limited to a single locality and occasionally to specific states. Lloyd-Jones reported results of a comprehensive survey in 1936 and 1937 of the statures and weights of 163,008 Los Angeles schoolchildren 5 to 18 years of age, including 121,820 white, 22,354 Mexican-American, 5,142 Afro-American, and 3,692 Japanese.[16] Although data for Mexican-Americans in the Ten-State Nutrition Survey 1968–70 are somewhat confusing, this survey provides a limited sample of heights and weights of Mexican-American children from Texas.

Lowenstein reviewed a number of published and unpublished local and statewide studies dealing with the nutritional status of U.S. Hispanics, primarily Mexican-Americans and Puerto Ricans, done between 1968 and 1978.[17] In those studies anthropometric data were briefly considered, with the focus primarily on weight and stature. Data for other anthropometric measures were occasionally reported, but these were generally related to overall body size (i.e., if the child is small in stature, he or she will also be smaller in skeletal and muscular dimensions). Measures of fatness are included in only the more recent studies. This undoubtedly reflects the fact that the early studies were more concerned with undernutrition and stunted growth, whereas recent studies often have overnutrition or excess fatness as a primary focus.

Data for representative samples of Hispanic children and youths in the United States were not available until the first and second phases of the National Health and Nutrition Examination Surveys (NHANES), which were conducted between 1971 and 1973 (NHANES I) and 1976 and 1980 (NHANES II). These surveys include anthropometric information for a complex, national probability sample of the U.S. population. Children and youth of Hispanic origin were included in proportion to their representation in the general population but were classified as white. This was also true in earlier health surveys, for example, cycles II and III of the U.S. Health Examination Survey of children and youths 6 to 17 years of age between 1963 and 1970. With the exception of Mendoza and Castillo[18] and Martorell et al.,[19] investigators have not identified those subjects claiming to be of Mexican ancestry in NHANES I and II. The major problem with these surveys is limited sample size (346 boys and 309 girls 2 to 17 years of age) because Hispanics made up only a small portion of the U.S. population.

At present, the best source of data is the Hispanic Health and Nutrition Examination Survey conducted between 1982 and 1984. The undertaking of the HHANES was no doubt motivated by the increasing visibility of the Hispanic presence in the United States. Bean and Tienda have emphasized three features in assessing demographic and socioeconomic changes in this growing segment of the U.S. population over the last two decades: rapid growth, regional concentration, and extensive demographic and socioeconomic variation according to national origin.[20] A second motivation for HHANES was the recognition that not enough was known about the health and nutrition of American Hispanics.

The sample design of HHANES was similar to that for NHANES I and II, but HHANES focused on three subgroups: Mexican-Americans in the Southwest, primarily California and Texas (N = 7462), Puerto Ricans in the

New York City metropolitan area (N = 2834), and Cuban-Americans in Dade County, Florida (N = 1357). Anthropometric measures included skeletal breadths (biacromial, biliac crest, bitrochanteric, and elbow); skinfolds (triceps, subscapular, iliac crest, and medial calf); circumferences (medial calf, chest, head, and mid-upper arm); and height, length, and weight (sitting and standing height, recumbent and crown rump length and weight). In addition, information on the secondary sex characteristics based on assessments of sexual maturation for hair and genitalia (males) or breasts (females) proposed by Tanner[21] of youths 10 to 17 years of age was also collected.

LINEAR GROWTH PATTERNS

To examine Hispanic growth patterns, data collected during NHANES I (1971–74) and II (1976–80) on the general U.S. population were used as reference standards. These data included all subjects measured and were reported by Frisancho.[22] Data on height, weight, and triceps and subscapular skinfolds were used in this analysis. Unpublished reference data for the subscapular-to-triceps skinfolds ratio were supplied by Frisancho.[23] Medians were estimated using sample weights at each age and compared to reference curves for the U.S. population (25th, 50th, and 75th percentiles). (Because the HHANES sample is not a simple random one, it is necessary to incorporate *sample weights* for proper analysis of the data. These sample weights are a composite of individual selection probabilities, adjustments for noncoverage and nonresponse, and poststratification adjustments.) A minimum of 20 subjects was needed to estimate a median value. For individuals younger than 18 years of age, this comparison was made yearly between Mexican-Americans, Cuban-Americans, and Puerto Ricans and U.S. reference values. Subjects older than 18 years, the age at which stature has been achieved, were compared to 18 to 24.9 year olds in the reference population.

Basic Pattern

Median values for height for Mexican-Americans and Puerto Ricans, plotted and compared to the U.S. reference population,[24] are shown in Figure 7.1, panels A and C for boys and girls 2 to 10 years of age, respectively, and panels B and D for boys and girls 10 to 24 years of age, respectively. Cuban-Americans were not included because sample sizes were small, usually less than 20 per year. Differences between Hispanic and reference medians in the case of both Mexican-Americans and Puerto Ricans were minor during early and middle childhood. In boys, differences became larger late in adolescence, and by adulthood, median heights were near the 25th percentile of the U.S. reference population. The pattern in girls was similar except that the differences appear earlier in adolescence because of earlier physical maturation.

Differences in the stature of Mexican-American and Puerto Rican children relative to that of reference children are shown in Figure 7.2, panels A

FIGURE 7.1 Height medians for Hispanic boys and girls compared to U.S. reference curves

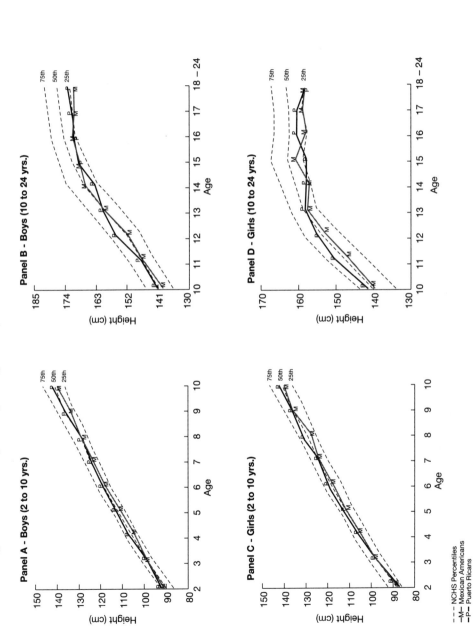

FIGURE 7.2   Difference between height medians for Hispanic boys and girls and U.S. reference values

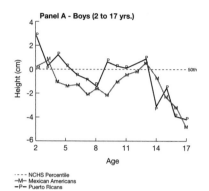
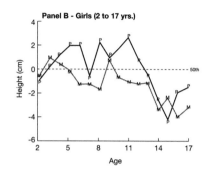

and B. Median values for height were subtracted from the appropriate age- and sex-specific U.S. reference medians such that positive differences indicate that Hispanic children were taller and negative differences indicate that they were shorter than the U.S. reference median. Until 14 years of age for boys and 12 years for girls, differences with respect to U.S. medians were minor (less than 2 cm). Later in adolescence, differences increased markedly and reached 4 cm and 3 cm in Mexican-American and Puerto Rican boys, respectively, and 4 cm in both Mexican-American and Puerto Rican girls. Similar analyses for children from rural areas of Mexico and Central America revealed even larger differences, typically 10 to 16 cm.[25]

Secular Trend in Child Stature

The U.S. Hispanic population is racially diverse, and in evaluations of the appropriateness of the U.S. reference growth norms, the ancestral origin of each of its major subpopulations should be taken into account. There are several reasons for focusing on the Mexican-American component of HHANES in order to examine the change over time, known as the *secular trend* in growth. (*Secular trend* is the process over time by which children have been getting larger and growing to maturity more rapidly, particularly in industrialized countries and recently in some developing ones. Factors such as improved nutrition, control of infectious disease through immunizations and sanitation, reduced family size, more widespread health and medical care, and population mobility appear to be responsible.) First, Mexican-Americans are the largest ethnic group in the U.S. Hispanic population (63% of all U.S. Hispanics, according to the Bureau of the Census.[26] Second, more anthropometric studies are available for Mexican-Americans over the last 50 years than is the case for Puerto Ricans or Cuban-Americans, a fact that facilitates the interpretation of the anthropometric data available for Mexican-Americans in HHANES. Finally, sample sizes are much larger for Mexican-Americans than for Puerto Ricans and Cuban-Americans in the HHANES data set. Thus the issue of the relative importance of genetics and environment as explanatory factors of body size differences with respect to the U.S. reference growth norms can be addressed more thoroughly for the Mexican-American component of HHANES.

Previous studies include the Los Angeles Study from 1936 to 1937 in which mean statures and weights for children of Mexican ancestry were consistently less than for black and white children but greater than for Japanese children. The general sequence of size variation was, from largest to smallest, white, black, Mexican, and Japanese. Weight for height relationships did not differ between white and Mexican-American children in this large sample (N = 11,014 boys and N = 10,629 girls). Statures and weights for Mexican-Americans from Texas within the Ten State Nutrition Survey conducted between 1968 and 1970 were grouped into 2 year age categories from 6 to 18 years. Mean statures and weight of school-age children in Texas (N = 558 males and 581 females) were consistently less than the medians reported in the first set of data for all Hispanic-Americans in the Ten-State Nutrition Survey.

The Mexican-American children measured in HHANES were markedly larger than children of similar ancestry measured nearly two or more decades ago. This is illustrated in Figure 7.3, panels A and B, in which Mexican-American boys and girls from HHANES, from the Los Angeles study, 1936–1037,[27] and from the Ten-State Nutrition Survey, 1968–1970,[28] were compared to the U.S. reference 50th percentile.

Secular Trend in Adult Stature

A secular trend of increasing stature in adults has been observed in developed countries over the last century.[29] This increase in height has been attributed to general improvements in socioeconomic conditions, environmental sanita-

FIGURE 7.3 Differences in height medians with respect to U.S. reference values in various surveys of Mexican-American boys and girls

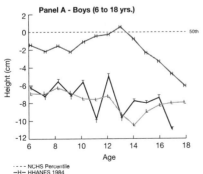
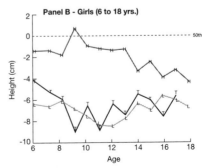

tion, and health care associated with industrialization, which led to improved nutrition and decreased morbidity. Cross-sectional data on adults may be used to infer secular trends in conjunction with appropriate adjustment for the phenomenon of "shrinkage associated with aging."[30] (Shrinkage is the process by which the vertebrae are gradually compressed with age.)

Trends in adults' stature in American Hispanics had not been examined. Therefore the secular trend was analyzed using the cross-sectional method employed by Ruel et al.[31] The method is based on the high correlation between subischial height (difference between stature and sitting height) and stature.[32] The rationale behind this method is that the length of certain long bones is highly correlated with stature and is influenced by secular trends but not by age-associated shrinkage. For example, stature and sitting height are assumed to reflect the effects of both aging and secular trends, whereas subischial height reflects only the effects of secular trends.[33] The partial regression coefficient of stature on age (b_1), controlling for subischial length, is interpreted as being the rate of shrinkage per year (aging effect), and is used to compute the age-adjusted height for each individual.

$$\text{age-adjusted height} = \text{observed height} + b_1 \, (\text{age} - 30)$$

Because shrinkage is assumed not to occur before the age of 30, the age used in the equation is the difference between actual age and 30 years. The age-adjusted height is then regressed against year of birth to test for the effect of secular trends.

The regression of age-adjusted height on birth year demonstrated a secular trend in increasing adult height between birth cohorts from the 1910s to the 1950s. *Cohort* is defined as people within a geographically or otherwise delineated population who experienced the same significant life event within a given period of time. Note that although the term *cohort* is almost always used to refer to *birth* cohorts (those born in a particular year or period), one may also define cohorts in terms of *event* (year of occurrence of any number of events). The coefficients obtained for the aging effect were –0.07/year and –0.10/year, and the coefficients for subischial height were 1.38 cm/year and 1.32 cm/year for Mexican-American males and females, respectively. Similar results were obtained for Cuban-Americans and Puerto Ricans. As shown in Table 7.1, the mean stature for adults over 10-year periods increased with age. Figure 7.4, panels A and B, presents the change in age-adjusted height by birth cohort and clearly shows an increase in height over time for both sexes in the three groups. One possible explanation is improvements in socioeconomic conditions; environmental sanitation and health care during childhood in the United States resulted in better nutrition and decreased morbidity and therefore increased growth. However, for lack of nationally representative data over time, these conclusions cannot be made at present.

TABLE 7.1   Height Uncorrected and Corrected for Age-Associated Shrinkage in U.S. Hispanics

Birth Cohort	N	Uncorrected Stature, cm ($\bar{X} \pm SD$)			Corrected Stature, cm ($\bar{X} \pm SD$)		
Males							
Mexican-American							
1910s	201	169.29	±	7.08	167.45	±	7.43
1920s	226	168.56	±	5.69	166.72	±	5.76
1930s	270	170.88	±	5.65	169.71	±	5.70
1940s	313	170.62	±	7.81	170.15	±	7.81
1950s	149	171.05	±	7.49	170.91	±	7.45
Cuban-American							
1910s	208	169.51	±	6.06	167.95	±	6.23
1920s	63	170.54	±	6.42	168.57	±	6.73
1930s	88	169.92	±	6.12	168.48	±	6.20
1940s	40	174.55	±	7.24	172.70	±	7.50
1950s	30	174.83	±	8.47	174.16	±	8.88
Puerto Rican							
1910s	201	169.50	±	7.18	167.85	±	7.82
1920s	60	166.98	±	6.55	164.60	±	6.69
1930s	100	169.45	±	6.41	167.70	±	6.54
1940s	77	169.04	±	7.12	167.93	±	7.11
1950s	66	171.90	±	6.88	171.04	±	6.97
Females							
Mexican-American							
1910s	244	155.13	±	6.39	152.18	±	6.95
1920s	262	155.98	±	5.17	153.22	±	5.23
1930s	323	156.01	±	5.23	154.22	±	5.31
1940s	404	157.69	±	6.31	156.92	±	6.30
1950s	167	158.49	±	6.18	158.29	±	6.29
Cuban-American							
1910s	269	156.54	±	5.33	155.00	±	5.65
1920s	85	156.79	±	4.67	155.02	±	4.70
1930s	94	156.56	±	4.66	155.35	±	4.76
1940s	83	156.76	±	6.04	155.89	±	6.27
1950s	50	157.98	±	4.79	157.23	±	5.07
Puerto Rican							
1910s	385	155.95	±	5.79	154.48	±	6.25
1920s	94	155.57	±	5.37	153.41	±	5.40
1930s	129	155.79	±	6.07	153.96	±	6.17
1940s	121	156.59	±	7.15	155.46	±	7.30
1950s	88	157.46	±	6.88	156.62	±	7.07

SOURCE: National Center for Health Statistics, *Plan and operation of the Hispanic Health and Nutrition Examination Survey, 1982–84.* DHHS Publication no. (PHS) 85-1321, Vital Health Statistics Ser.1 (Washington, DC, 1985).

FIGURE 7.4   Change in height corrected for age-associated shrinkage in U.S. Hispanic males and females

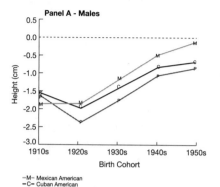
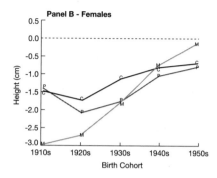

−M− Mexican American
−C− Cuban American
−P− Puerto Rican

Causes of Short Stature in Hispanics

Earlier analyses were done to explain the extent to which genetic and environmental determinants influenced the differences in body size between Mexican-Americans and non-Hispanic Whites.[34] In confirmation of other analyses performed using NHANES data,[35] differences in stature prior to adolescence were minor and practically disappeared after adjustment for differences in income levels. Differences during adolescence, on the other hand, remained largely unchanged after controlling for income levels.

In addition, Mexican-Americans were moderately delayed in terms of the development of secondary sexual characteristics when compared with populations from around the world.[36] However, secondary sexual characteristics are difficult data to standardize, and the possibility of systematic differences exists across studies. Also, there are no U.S. reference data for secondary sexual characteristics. Thus the possibility was considered that growth continues beyond 17 years in the Mexican-American sample and that some of the differences in stature with respect to the NCHS curves are lessened later through catch-up growth. (The higher than normal growth velocity for age and/or skeletal maturity experienced after a child suffers an insult for a short period of time has been called "catch-up growth." During this period the child is able to return to, or at least approach, his or her regular course of growth when conditions improve.) However, this was not the case for boys or girls. Mean height was similar for age 17 through 25 years, whereas body mass index increased substantially in both sexes throughout this age range.

Furthermore, the largely poor Mexican-American sample was almost as tall at 17 years of age as two elite samples from cities in Guatemala[37] and Mexico.[38] Again, one possible interpretation of these findings is that the reduced stature observed in late adolescence relative to the NCHS reference population is genetic in origin because the same pattern is shown in elite samples of similar ethnic origin. Specifically Mexican-Americans differ from other Hispanic groups in being of Spanish/Indian ancestry similar to Guatemalans and Mexicans. However, a Spanish/black admixture is characteristic among mainland and island Puerto Ricans and, to a much lesser extent, among Cuban-Americans. (*Admixture* is defined by Webster as "the fact of being mixed." In this case racial admixture is the result of multiple blood lines.) Yet all three Hispanic groups have similar heights.

It is not certain that the elite samples from Mexico and Guatemala provide good measures of growth potential. Both the Guatemalan and Mexican studies were published in the mid-1970s. It may be that these populations, in spite of their economic status, had not yet exhibited their full genetic potential in growth.

There is a strong possibility that the Mexican-American population in HHANES had not yet reached its height potential as well. Subjects from HHANES 1982–84 were much larger than those included in the Ten State Nutrition Survey, 1968–70 and the Los Angeles study, 1936–37. And the height of Hispanic adults increased with each birth cohort from 1910 to 1950. Regardless of issues of comparability among surveys, it is clear that a rapid trend toward increased size has taken place in the Hispanic-American population. Whether more changes will occur is an issue that can be addressed only through future surveys, for example, NHANES III, which began in 1988 and will continue for approximately 6 years at 88 locations in the United States. Although there is no planned HHANES II, NHANES III is oversampling U.S. Hispanics and will be released in the late 1990s.

If the possibility of a continuing secular trend in stature is accepted, then caution must be exercised in attributing the shorter stature of Mexican-American adolescents entirely to genetic factors. Cohort effects could explain the apparent growth retardation observed during adolescence. Thus adolescents measured in HHANES may have developed under conditions less favorable in early childhood than those that occur today. Because HHANES is a cross-sectional survey, it is impossible to pinpoint when the growth of the adolescents may have been adversely affected. A possibility that must be seriously entertained is that the growth retardation in HHANES Mexican-American adolescents may have occurred in early childhood. Health and nutrition may have improved such that Mexican-American young children now grow at a better rate than Mexican-American adolescents did as young children 10 or more years earlier. Such a view is entirely compatible with the growth patterns observed in HHANES adults. This view also suggests that the HHANES indices of the family today is an inappropriate measure to use in controlling for differences between Mexican-American and non-Hispanic adolescents; a more appropriate but unavailable measure would be family status when the adolescents were infants and young children. This may explain why the HHANES poverty index is an important predictor of growth in early and middle childhood but not in adolescence.

Implications of Short Stature

Pediatricians and public health nutritionists should expect similar heights in Hispanic and in non-Hispanic white pre-adolescent children; deviations should be interpreted as indicative of poor nutritional status and not as an ethnic marker. For Hispanic adolescents, the interpretation of small stature is not clear, because genetic potential for growth or cohort effects may account for the difference. Heights are not likely to be a problem for reproductive risk in most women, as few of the 18 to 24.9 year olds are less than 150 cm, a widely used risk indicator of obstetric risk and delivery complications.[39] Specifically, 8.9, 6.7, and 5.5% of Mexican-American, Cuban-American, and Puerto Rican women were less than 150 cm in height; in many populations from Mexico and Central America, the corresponding proportion often exceeds 50%.

Many industries—airlines, fire departments, and police departments—have minimum height entrance requirements. Regardless of the cause of these requirements, these practices discriminate against Hispanics. For example, if a job has a height requirement of 6 feet (180 cm) or more, 89.0% of Mexican-American, 81.4% of Cuban-American, and 86.6% of Puerto Rican males 18 to 24 years of age would be turned away, compared to approximately 71% of non-Hispanic whites the same age. How well height correlates with performance in these occupations is unclear. Certain sports, such as basketball, are not as open to Hispanics due to their short stature, but in these instances size is more clearly related to performance.

OVERWEIGHT AND OBESITY

Measuring Overweight and Obesity

The physical measurement of obesity ranges from the relatively simple and inexpensive, such as weight, skinfolds, and circumferences, which have been used extensively in large population-based studies, to the complex and expensive, such as underwater weighing, labeled water, bioelectrical impedance, computerized tomography, and magnetic resonance imaging, which have been used in smaller clinical studies.[40] These latter methods have been invaluable in determining more precise estimates of body composition, including both the amount and distribution of body fat, but have limited use for large population-based studies. Questions remain about how the commonly used measures of weight for height, skinfolds, and circumferences and their ratios correlate to body composition estimates derived from more precise methods, such as computerized tomography and underwater weighing, and which of these measures can be applied in the measurement of obesity across population groups and the appropriateness of applying standards derived from the general population to individual subpopulation groups.

Two derived indicators that have been generally accepted to assess overweight, obesity, and fat distribution in population-based surveys are the body mass index (kilograms per meters squared) and the ratio of subscapular to triceps skinfolds thickness. These are used as indicators of overweight and/or obesity and of centralized fat distribution, respectively. An individual is defined as overweight if the particular anthropometric variable is greater than or equal to the 85th percentile of the reference population, and obese if greater than or equal to the 95th percentile. The reference source used here is that of Frisancho, who combined data collected during the first and second National Health and Nutrition Examination Surveys, 1971–74 and 1976–80, creating the largest nationally representative sample available today.[41] For individuals younger than 18 years of age, comparisons were made yearly between each Hispanic ethnic group and U.S. populations. Subjects older than 18 years were defined as overweight or obese if they met or exceeded the 85th or 95th percentile for the youngest adult group for which national reference standards were provided, in this case 18 to 24.9 years. The rationale for using young adults as the reference group is that they are leaner than older adults. A similar rationale was followed by Najjar and Rowland,[42] who used a 20 to 29 year age group, and Pawson et al.,[43] who used an 18 to 24.9 year age group.

Patterns of Overweight and Obesity

Historically, Mexican-Americans have exhibited increasing median body mass index (BMI) values in respect to U.S. references, as shown in the comparison of the Los Angeles study, 1936–37, the Ten-State Nutrition Survey, 1968–70, and the HHANES, 1982–84 (Figure 7.5, panels A and B). Among HHANES male Mexican-Americans age 18 to 24.9 years, the prevalence of overweight and obesity conformed to expected values but exceeded them to

FIGURE 7.5   Differences in body mass index medians with respect to U.S. reference values in various surveys of Mexican-American boys and girls

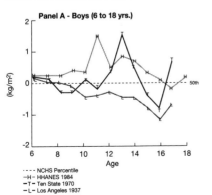
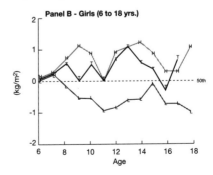

TABLE 7.2   Prevalence of Overweight and Obesity in U.S. Hispanics

Age Category (yr)	Overweight			Obese		
	Mexican-American	Cuban-American	Puerto Rican	Mexican-American	Cuban-American	Puerto Rican
Males						
2–4.9	21.8	30.3	26.1	7.2	12.1	12.6
5–11.9	23.6	42.3	28.2	10.5	16.9	12.9
12–17.9	21.3	20.5	21.5	6.8	5.7	11.4
18–24.9	17.7	19.3	14.3	5.3	7.0	4.0
25–29.9	28.0	18.1	17.2	11.4	18.8	6.2
30–39.9	39.2	29.5	32.4	12.0	4.9	9.5
40–49.9	46.6	44.0	40.4	12.4	8.3	8.1
50–59.9	43.7	38.6	46.4	16.8	12.3	15.2
60+	38.5	35.6	37.7	11.2	9.6	13.2
Females						
2–4.9	20.8	40.9	24.5	8.8	22.7	15.1
5–11.9	24.5	37.0	29.9	9.0	13.7	13.1
12–17.9	21.6	10.5	23.6	6.0	2.6	6.9
18–24.9	23.1	13.3	24.6	7.5	1.7	9.8
25–29.9	30.8	27.3	26.0	9.7	0.0	7.0
30–39.9	45.2	33.0	41.4	14.9	7.8	16.1
40–49.9	54.2	49.1	53.3	21.9	12.0	17.4
50–59.9	58.2	50.4	58.9	22.4	15.7	19.9
60+	62.4	49.5	62.4	22.4	5.6	26.7

NOTE: Overweight and obesity are defined using the age- and sex-specific 85th and 95th percentiles of NHANES I and II tabulated by Frisancho.

SOURCE: National Center for Health Statistics, *Plan and operation of the Hispanic Health and Nutrition Examination Survey 1982–84.* DHHS Publication no. (PHS) 85-1321, Vital Health Statistics Ser. 1 (Washington, DC 1985).

various degrees in other age cohorts (Table 7.2). Older males exhibited a substantially greater prevalence of overweight and obesity, reaching 46.6% overweight in individuals age 40 to 49.9 years. In terms of relative risk or the actual percentage divided by the expected percentage, males exhibited increasing relative risk of overweight as children and adolescents, decreased levels as young adults, and strongly increased risk as older adults (Table 7.3). (*Relative risk* is defined as the actual percentage divided by the expected percentage.) The data for Puerto Rican and Cuban subgroups showed similar trends, although many of the cohorts for the latter group were too small to make cohort-specific comparisons.

Female Mexican-Americans exhibited moderate levels of overweight and obesity as children and young adults but strongly increasing levels as older adults (Table 7.2). Generally 50% or more of Mexican-American, Cuban-American, and Puerto Rican females older than 40 years exceeded the criteria for overweight. Rates of overweight and obesity were lower for Cuban females, although all cohorts older than 25 years had approximately twice the relative risk of overweight compared with the reference population (Table 7.3).

TABLE 7.3   Relative Risk of Overweight and Obesity in U.S. Hispanics

Age Category (yr)	Overweight			Obese		
	Mexican-American	Cuban-American	Puerto Rican	Mexican-American	Cuban-American	Puerto Rican
Males						
2-4.9	1.45	2.02	1.74	1.44	2.42	2.52
5-11.9	1.57	2.82	1.88	2.10	3.38	2.58
12-17.9	1.42	1.37	1.43	1.36	1.14	2.28
18-24.9	1.18	1.29	.95	1.06	1.40	.80
25-29.9	1.87	1.87	1.15	2.28	3.76	1.24
30-39.9	2.61	1.97	2.16	2.40	.98	1.90
40-49.9	3.11	2.93	2.69	2.48	1.66	1.62
50-59.9	2.91	2.57	3.09	3.36	2.46	3.04
60+	2.57	2.37	2.51	2.24	1.92	2.64
Females						
2-4.9	1.38	2.73	1.63	1.76	4.54	3.02
5-11.9	1.63	2.47	1.99	1.80	2.74	2.62
12-17.9	1.44	.70	1.57	1.20	.52	1.38
18-24.9	1.54	.89	1.64	1.50	.34	1.96
25-29.9	2.05	1.82	1.73	1.94	.00	1.40
30-39.9	3.01	2.20	2.76	2.98	1.56	3.22
40-49.9	3.61	3.27	3.55	4.38	2.40	3.48
50-59.9	3.88	3.36	3.93	4.48	3.14	3.98
60+	4.16	3.30	4.16	4.48	1.12	5.34

NOTE: Relative Risk is defined as actual percentage divided by expected percentage. Overweight and obesity are defined using the age- and sex-specific 85th and 95th percentiles of NHANES I and II tabulated by Frisancho.

SOURCE: National Center for Health Statistics, *Plan and operation of the Hispanic Health and Nutrition Examination Survey 1982–84.* DHHS Publication no. (PHS) 85-1321, Vital Health Statistics Ser. 1 (Washington, DC 1985).

As noted in studies in which NHANES data have been used and in many regional and local investigations (see review by Malina et al.,[44] Mexican-American children tended to have greater weight for height values than the average American child. Shown in Figure 7.6, panels A and B, Mexican-American and Puerto Rican children had BMI greater than or equal to the median BMI for U.S. reference values. This pattern continued through adulthood for Mexican-Americans, Cuban-Americans, and Puerto Ricans, particularly for women (Figure 7.6, panels C and D).

Results not shown here indicate that much of this overweight represents increased levels of fatness, particularly in the trunk.[45] Studies have shown that centralized adiposity in Mexican-Americans is associated with increased risk for noninsulin dependent diabetes mellitus[46] and a number of cardiovascular risk indicators, including high-density lipoprotein cholesterol, total cholesterol, and blood glucose.[47] Centralized distribution of adipose tissue has been shown in numerous population-based studies to be associated with increased risk for the development of diabetes, hypertension, hyperlipidemia, and coronary heart disease.[48]

FIGURE 7.6   Differences in body mass index medians for Hispanic males and females and U.S. reference values

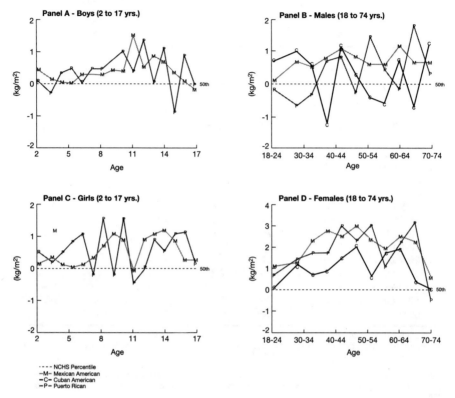

In a more detailed analysis of fat patterning in children,[49] Kaplowitz et al. showed that the ratio of subscapular to triceps skinfolds in Mexican-American boys and girls was higher than average, falling between the 50th and 75th percentiles of reference curves. This suggests that the development of centralized obesity may begin at an early age in this population. Baumgartner et al. reached a similar conclusion using principal-component analyses of skinfolds from the Mexican-American portion of HHANES.[50]

In HHANES, males had a higher proportion of centralized obesity than did females, even though the latter were, in absolute terms, fatter. Specifically, peripheral fat patterning as measured by triceps skinfolds was higher than average, generally between the 50th and 75th percentiles of U.S. reference values for Hispanic adults (Figure 7.7, panels A and B) and truncal fat patterning as measured by subscapular skinfolds was also high, between the 50th and 75th percentiles. But for all ages, subscapular skinfolds were higher for Hispanic females than males (Figure 7.8, panels A and B).

Centralized obesity is measured by the ratio of truncal (subscapular) to peripheral (triceps) fat patterning. In adults the median subscapular to triceps

FIGURE 7.7   Triceps skinfolds medians for Hispanic males and females compared to U.S. reference curves

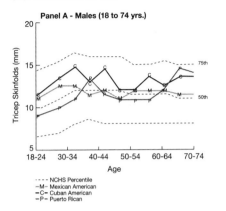
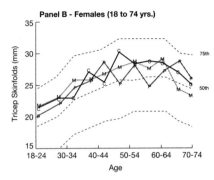

skinfolds ratio in Hispanics was higher than average from early adulthood with a slight decline in later life (Figure 7.9, panels A and B, males and females, respectively). Pawson et al. also reported that adult males age 18 to 60 years exhibited a pronounced tendency of greater relative amounts of centralized fat compared with that of females.[51] The proportion of individuals who met or exceeded the 85th and 95th percentiles diminished after 60 years of age, particularly in Mexican-Americans and Puerto Ricans.

Correlates of Overweight and Obesity

Current knowledge of human obesity has progressed beyond the simple generalizations of the past. Formerly, obesity was considered fully explained by the single adverse behavior of inappropriate eating. The study of animal models of obesity, biochemical alterations in humans and experimental animals,

FIGURE 7.8   Subscapular skinfolds medians for hispanic males and females compared to U.S. Referemnce Curves

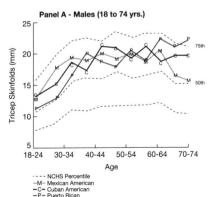
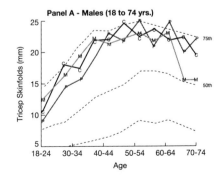

FIGURE 7.9 Subscapular to triceps skinfolds ratio medians for Hispanic males and females compared to U.S. reference curves

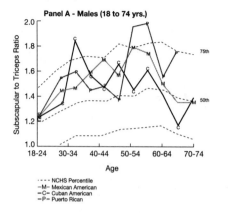

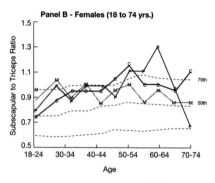

---- NCHS Percentile
−M− Mexican American
−C− Cuban American
−P− Puerto Rican

and the complex interactions of psychosocial and cultural factors that create susceptibility to human obesity indicate that this disease in humans is complex and deeply rooted in biological systems. Regional studies of Hispanics have demonstrated that sociocultural and socioeconomic factors may influence the health status of these populations. Thus it is almost certain that obesity within this population has multiple predisposing factors and associated risk factors, such as genetic predisposition, fat distribution, environmental influences, energy balance, and health behaviors.

Genetic Predisposition Because members of the same family share many dietary and other environmental exposures, the identification of genetic factors is complex: "The specific genes involved in obesity are still unknown."[52] Borjeson estimated heritability of obesity to be 88%.[53] (*Heritability* is defined as the extent to which an individual acquires the sum of the qualities and potentialities genetically derived from an ancestor.) Several studies have shown that Mexican-Americans exhibit increased rates of diabetes,[54] although the extent to which this increased risk is directly attributable to obesity is uncertain. Findings from the San Antonio Heart Study indicate that lean Mexican-Americans are at higher risk for NIDDM than are equally lean anglo Americans and may share the same genetic predisposition to the disease as do Native Americans.[55] Additional evidence for a hereditary component similar to Native Americans is derived from comparisons of prevalence rates for diabetes, gallbladder disease, obesity, and hypertension among Mexican-Americans in New Mexico.[56]

Body Fat Distribution Clinical data[57] and epidemiologic studies[58] indicate that a major factor in the correlation between obesity and morbidity is not obesity per se but the distribution of adipose tissue in the body. Individuals with a predominantly central ("android" or "apple") distribution of fat will experience higher rates of atherosclerotic heart disease, stroke, hypertension, hyperlipidemia, and diabetes mellitus than will similarly obese individuals with peripherally distributed adipose tissue ("gynoid" or "pear"). Studies have shown that centralized adiposity in Mexican-Americans is associated with increased risk for NIDDM,[59] gallbladder disease,[60] and a number of cardiovascular risk indicators, including high-density lipoprotein cholesterol, total serum cholesterol, and blood glucose.[61] Hispanic men in HHANES had a higher proportion of centralized adiposity than did women.[62]

Environmental Influences Many physical factors are important in the etiology of obesity, but, as Stunkard notes, social factors must be considered as among the most important, if not the most important, influence upon the prevalence of obesity today.[63] There has been substantial research on socioeconomic status, usually measured by educational and income levels, and obesity;[64] a review by Sobal and Stunkard found more than 130 studies.[65] However, other social variables have rarely been considered in relationship to obesity. Stern et al. found that obesity decreased with increasing socioeconomic status in Mexican-American women but not in men.[66] The influence of poverty on obesity levels in Hispanics is relatively minor when compared with other social determinants. Overweight was found to be unrelated to the HHANES poverty index, which suggests the influence of factors that operate at all levels of income such as diet and physical activity patterns peculiar to the Mexican-American population or a genetic predisposition to greater fat deposition. In a comparison of nutrient intake in two Mexican-American populations, one rural and one urban, there were higher calorie intakes in the rural population compared with the urban population.[67] In addition, the diet in the rural population, based on higher levels of the Keys score, was more atherogenic than that of the urban population.

Separate from attained social influences, cultural background in particular is being recognized as an important potential influence on health (as demonstrated by the *American Journal of Public Health,* December 1990, supplemental issue, being dedicated to acculturation and various aspects of health, the majority of which used HHANES data). *Acculturation* is the process of change that occurs as a result of contact between cultural groups. Change may occur along several dimensions (beliefs, values, behavioral practices). Researchers have distinguished between modes of acculturation, such as assimilation, integration, marginalization, or separation.

Acculturation, as measured by integration into mainstream U.S. society and the maintenance of traditional cultural values, was associated with a significant linear decline in both obesity and diabetes in Mexican-Americans in the San Antonio Heart Study. Massara suggests that levels of fatness in Hispanic groups may reflect cultural preferences and that, in some cases, individuals may consciously seek to attain a certain level of fatness in keeping with culturally perceived norms.[68] Using principal language spoken as an indicator of acculturation within HHANES, Pawson et al. found an insignificant relationship to obesity or fat distribution. Considering the ramifications of possible limited health care utilization of minorities as shown by Quesada,[69] the high prevalence of obesity in Hispanic populations and the extent to which an individual's self-perception is influenced by cultural norms may be an important predisposing factor to obesity and related disease within a westernized society that discriminates against overweight.

Energy Balance Numerous studies of Hispanics have demonstrated that sociocultural and socioeconomic factors may influence health status through differentiation in the diet. Bartholomew et al.[70] found that Mexican-Americans 60 to 96 years of age used saturated fats in cooking more frequently than did non-Hispanic whites. Dietary fat, particularly saturated fat consumption, was found to be an important correlate of blood lipid levels in Hispanic children.[71] Haffner et al.[72] were unable to confirm an effect of dietary variables or level of physical exercise in predicting obesity in Mexican-Americans in the San Antonio Heart Study. However, in relation to diabetes, based on cross-sectional data, Regensteiner et al.[73] concluded that higher levels of habitual physical activity were associated with lower fasting insulin and C-peptide levels in Hispanic and non-Hispanic white men. The just-released HHANES 24-hour food recall data should provide information on total dietary fat and dietary consumption patterns in relation to overweight and obesity in Hispanics.

Health Behaviors Cigarette smoking is correlated with a number of deleterious health outcomes; in particular, smoking has an inverse relationship with obesity.[74] Overall, smoking rates among Mexican-American men are comparable to estimates for black American males (44% versus 41%) and rates for Mexican-American women are comparable to those for white women (25% versus 27%)[75] In two recent analyses of HHANES, Lee and Markides[76] found that smokers generally weighed less than nonsmokers and younger male smokers reported greater activity limitation due to poor health, and Perez-Stable et al.[77] suggested that Mexican-American light smokers may truly be moderate to heavy smokers. Escobedo et al.[78] found that smoking rates for Hispanic women are beginning to converge with those of Hispanic men. More important, the reference population itself may be biased in that HHANES contains a significant number of overweight subjects and therefore the results may be underestimating the problem in Hispanics.

Implications of Overweight and Obesity

A serious public health problem is clearly evident. Significant proportions of Hispanic adults are overweight ($\geq$ 85th percentile) or obese ($\geq$ 95th percentile), regardless of the anthropometric indicator selected (body mass index, triceps skinfolds thickness, subscapular skinfolds thickness). Also clear is the greater tendency among Hispanics for fat to be deposited in the trunk. Most disturbing is the finding that children are also fatter than the general population, and that this difference is increasing over time.

The increasing levels of obesity among adults are associated with elevated risk of degenerative cardiovascular and metabolic disease, including coronary heart disease, hypertension, stroke, and adult-onset diabetes. Several studies show that Mexican-Americans exhibit increased rates of diabetes, although the extent to which this increased risk is directly attributable to obesity is uncertain. Findings from the San Antonio Heart Study indicate that lean Mexican-Americans are at higher risk for diabetes than are equally lean Anglo-Americans[79] and may share the same genetic predisposition to the disease as do Native Americans. Evidence for a hereditary component in the obesity-related risk patterns in Mexican-Americans because of Native American or Indian admixture has been further supported from comparisons of prevalence rates for diabetes, gallbladder disease, obesity, and hypertension among Hispanics in New Mexico.[80] This has been suggested as evidence of the origin of the "thrifty genotype" of American Indians and Mexican-Americans in contrast to that of Puerto Ricans and Cuban-Americans, who do not share this genetic admixture.

The Hispanic population in the United States is the second largest minority group and among the fastest growing. Because of the relatively low median age of this population at the time HHANES was conducted, the health risk exhibited by Hispanic adults who participated in the survey can be expected to increase in absolute prevalence as the population ages. As a result, obesity-linked diseases will assume greater significance in areas that support large Hispanic populations and place a greater burden on public health resources and facilities that cater to the needs of minorities, in particular, urban minorities.

The tendency for overweight and obesity observed in U.S. Hispanics might be the result of a combination of factors: high energy intakes, low energy expenditures, and/or genetic predisposition. There are few data on the physical activity patterns of Mexican-Americans, but the recently released 24-hour food recall HHANES data should provide extensive dietary information needed to answer this question in part. A possibility is that the energy imbalance, if it exists, is aggravated by a genetic predisposition to store excess energy as fat, particularly in the trunk. Any effective national intervention requires implementation that provides dietary and lifestyle or behavioral recommendations to the public in languages and formats that are relevant and comprehensible to them, given their diversities. The information provided must identify the components of a healthful diet and lifestyle and link such information to a life relatively freer of disease and disability. The nature of any proposed program or intervention should be culturally appropriate. Specifically, the multicultural nature of this population requires the use of terminology suitable for each ethnic group. Also, intervention should start early in life, as Hispanic children are already heavy.

SUMMARY

When HHANES data are compared with U.S. reference data, a number of interesting findings are seen. Mexican-American children of both sexes are shorter than the general population but differences are a function of age. Similar analyses for children from rural areas of Mexico and Central America reveal larger differences. Differences in stature between Mexican-Americans in HHANES and the U.S. reference data increase in later adolescence; at 17 years of age, the average Mexican-American child is at or less than the 25th percentile of the U.S. reference curves.

The Mexican-American children measured in HHANES are markedly taller than children of similar ancestry measured nearly two or more decades ago. Furthermore, the mean stature of adults over 10-year periods has increased with time as well. In particular, the regression of age-adjusted height on birth year demonstrated the presence of a secular trend of increased adult height between birth cohorts from the 1910s to the 1950s. In addition, the change in height over time was present for both sexes in all Hispanic ethnic groups.

Among male Mexican-Americans, Cuban-Americans, and Puerto Ricans aged 18 to 24.9 years, the prevalence of overweight and obesity conformed to expected values but exceeded them to various degrees in other age cohorts. Older males exhibited a substantially higher prevalence of overweight and obesity. In general, Hispanic males exhibited increasing levels of overweight as children and adolescents, decreased levels as young adults, and strongly increased levels as older adults. Female Mexican-Americans, Cuban-Americans, and Puerto Ricans exhibited moderate levels of overweight and obesity as children and young adults but strongly increasing levels as older adults. Overall, adult Hispanic males and females exceeded expected levels of overweight and obesity, with Mexican-Americans generally exhibiting the highest rates.

The role of acculturation, as measured by integration into mainstream society and the maintenance of traditional cultural values, and socioeconomic factors in the etiology of obesity in Mexican-Americans are negatively associated with both obesity and diabetes. These findings are consistent with studies that suggest that levels of fatness in Hispanic groups may reflect cultural preferences and that, in some cases, individuals may consciously seek to attain a certain level of fatness in keeping with culturally perceived norms. The role of poverty as an independent influence on obesity levels in Hispanics seems relatively minor when compared with other cultural determinants.

NOTES

1. J. M. Chapman and F. J. Massey, The interrelationship of serum cholesterol, hypertension, body weight, and risk of coronary disease, results of the first ten years' follow-up in the Los Angeles Heart Study. *Journal of Chronic Diseases, 17* (1964), 933–949.

2. National Institutes of Health, *Report of the Hypertension Task Force*, Vol. 9, NIH Publication no. 79-1631. (Washington, DC:

U.S. Department of Health, Education and Welfare, 1979.)

3. M. Toeller, F. A. Gries, and K. Dannehl, Natural history of glucose intolerance in obesity: A ten year observation. *International Journal of Obesity, 6* (Suppl. 1) (1982), 145–40.

4. G. A. Bray, Complications of obesity. *Annals of Internal Medicine, 103* (1985), 1052–1062.

5. E. A. Lew and L. Garfinkel, Variations in mortality by weight among 750,000 men and women. *Journal of Chronic Diseases, 32* (1979), 561–576.

6. C. S. Ray, D. Y. Sue, A. Bray, J. E. Hansen, and K. Wasserman, Effect of obesity on respiratory function. *American Review of Respiratory Diseases, 128* (1983), 501–506.

7. S. M. Garn and A. S. Ryan, The effect of fatness on hemoglobin levels. *American Journal of Clinical Nutrition, 36* (1982), 189–192.

8. Bray, Complications of obesity.

9. R. L. Naeye, Maternal body weight and pregnancy outcome. *American Journal of Clinical Nutrition, 52* (1990), 273–279.

10. G. A. Bray, *The obese patient: Major problems in internal medicine*, Vol. IX (Philadelphia: Saunders, 1976).

11. S. Kumanyika, Diet and chronic disease issues for minority populations. *Journal of Nutrition Education, 22* (1990), 89–96.

12. Centers for Disease Control, Prevalence of overweight for Hispanics—United States, 1982–1984. *Morbidity and Mortality Weekly Report;* S. P. Gaskill, C. R. Allen, V. Garza, J. L. Gonzales, and R. H. Waldrop, Cardiovascular risk factors in Mexican Americans in Laredo, Texas. I. Prevalence of overweight and diabetes and distributions of serum lipids. *American Journal of Epidemiology, 113* (1981), 546–555; J. M. Samet, D. A. Coultas, C. A. Howard, B. J. Skipper, and C. L. Hanis, Diabetes, gallbladder disease, obesity, and hypertension among Hispanics in New Mexico. *American Journal of Epidemiology, 128* (1988), 1302–1311; C. L. Hanis, R. E. Ferrell, B. R. Tulloch, and W. J. Schull, Gallbladder disease epidemiology in Mexican Americans in Starr County, Texas. *American Journal of Epidemiology, 122* (1985), 820–829.

13. M. P. Stern, M. Rosenthal, S. M. Haffner, H. P. Hazuda, and L. J. Franco, Sex difference in the effects of sociocultural status on diabetes and cardiovascular risk factors in Mexican-Americans. The San Antonio Heart Study. *American Journal of Epidemiology, 120* (1984), 834–851; K. G. Dewey, M. N. Chávez, C. L. Gauthier, L. B. Jones, and R. E. Ramirez, Anthropometry of Mexican-American migrant children in northern California. *American Journal of Clinical Nutrition, 37* (1983) 828–833; A. N. Zaveleta and R. M. Malina, Growth, fatness, and leanness in Mexican-American children. *American Journal of Clinical Nutrition, 33* (1980),

2008–2020; H. P. Hazuda, S. M. Haffner, M. P. Stern, and C. W. Eifler, Effects of acculturation and socioeconomic status on obesity and diabetes in Mexican-Americans. The San Antonio Heart Study. *American Journal of Epidemiology, 128* (1988), 1289–1301; S. M. Haffner, M. P. Stern, H. P. Hazuda, M. Rosenthal, and J. A. Knapp, The role of behavioral variables and fat patterning in explaining ethnic differences in serum lipids and lipoproteins. *American Journal of Epidemiology, 123* (1986), 830–839.

14. Gaskill et al., Cardiovascular risk factors; S. P. Gaskill, H. P. Hazuda, L. I. Gardner, and S. M. Haffner, Does obesity explain excess prevalence of diabetes among Mexican-Americans? Results of the San Antonio Heart Study. *Diabetologia, 24* (1983), 272–277.

15. National Center for Health Statistics, *Plan and operation of the Hispanic Health and Nutrition Examination Survey, 1982–84*. DHHS Publication no. (PHS) 85–1321, Vital Health Statistics (Washington, DC, 1985).

16 O. Lloyd Jones, Race and stature: Study of Los Angeles school children. *Research Quarterly, 12* (1941), 83–97.

17. F. W. Lowenstein, Review of the nutritional status of Spanish Americans based on published and unpublished reports between 1968 and 1978. *World Review of Nutrition and Dietetics, 37* (1980), 1–37.

18. F. S. Mendoza and R. O. Castillo, Growth abnormalities in Mexican-American children in the United States: The NHANES study. *Nutrition Research, 6* (1986), 1247–1257.

19. R. Martorell, F. S. Mendoza, R. O. Castillo, I. G. Pawson, and C. C. Budge, Short and plump physique of Mexican-American children. *American Journal of Physical Anthropology, 73* (1987), 475–487.

20. F. D. Bean and M. Tienda, *The Hispanic population of the United States* (New York: Russell Sage Foundation, 1987).

21. J. M. Tanner, The secular trend towards earlier physical maturation. *Tijdschrift voor Sociale Geneeskunde, 44* (1966), 524–539.

22. A. R. Frisancho, *Anthropometric standards for the assessment of growth and nutritional status* (Ann Arbor: University of Michigan Press, 1990).

23. A. R. Frisancho, personal communication, 1990.

24. Frisancho, *Anthropometric standards.*

25. R. Martorell and J. P. Habicht, Growth in early childhood in developing countries. In F. Falkner and J. M. Tanner (eds.), *Human growth: A comprehensive treatise, 2nd ed., Vol. 3: Methodology, ecological, genetic, and nutritional Effects on growth* (New York: Plenum Press, 1986).

26. Bureau of the Census, U.S. Department of Commerce, The Hispanic population in the United States: March 1986 and 1987 (advance report). *Current Population Reports*, Series P-20, no. 416, 1987.

27. Lloyd Jones, Race and stature.

28. Center for Disease Control, *Ten-State Nutritions Survey, 1968–1970. III. Clinical anthropometry, dental.* DHEW Publication no. (HSM) 72–8131 (Atlanta, 1972).

29. J. C. Van Wieringen, Secular growth changes. In F. Falkner and J. M. Tanner (eds.), *Human growth: A comprehensive treatise, 2nd ed., Vol. 2: Postnatal Growth* (New York: Plenum Press, 1978); also Tanner, Secular trends.

30. M. G. Cline, K. E. Meredith, J. T. Boyer, and B. Burrows, Decline of height with age in adults in a general population sample: Estimating maximum height and distinguishing birth cohort effects from actual loss of stature and aging. *Human Biology, 61* (1989), 415–425.

31. M. T. Ruel, J. Rivera, H. Castro, J. P. Habicht, and R. Martorell, Secular trends in adult and child anthropometry in four villages in Guatemala. *Food and Nutrition Bulletin* (1992). (In press).

32. J. H. Himes and W. H. Mueller, Aging and secular change in adult stature in rural Colombia. *American Journal of Physical Anthropology, 46* (1977), 275–279.

33. J. H. Relethford and F. C. Lees, The effects of aging secular trends on adult stature in rural western Ireland. *American Journal of Physical Anthropology, 55* (1981), 81–88.

34. R. Martorell, F. S. Mendoza, and R. O. Castillo, Genetic and environmental determinants of growth in Mexican-Americans. *Pediatrics, 84*(5) (1989), 864–871.

35. Martorell et al., Short and plump physique.

36. S. F. Villarreal, R. Martorell, and F. S. Mendoza, Sexual maturation of Mexican-American adolescents. *American Journal of Human Biology, 1* (1989), 87–95.

37. F. E. Johnston, M. Borden, and R. B. MacVean, Height, weight, and their growth velocities in Guatemalan private school children of high socioeconomic class. *Human Biology, 45* (1973), 627–641; F. E. Johnston, H. Wainer, D. Thissen, et al., Hereditary and environmental determinants of growth in height in a longitudinal sample of children and youth of Guatemalan and European ancestry. *American Journal of Physical Anthropology, 44* (1976), 469–476.

38. R. Ramos-Galván, Somatometría pediátrica. Estudio semilongitudinal en niños de la ciudad de México. *Archivos de Investigación Medica, 6* (Suppl. 1) (1975), 1–396.

39. K. Krasover and M. A. Anderson, (eds)., *Maternal nutrition and pregnancy outcomes: Anthropometric risk.* Pan American Health Organization, Scientific Publication no. 529, 1991.

40. H. C. Lukaski, Methods for the assessment of human body composition: traditional and new. *American Journal of Clinical Nutrition, 46* (1987), 537–556.

41. Frisancho, Anthropometric standards.

42. M. F. Najjar and M. Rowland, *Anthropometric reference data and prevalence of overweight, United States, 1976–80.* Vital Health Statistics, DHHS Publication no. (PHS) 87–1688 (Washington, DC, 1987).

43. I. G. Pawson, R. Martorell, and F. E. Mendoza, Prevalence of overweight and obesity in U.S. Hispanic populations. *American Journal of Clinical Nutrition, 53* (1991), 1522s–1528s.

44. R. M. Malina, R. Martorell, and F. S. Mendoza, Growth status of Mexican-American children and youths: Historical trends and contemporary issues. *Yearbook of Physical Anthropology, 29* (1986) 45–79.

45. H. Kaplowitz, R. Martorell, and F. S. Mendoza, Fatness and fat distribution in Mexican-American children and youths from the Hispanic Health and Nutrition Examination Survey. *American Journal of Human Biology, 1* (1989), 631–648.

46. S. M. Haffner, M. P. Stern, B. D. Mitchell, H. P. Hazuda, and J. K. Patterson, Incidence of type II diabetes in Mexican-Americans predicted by fasting insulin and glucose levels, obesity, and body-fat distribution. *Diabetes, 39* (1990), 283–288.

47. K. B. Reichley, W. H. Mueller, C. L. Hanis, et al., Centralized obesity and cardiovascular disease risk in Mexican-Americans. *American Journal of Epidemiology, 125* (1987), 373–386.

48. P. Bjorntrop, The associations between obesity, adipose tissue distribution, and disease. *Acta Medica Scandinavica Supplement, 723* (1988), 121–134.; J. P. Despes, S. Moorjani, P. J. Lupien, A. Tremblay, A. Nadeau, and C. Bouchard, Regional distribution of body fat, plasma lipoproteins, and cardiovascular disease. *Arteriosclerosis, 10* (1990), 497–511; A. H. Kissebah and A. N. Peiris. Biology of regional fat distribution: Relationship to non-insulin-dependent diabetes mellitus. *Diabetes Metabolism Reviews, 5* (1989), 83–109.

49. Kaplowitz et al., Fatness and fat distribution.

50. R. N. Baumgartner, A. F. Roche, S. Guo, W. C. Chumlea, and A. S. Ryan, Fat patterning and centralized obesity in Mexican-American children in the Hispanic Health and Nutrition Examination Survey (HHANES 1982–84). *American Journal of Clinical Nutrition, 51* (Suppl.) (1990), 736s–743s.

51. Pawson et al., Prevalence of overweight.

52. National Research Council, Obesity and eating disorders. In *Diet and health: Implications for reducing chronic disease risk*, ed. Committee on Diet and Health, Food and Nutrition Board, Commission on Life Sciences, (Washington, DC: National Academy Press, 1989).

53. M. Borjeson, The aetiology of obesity in children. A study of 101 twin pairs. *Acta Paediatrica Scandinavica, 65* (1976), 279–287.

54. Haffner et al., Incidence of type II diabetes.

55. Stern et al., Sex difference.

56. Samet et al., Diabetes, gallbladder disease.

57. J. Vague, The degree of masculine differentiation of obesity: A factor determining predisposition to diabetes, atherosclerosis, gout, and uric calculous disease. *American Journal of Clinical Nutrition, 4* (1956), 20–34; R. Feldmen, A. J. Sender, and A. B. Siegelaub, Differences in diabetic and nondiabetic fat distribution patterns by skinfolds measurements. *Diabetes, 18* (1969), 478–486.

58. Bjorntrop, Associations between obesity, adipose tissue distribution, and disease; Despes et al. Regional distribution of body fat; Kissebah and Peiris, Biology of regional fat distribution.

59. Haffner et al., Incidence of type II diabetes.

60. S. M. Haffner, A. K. Diehl, M. P. Stern, and H. P. Hazuda. Central adiposity and gallbladder disease in Mexican-Americans. *American Journal of Epidemiology, 129* (1989), 587–595.

61. Reichley et al., Centralized obesity.

62. Pawson et al., Prevalence of overweight.

63. A. J. Stunkard, From explanation to action in psychological medicine: the case of obesity. *Psychosomatic medicine, 37* (1975), 195–236. A. J. Stunkard, *Obesity* (Philadelphia: Saunders, 1980), pp. 438–462.

64. M. Moore, A. Stunkard, and L. Srole, Obesity, social class and mental illness. *JAMA, 181* (1962), 962–966; S. Garn, S. Bailey, P. Cole, and I. Higgins. Level of education, level of income and level of fatness in adults. *American Journal of Clinical Nutrition, 30* (1977), 721–725; P. Goldblatt, M. Moore, and A. Stunkard. Social factors in obesity. *JAMA, 152* (1965), 1039–1042.

65. J. Sobal and A. Stunkard, Socioeconomic status and obesity: A review of the literature. *Psychological Bulletin, 105(2)* (1989), 260–275.

66. Stern et al., Sex difference.

67. M. Z. Nichaman and G. Garcia, Obesity in Hispanic Americans. *Diabetes Care, 14* (7) (1991), 691–694.

68. E. B. Massara, *Qúe gordita! A study of weight among women in a Puerto Rican community* (New York: AMS Press, 1989).

69. G. M. Quesada, Language and communication barriers for health delivery to a minority group. *Social Science and Medicine, 10* (1976), 323–327.

70. A. M. Bartholomew, E. A. Young, H. W. Martin, and H. P. Hazuda. Food frequency intakes and sociodemographic factors of elderly Mexican Americans and non-Hispanic whites. *Journal of the American Dietetic Association, 90* (1990), 1693–1696.

71. S. Shea, C. E. Basch, M. Irigoyen, P. Zybert, J. L. Rips, I. Contento, and B. Gutin, Relationships of dietary fat consumption to serum total and low-density lipoprotein. *Preventive Medicine, 20(2)* (1991), 237–249.

72. S. M. Haffner, M. P. Stern, B. D. Mitchell, and H. P. Hazuda. Predictors of obesity in Mexican Americans. *American Journal of*

Clinical Nutrition, 53 (6 Suppl.) (1991), 1571s–1576s.

73. J. G. Regensteiner, E. J. Majer, S. M. Shetterly, R. H. Eckel, W. L. Hakell, J. A. Marshall, et al., Relationship of habitual physical activity and insulin levels among non-diabetics. *Diabetes Care, 14*(11) (1991), 1066–1074.

74. R. C. Klesges, A. W. Meyers, L. M. Klesgess, and M. E. La Vasque, Smoking, body weight, and their effects on smoking behavior: A comprehensive review of the literature. *Psychological Bulletin, 106* (1989), 204–230.

75. L. G. Escobedo and P. L. Remington, Birth cohort analysis of prevalence of cigarette smoking among Hispanics in the United States. *JAMA, 261* (1989), 66–69.

76. D. J. Lee and K. S. Markides, Health behaviors, risk factors, and health indicators associated with cigarette use in Mexican-Americans: Results from the Hispanic HANES. *American Journal of Health, 81*(7) (1991), 859–864.

77. E. J. Perez-Stable, B. Vanoss Marin, G. Marin, D. J. Brody, and N. L. Benowitz, Apparent under-reporting of cigarette consumption among Mexican American smokers. *American Journal of Health, 80*(9) (1990), 1057–1061.

78. L. G. Escobedo, P. L. Remington, and R. F. Anda, Long-term age-specific prevalence of cigarette smoking among Hispanics in the United States. *Journal of Psychoactive Drugs, 21*(3) (1989), 307–318.

79. Hazuda et al., Effects of acculturation and socioeconomic status.

80. Samet et al., Diabetes, gallbladder disease.

8

Applying the United States Dietary Guidelines to Hispanic Diets

The U.S. Dietary Guidelines
Eat a Variety of Foods
Maintain Healthy Weight
Choose a Diet Low in Fat, Saturated Fat, and Cholesterol
Choose a Diet with Plenty of Vegetables, Fruits, and Grain Products
Use Sugars Only in Moderation
Use Salt and Sodium Only in Moderation
If You Drink Alcoholic Beverages, Do So in Moderation

Dietary Data from Hispanic HANES
Macronutrient Contribution to Energy Intake
Frequency of Consumption of Food Groups
Patterns of Micronutrient Intake

Samples of Menus at Three Caloric Levels and Menus That Meet the U.S. Dietary Guidelines

The U.S. government has advocated a particular pattern of food choices for Americans since 1956, when the concept of the Basic Four Food Groups was instituted. In a thought-provoking essay, Perkin and McCann argue that it is inappropriate to assume dietary and cultural homogeneity of an American population that includes many subcultural groups with strong ethnic identifications and food traditions.[1] The authors rightly argue that the United States has a rich cultural heritage of foodways. Despite some modifications, traditional food choices have persisted over generations. At the same time, Americans are sharing ethnic foods at home and in cafeterias, restaurants, and other places where food is served. Thus, Perkin and McCann argue, the U.S. government is misguided when it advocates a "food groups concept" that fails to address the cultural diversity of the American population.

Perkin and McCann note that there are two inherent conflicts between dietary recommendations based on the concept of food groups and acknowledgment of cultural diversity. First, although designed to provide key nutrients and ensure an adequate diet, the Basic Four (or Seven) Food Groups has never fully utilized knowledge of food composition or acknowledged alternative food sources among ethnic groups.[2] As an illustration, Perkin and McCann give the following example:

> Inclusion of the milk and dairy product group as a must for good eating ignores the fact that among some U.S. ethnic groups (Afro-Americans, Chinese-Americans, and Mexican-Americans), there is a large percentage of the population that is unable to digest lactose, the sugar found in milk. . . .
>
> Since the major nutrient provided by the milk and dairy product group is calcium, seeking alternative calcium sources such as turnip greens (Afro-Americans), soybeans, soy sauce, and green vegetables (Chinese-Americans), and tortillas prepared with lime (Mexican-Americans) which have evolved as culturally acceptable for these ethnic groups makes more sense. Furthermore, the notion of biological adaptation to various levels of calcium intake is possible and has, in fact, occurred in some ethnic groups.[3]

Second, Whitney and Hamilton,[4] as cited by Perkin and McMann, note that the Basic Four Food Groups concept has failed to guide ethnic Americans in the choice of foods as they are actually prepared and consumed. (More on methodological problems in counseling and assessing ethnic diets is presented in Chapters 9 and 10.) Individual subcultural groups often eat one-dish combination foods with many ingredients, such as the Mexican *enchiladas*, Cuban *ajiaco*, or Puerto Rican *asopao*. Guidance, Perkin and McCann argue, would be more useful if recommendations were based on what people *eat* rather than on what people *buy*.

In recent years, the U.S. government has begun to address the relationship of nutrition to health and prevention of disease. In 1977, the Select Committee on Nutrition and Human Needs of the U.S. Senate published *Dietary Goals for the United States*.[5] These goals were meant to provide guidelines for consumption of a diet that, unlike the average American diet, did not have too much fat or too much sugar or salt, and to address specific health and disease issues, including obesity, heart disease, stroke, and cancer. Then, in 1980, the U.S. Department of Agriculture and U.S. Department of Health, Education, and Welfare published *Nutrition and Your Health: Dietary Guidelines for Americans* that provided additional guidance for food selection.[6]

THE U.S. DIETARY GUIDELINES

Over the last 40 years, advice to consumers about nutrition has promoted consumption of appropriate amounts of energy, balanced protein, and sufficient vitamins and minerals to prevent nutritional deficiency diseases. Since the late 1970s, however, there has been a growing consensus that nutritional recommendations should consider diet composition in somewhat different ways. This change in the focus of dietary advice was based on evidence that certain dietary patterns were associated with the development of chronic disease, notably heart disease, stroke, and cancer. The consumption of a high proportion of dietary energy as fat, especially saturated fat, was identified as a risk factor for coronary heart disease and cancer. High-fat diets were also associated with obesity, a risk factor for hypertension and diabetes.

In 1980, the U.S. Departments of Agriculture (USDA) and of Health and Human Services (USDHHS) jointly issued the first edition of *Nutrition and Your Health: Dietary Guidelines for Americans*. This publication listed seven guidelines that considered primarily the dietary sources of energy and other dietary components rather than individual nutrients. *The Dietary Guidelines Bulletin* was last revised in 1990, when the third edition was published.[7] The third edition followed two major reports on diet and health that evaluated current evidence relating dietary practices to health: the surgeon general's 1988 report *Nutrition and Health*[8] and the National Research Council's 1989 report *Diet and Health: Implications for Reducing Chronic Disease Risk*.[9]

The 1990 Dietary Guidelines are as follows:

Eat a variety of foods.

Maintain healthy weight.

Choose a diet low in fat, saturated fat, and cholesterol.

Choose a diet with plenty of vegetables, fruits, and grain products.

Use sugars only in moderation.

Use salt and sodium only in moderation.

If you drink alcoholic beverages, do so in moderation.

These relatively simple statements promote consumption of a varied diet, with moderate amounts of energy from fats, adequate amounts of fruits, vegetables, and grain products, and moderate amounts of sodium, sugar, and alcohol. The importance of prevention of obesity is also stressed in the guidelines.

Since first publication of the Dietary Guidelines, other countries have also published similar dietary recommendations. Those from Canada are as follows:[10]

> The Canadian diet should provide energy consistent with the maintenance of body weight within the recommended range.
>
> The Canadian diet should include essential nutrients in amounts recommended in this report.
>
> The Canadian diet should include no more than 30% of energy as fat (33 g/1000 kcal) and no more than 10% as saturated fat (11 g/1000 kcal).
>
> The Canadian diet should provide 55% of energy as carbohydrate (138 g/1000 kcal) from a variety of sources.
>
> The sodium content of the Canadian diet should be reduced.
>
> The Canadian diet should include no more than 5% of total energy as alcohol, or two drinks daily, whichever is less.
>
> Community water supplies containing less than 1 mg/liter should be fluoridated to that level.

The most recent United Kingdom Recommendations stress moderate fat intake (30% of energy consumed or less) and recommend an intake of at least 22 grams per day of dietary fiber.[11]

The U.S. Surgeon's General's report also includes a set of guidelines very similar to the U.S. Dietary Guidelines, with the exception of a specific statement about sugar. In the National Research Council's report, additional guidelines were suggested:[12]

> Maintain adequate calcium intake.
>
> Maintain an optimal intake of fluoride, particularly during the years of primary and secondary tooth formation and growth.
>
> Maintain protein intake at moderate levels.
>
> Avoid taking dietary supplements in excess of the RDA in any one day.

In the United Kingdom and Canada, a single publication encompasses general dietary guidelines as well as recommended dietary allowances (RDAs) for individual nutrients; in the United States these are prepared as separate recommendations. The RDAs in the United States discuss fluoride intake, suggest a limit for protein intake, and recommend consumption of adequate calcium. In the future, it is likely that the United States will merge the Dietary Guidelines with the RDAs in a single publication.

Though there are variations in dietary guidelines from nation to nation or among expert groups, all of the current guidelines emphasize reduction of dietary fat, maintenance of body weight, and consumption of a varied diet, with plenty of vegetables, fruits, and cereal products. It might be useful to review the individual guidelines in some detail prior to considering how they might be adapted to food patterns of specific population groups.

Eat a Variety of Foods

Most dietary recommendations stress the desirability of consuming essential nutrients from foods rather than from special nutritional supplements (see the NRC's *1989 Recommended Dietary Allowances*, 10th ed.). By eating a varied diet, one is more likely to consume sufficient quantities of the known essential nutrients than if a diet contains limited foods. This is the basis for various food guides devised as nutrition education tools for the public. The 1990 edition of the U.S. Dietary Guidelines recommends consuming specific numbers of servings from five food groups to ensure intake of a varied diet. The U.S. Dietary Guidelines provide the following daily food guide:

> Eat a variety of foods daily, choosing different foods from each suggested food group. Most people should have at least the lower number of servings suggested from each food group. Some people may need more because of their body size and activity level. Young children should have a variety of foods but may need small servings.

FOOD GROUP	SUGGESTED SERVINGS
Vegetables	3–5
Fruits	2–4
Breads, cereals, rice, and pasta	6–11
Milk, yogurt, and cheese	2–3
Meats, poultry, fish, dry beans and peas, eggs, and nuts	2–3

Maintain Healthy Weight

The 1990 edition of the U.S. Dietary Guidelines recognizes that certain health problems are associated with excessive body fat and, to a lesser degree, with extreme thinness. It identifies "healthy" ranges of body weight rather than "ideal" or "desirable" weight, as in earlier versions of dietary guidelines. In the judgment of the Dietary Guidelines Committee, the weight ranges listed in Table 8.1 (see p. 252) represent the current best estimates of healthy weights for men and women. More data are needed linking body weight to health outcomes, and estimates of healthy weight are likely to change as more data are examined. The weight ranges in Table 8.1 are higher for adults over 35 years of age because body weight tends to increase with age.

TABLE 8.1 Suggested Weights for Adults

Height	Weight (lb.)	
	19 to 34 Years	35 Years and Over
5'0"	97–128	108–138
5'1"	101–132	111–143
5'2"	104–137	115–148
5'3"	107–141	119–152
5'4"	111–146	122–157
5'5"	114–150	126–162
5'6"	118–155	130–167
5'7"	121–160	134–172
5'8"	125–164	138–178
5'9"	129–169	142–183
5'10"	132–174	146–188
5'11"	136–179	151–194
6'0"	140–184	155–199
6'1"	144–189	159–205
6'2"	148–195	164–210
6'3"	152–200	168–216
6'4"	156–205	172–222
6'5"	160–211	177–228
6'6"	164–216	182–234

NOTES: Weight is measured with clothes; height, without shoes. The higher weights in the ranges generally apply to men, who tend to have more muscle and bone; the lower weights more often apply to women, who have less muscle and bone.

SOURCE: U.S. Department of Agriculture and U.S. Department of Health and Human Services, *Nutrition and your health—Dietary Guidelines for Americans,* 3rd ed. Home and Garden Bulletin no. 232. (Washington, DC: U.S. Government Printing Office, 1990).

The guidelines also define a "healthy" weight as a waist-to-hip ratio of less than 1 and the absence of a medical condition for which a physician might recommend weight gain or loss. The concept of waist-to-hip ratio is introduced because of evidence that excessive fat deposition in the abdominal area is a risk factor for several chronic diseases. Furthermore, the Dietary Guidelines recommend that sedentary people increase their level of regular exercise. For overweight individuals weight loss is recommended as no more than one half to one pound a week. This rate of weight reduction is considered "practical and sustainable."

Choose a Diet Low in Fat, Saturated Fat, and Cholesterol

The association of high intakes of fat, especially saturated fat, with increased risk of some types of cancer and obesity was deemed especially strong by both the NRC and the Surgeon General. Similarly, strong evidence links the consumption of saturated fat and cholesterol with increased risk of coronary heart disease. The Dietary Guidelines call for consuming a diet low in fat, saturated fat, and cholesterol. In this case low is defined as less than 30% of total daily energy from fat, with no more than 10% of energy from saturated fat. This guideline does not apply to children under 2 years of age.

Although no goal was established for cholesterol consumption, it was expected that a reduction in foods containing saturated fats would also result in lowered cholesterol consumption. The NRC committee recommended that no more than 300 mg of cholesterol be consumed per day. The U.S. Dietary Guidelines suggest the following to limit fat, saturated fat, and cholesterol in the diet.

FATS AND OILS

Use fats and oils sparingly in cooking.

Use small amounts of salad dressings and spreads, such as butter, margarine, and mayonnaise. One tablespoon of most of these spreads provides 10 to 11 g of fat.

Choose liquid vegetable oils most often because they are lower in saturated fat.

Check labels on foods to see how much fat and saturated fat are in a serving.

MEAT, POULTRY, FISH, DRY BEANS, AND EGGS

Have two or three servings, with a daily total of about 6 oz. Three ounces of cooked lean beef or chicken without skin—the size of a deck of cards—provides about 6 g of fat.

Trim fat from meat; take skin off poultry.

Have cooked dry beans and peas instead of meat occasionally.

Moderate the use of egg yolks and organ meats.

MILK AND MILK PRODUCTS

Have two or three servings daily. (Count as a serving: 1 cup of milk or yogurt or about 1 1/2 oz of cheese.)

Choose skim or low-fat milk and fat-free or low-fat yogurt and cheese most of the time. One cup of skim milk has only a trace of fat, 1 cup of 2% fat milk has 5 g of fat, and 1 cup of whole milk has 8 g of fat.

Note that these recommendations call for consumption of small servings of meat and low-fat milk products and limited use of cooking and salad oils. These recommendations affect food preparation practices.

Choose a Diet with Plenty of Vegetables, Fruits, and Grain Products

Earlier guidelines had stressed increased consumption of dietary fiber because evidence suggested that populations who consumed diets low in complex carbohydrates and dietary fiber had greater prevalence of heart disease, obesity, and some types of cancer. In evaluating this evidence, the NRC panel indicated that the strongest evidence linked diets rich in certain types of foods rather that fiber per se with lower prevalence of disease. Therefore this guideline stresses consumption of vegetables, fruits, and grain products. Quantitative guidelines for consumption of these foods are as follows. Have *daily*:

> *Three or more servings of various vegetables* (Count as a serving: 1 cup of raw leafy greens, 1/2 cup of other kinds):
>
> Have dark-green leafy and deep-yellow vegetables often.
>
> Eat dry beans and peas often. (Count 1/2 cup of cooked dry beans or peas as a serving of vegetables or as 1 oz of the meat group.)
>
> Also eat starchy vegetables, such as potatoes and corn.
>
> *Two or more servings of various fruits* (Count as a serving: 1 medium apple, orange, or banana; 1/2 cup of small or diced fruit; 3/4 cup of juice):
>
> Have citrus fruits or juices, melons, or berries regularly.
>
> Choose fruits as desserts and fruit juices as beverages.
>
> *Six or more servings of grain products* (breads, cereals, pasta, and rice) (Count as a serving: 1 slice of bread; 1/2 bun, bagel, or English muffin; 1 oz of dry ready-to-eat cereal; 1/2 cup of cooked cereal, rice, or pasta):
>
> Eat products from a variety of grains, such as wheat, rice, oats, and corn.
>
> Have several servings of whole-grain breads and cereals daily.
>
> Vegetables, fruits, and grain products are generally low in calories if fats and sugars are used sparingly in their preparation and at the table.

Following these guidelines will ensure consumption of foods that contain significant amounts of dietary fiber. These guidelines should be useful in giving specific recommendations for use in nutrition education programs.

Use Sugars Only in Moderation

Foods today may contain several types of sugars that are principally sources of energy but few other nutrients. Sugars are added to foods to impart sweet taste or to act as natural preservatives, thickeners, or aids in baking. The principal reason for this dietary guideline is that foods high in sugars may contain few other nutrients. Thus a diet high in sugars may be low in other essential nutrients.

Simple sugars and starches also contribute to the development of tooth decay because they are good substrates for mouth bacteria that produce dental plaque and the acid products of fermentation that may dissolve portions of the tooth enamel. Although some researchers have linked sugar consumption with heart disease, the evidence is weak and was not considered convincing by the Surgeon General or the NRC panel. Similarly, diets high in sugar have not been shown to cause diabetes. Consumer advice relative to sugar consumption has often concentrated on proper dental hygiene. The following advice is provided by the 1990 edition of the Dietary Guidelines:

Moderate the use of foods containing sugars and starches between meals.

Brush and floss teeth regularly.

Use a fluoride toothpaste.

Ask your dentist or doctor about the need for supplemental fluoride, especially for children.

Do not use a nursing bottle with any beverage other than water as a pacifier.

Use Salt and Sodium Only in Moderation

This guideline calls for caution in use of salt and sodium in foods. The health issue involved is the relationship between salt consumption and hypertension. This relationship of complex. In populations consuming rather low levels of salt and sodium, hypertension is rare. In populations consuming generous amounts of sodium, some individuals, perhaps as many as one-third, may lower their blood pressures with restriction of salt intake. For this reason the dietary guidelines have called for moderation in salt and sodium consumption. There is no established RDA for sodium. The tenth edition of Recommended Dietary Allowances estimates that an intake of about 500 mg of salt per day would provide a safe minimum intake of sodium. The NRC Committee on Diet and Health has also recommended that daily intake of salt (sodium chloride) be limited to 6 g or less.

The primary source of sodium in diets is sodium chloride. The highest salt intake comes from diets high in processed foods because considerable amounts of salt are often added during processing. There is relatively little sodium in fresh fruits, cereals, vegetables, and meats. Sources of dietary sodium other than table salt include sodium bicarbonate and monosodium glutamate, but relative to common salt, these sources are relatively minor.

Dietary Guidelines provide the following advice for moderating the use of salt and sodium:

Use salt sparingly, if at all, in cooking and at the table.

Fresh and plain frozen vegetables prepared without salt are lower in sodium than canned ones.

Cereals, pasta, and rice cooked without salt are lower in sodium than ready-to-eat cereals.

Milk and yogurt are lower in sodium than most cheeses.

Fresh meat, poultry, and fish are lower in sodium than most canned and processed ones.

Most frozen dinners and combination dishes, packaged mixes, canned soups, and salad dressings contain a considerable amount of sodium. So do condiments, such as soy and other sauces, pickles, olives, catsup, and mustard.

Use salted snacks, such as chips, crackers, pretzels, and nuts sparingly. Check labels for the amount of sodium in foods. Choose those lower in sodium most of the time.

If You Drink Alcoholic Beverages, Do So in Moderation

This guideline recognizes that alcoholic beverages are a significant source of energy in the U.S. diet. The gallons per capita of beer, wine, and spirits in the U.S. adult population in 1985 was:

Beer	34.5
Wine	3.8
Distilled spirits	2.5
Total	40.8

Alcoholic beverages provide few other nutrients than energy. The guideline defines moderate drinking as no more than one drink a day for women and two drinks a day for men. A drink is considered 12 oz of regular beer, 5 oz of wine, or 1 oz of distilled spirits (80 proof).

The different recommendations for men and women are related to differences in body size, body water content, and evidence that shows that women absorb alcohol more rapidly than men.[13] The Dietary Guidelines committee also recommended that the following categories of people not drink alcoholic beverages:

Women who are pregnant or trying to conceive: Major birth defects have been attributed to heavy drinking by the mother while pregnant. Women who are pregnant or trying to conceive should not drink alcoholic beverages. However, there is no conclusive evidence that an occasional drink is harmful.

Individual who plan to drive or engage in other activities that require attention or skill: Most people retain some alcohol in the blood three to five hours after even moderate drinking.

Individuals using medicines, even over-the-counter kinds: Alcohol may affect the benefits or toxicity of medicines. Also, some medicines may increase blood alcohol levels or increase alcohol's adverse effect on the brain.

Individuals who cannot keep their drinking moderate: This is a special concern for recovering alcoholics and people whose family members have alcohol problems.

Children and adolescents: Use of alcoholic beverages by children and adolescents involves risks to health and other serious problems.

Dietary guidelines are intended to provide guidance for major components of consumers' diets. These guidelines, along with the RDAs, represent the principal standards of dietary advice. Unfortunately, the more constraints that nutritionists place on diets, the more difficult it becomes to devise menus that meet both dietary guidelines and the RDAs. Restriction of consumption of red meats, for example, to reduce intake of saturated fat, often makes it more difficult to meet the RDA for iron. As one adapts these dietary recommendations to the dietary patterns of different cultures, some compromises may need to be made. Fortunately, diets from several Hispanic traditions emphasize the consumption of cereals, vegetables, and legumes that are consistent with the dietary guidelines.

DIETARY DATA FROM HISPANIC HANES

The National Center for Health Statistics conducted the Hispanic Health and Nutrition Examination Survey (HHANES) in 1982 to 1984 to learn more about the health and nutritional status of Hispanics living in the United States. The survey collected data from three major groups of Hispanics—Mexican-Americans, Cuban-Americans, and Puerto Ricans—selected as follows:[14]

MEXICAN-AMERICANS

Resided in selected counties of Texas, Colorado, New Mexico, Arizona, and California

Surveyed between July 1982 and November 1983

9894 persons sampled; 8554 interviewed

CUBAN-AMERICANS

Resided in Dade County (Miami), Florida

Surveyed between January 1984 and April 1984

2244 persons sampled; 1766 interviewed

PUERTO RICANS

Resided in the New York City area, which included parts of New Jersey and Connecticut

Surveyed between May 1984 and December 1984

3786 persons sampled; 3369 interviewed

HHANES collected many kinds of data through dietary interviews, medical examinations, anthropometric measurements, laboratory tests, and selected diagnostic tests. The dietary data summarized in this section came from a single 24-hour recall that was part of HHANES interviews. Trained interviewers collected and recorded information about the foods that subjects consumed during the previous day. HHANES used many techniques to ensure that the dietary data collected was of high quality. However, because of the way it was designed, HHANES provides regional prevalence estimates for three Hispanic subgroups only, not national estimates for Hispanics in general.

Macronutrient Contribution to Energy Intake

Figures 8.1 and 8.2 show the percentage of energy that subgroups of Hispanic children and adults derived from fat. In general, Cuban-Americans and mainland Puerto Ricans consumed lower percentages of dietary energy as fat (33 to 35%) than did Mexican-Americans (36 to 38%). Although these differences may not be of statistical significance, they are consistent with dietary practices followed by members of these populations (discussed in previous chapters).

Before considering nutrition education for Hispanic groups, it is useful to compare the macronutrient intakes of Hispanics with intakes of the general U.S. population. According to the 1985 USDA Continuing Survey of Food Intake, as cited in the U.S. Surgeon General's Report,[15] adult men in the United States consume about 36% and women about 37% of their daily energy as fat. Both men and women derive 16% of their energy from dietary protein, and men get 45% and women 46% of their energy from carbohydrates. (Data were based on one-day dietary recall obtained by interviewing 658 men, 19–50 years of age, and 1459 women, 19–50 years of age, for the 1985 USDA Continuing Food Consumption Survey—Individual Intake.) Though the trends are not completely consistent, Figure 8.3 (see p. 260)

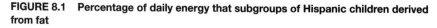

FIGURE 8.1   Percentage of daily energy that subgroups of Hispanic children derived from fat

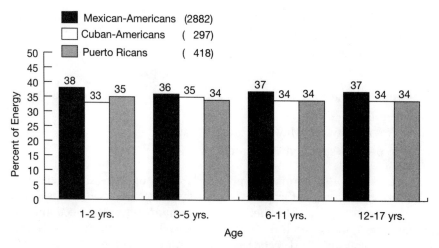

SOURCE: National Center for Health Statistics, *Hispanic Health and Nutrition Examination Survey (HHANES). Dietary practices, food frequency, and total nutrient intakes.* Tape no. 6525, version 3 (Hyattsville, MD, September 1991).

FIGURE 8.2 **Percentage of daily energy that subgroups of Hispanic adults derived from protein, fat, and carbohydrate**

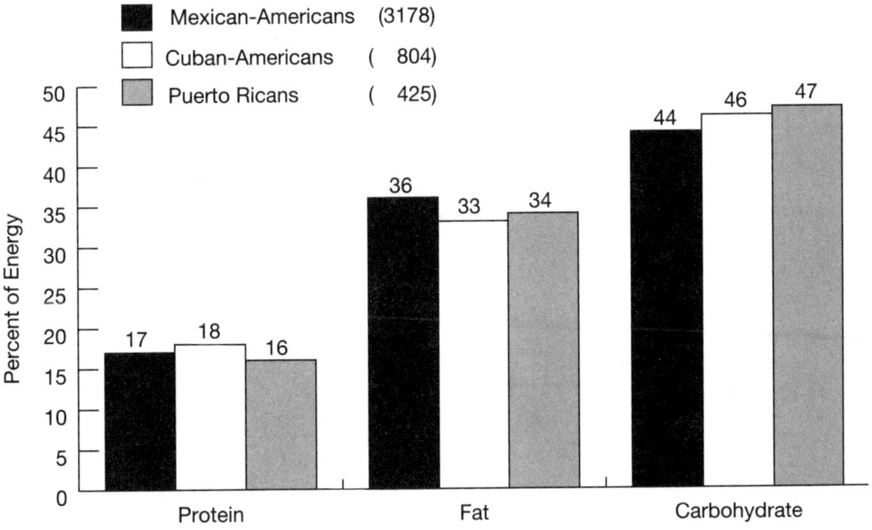

SOURCE: National Center for Health Statistics, *Hispanic Health and Nutrition Examination Survey (HHANES). Dietary practices, food frequency, and total nutrient intakes.* Tape no. 6525, version 3 (Hyattsville, MD, September 1991).

shows that younger Cuban-American and Puerto Rican women consumed a greater proportion of energy as fat than did older women in these subgroups. This difference might be due to a greater adherence by older women to traditional diets. However, as shown in Figure 8.4 (see p. 261), data to support this idea are not as clear among Hispanic men.

Frequency of Consumption of Food Groups

Data from HHANES also provide an opportunity to observe average daily consumption of food groups by children, men, and women (see Tables 8.2, 8.3, and 8.4, pp. 262–264). Although it is somewhat difficult to compare these observations with the numbers of servings recommended by the U.S. Dietary Guidelines, general trends were apparent. For example, Mexican-American men and women consumed more servings of meat each day than did Cuban-Americans or Puerto Ricans. This is consistent with the finding that Mexican-Americans also derived a greater proportion of energy from fat, because meat generally contributes significant amounts of fat to diets. On the other hand, the frequency of vegetable and fruit consumption appears relatively low for all subgroups.

FIGURE 8.3   Percentage of daily energy that subgroups of Hispanic women derived from fat

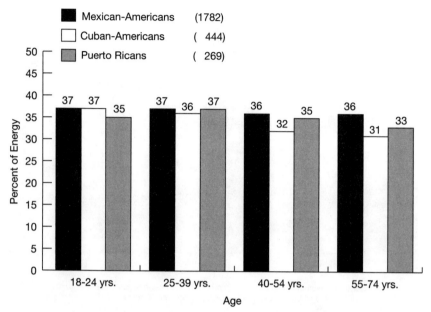

SOURCE: National Center for Health Statistics, *Hispanic Health and Nutrition Examination Survey (HHANES). Dietary practices, food frequency, and total nutrient intakes.* Tape no. 6525, version 3 (Hyattsville, MD, September 1991).

Patterns of Micronutrient Intake

Table 8.5 (see p. 265) shows micronutrient intake among U.S. Hispanic subgroups of Mexican-Americans, Cuban-Americans, and Puerto Ricans. The intakes are expressed as percentages of the levels recommended by the 1989 recommended dietary allowances (RDAs). Men consumed virtually all of the nutrients at levels equal to or greater than the RDAs. Only Cuba-American and Puerto Rican men had lower than recommended intakes of vitamin A.

Women's intakes were more problematic. All women had intakes of vitamin B, calcium, iron, and zinc that were below the RDAs. In addition, Puerto Rican and Cuban-American women had low intakes of vitamin A. These data show similar patterns as data on the micronutrient intake among the general U.S. adult population (Table 8.6, section B, p. 266). Men consumed almost all nutrients (except for vitamin B_6 and folacin) at levels equal to or exceeding the RDAs. Whereas women consumed vitamin B_6, folacin, calcium, iron, and zinc at levels significantly below the RDAs.

It is important to note that the data in Tables 8.5 and 8.6 cannot be directly compared, as Table 8.6 is based on the 1980 RDAs and Table 8.5 is based on the 1989 RDAs. These RDAs are not always the same. For exam-

FIGURE 8.4 Percentage of daily energy that subgroups of Hispanic men derived from fat

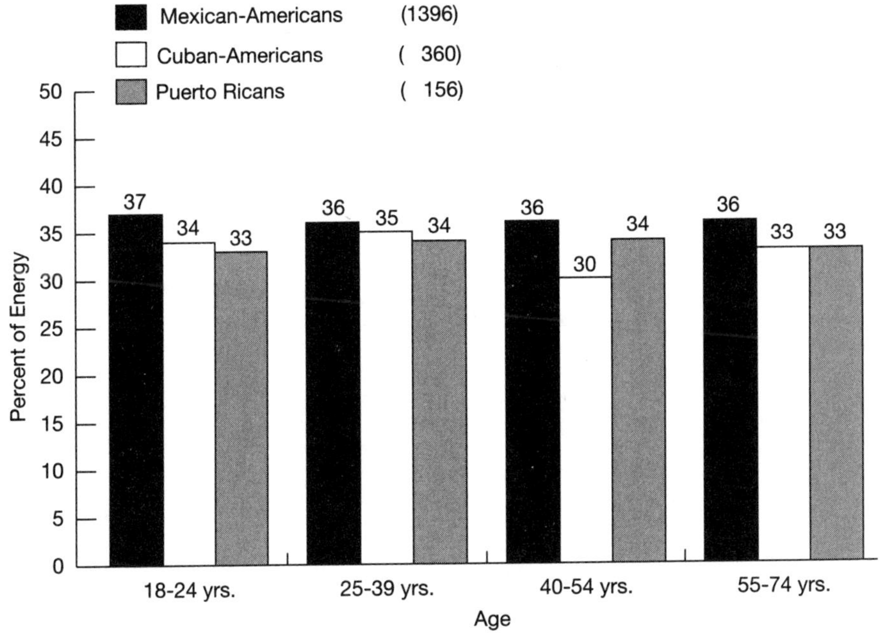

SOURCE: National Center for Health Statistics, *Hispanic Health and Nutrition Examination Survey (HHANES). Dietary practices, food frequency, and total nutrient intakes.* Tape no. 6525, version 3 (Hyattsville, MD, September 1991).

ple, the RDAs for iron and zinc for women were higher in 1980 than in 1989.

Obviously, dietary data alone do not enable one to make direct statements about the potential for dietary deficiency disease in these Hispanic subgroups. Preliminary examination of the HHANES data, beyond dietary data, indicates that the three Hispanic subgroups experienced similar patterns of iron deficiency, elevated serum cholesterol, hypertension, and overweight as the general U.S. population.[16] (Chapter 6 also focuses on issues related to health and disease prevalence among U.S. Hispanics.)

SAMPLES OF MENUS AT THREE CALORIC LEVELS AND MENUS THAT MEET THE U.S. DIETARY GUIDELINES

Tables 8.7 (see p. 267), for Mexican-Americans, and Table 8.8 (see p. 269), for Puerto Ricans, show typical diets for adults at three caloric levels. These sample diets could serve as useful tools for counseling Hispanic clients about diet modification in a culturally relevant context. (See Coll, Sánchez,

TABLE 8.2 Mean Daily Frequency of Consumption of Food Groups by Hispanic Children (24-Hour Recall)

Food Group	Age Group (years)			
	1–2 (N)	3–5 (N)	6–11 (N)	12–17 (N)
Mexican-American (N = 2882)	(388)	(555)	(1067)	(872)
Milk	3.56	3.01	2.80	2.22
Meat	3.06	3.10	2.97	2.73
Bread	2.88	3.12	2.94	2.75
Vegetable	0.72	0.71	0.61	0.52
Fruit	1.20	1.22	0.94	0.78
Fat	1.07	1.20	1.27	1.14
Sugar	1.71	1.93	1.93	2.29
Cuban-American (N = 297)	(39)	(40)	(101)	(117)
Milk	3.91	3.73	3.13	2.25
Meat	2.63	2.43	2.47	2.31
Bread	2.51	2.48	2.38	1.79
Vegetable	0.85	0.64	0.50	0.48
Fruit	1.51	1.41	0.91	0.85
Fat	0.76	1.01	1.21	0.99
Sugar	3.02	2.92	2.63	2.96
Puerto Rican (N = 418)	(55)	(74)	(144)	(145)
Milk	3.83	3.34	3.47	2.95
Meat	2.84	2.92	2.87	3.02
Bread	2.38	2.17	2.42	2.11
Vegetable	0.62	0.47	0.50	0.46
Fruit	1.50	1.11	1.05	0.94
Fat	0.81	1.03	1.28	1.19
Sugar	1.91	2.08	2.31	2.89

SOURCE: National Center for Health Statistics, *Hispanic Health and Nutrition Examination Survey (HHANES). Dietary practices, food frequency, and total nutrient intakes.* Tape no. 6525, version 3 (Hyattsville, MD, September 1991).

TABLE 8.3 Mean Daily Frequency of Consumption of Food Groups by Hispanic Men (24-Hour Recall)

Food Group	Age Group (years)			
	18–24 (N)	25–39 (N)	40–54 (N)	55–74 (N)
Mexican-American (N = 1396)	(307)	(521)	(334)	(234)
Milk	1.72	1.43	1.20	1.38
Meat	3.16	2.98	2.69	2.44
Bread	2.67	2.47	2.33	2.44
Vegetable	0.60	0.70	0.63	0.58
Fruit	0.66	0.68	0.68	0.77
Fat	1.28	1.37	1.41	1.20
Sugar	2.42	2.40	2.33	1.86
Cuban-American (N = 360)	(50)	(86)	(126)	(98)
Milk	2.04	1.75	1.41	1.76
Meat	2.88	2.25	1.91	1.73
Bread	1.72	1.74	1.69	1.79
Vegetable	0.62	0.68	0.63	0.58
Fruit	0.68	0.87	0.77	0.78
Fat	1.39	1.30	1.14	0.89
Sugar	3.12	2.69	2.68	2.18
Puerto Rican (N = 156)	(34)	(55)	(49)	(18)
Milk	2.59	2.00	1.68	1.90
Meat	3.03	2.40	2.10	1.70
Bread	1.86	1.75	1.52	1.40
Vegetable	0.48	0.54	0.67	0.82
Fruit	0.66	0.72	0.84	0.89
Fat	1.13	1.52	1.29	1.41
Sugar	3.04	3.27	2.64	2.52

SOURCE: National Center for Health Statistics, *Hispanic Health and Nutrition Examination Survey (HHANES). Dietary practices, food frequency, and total nutrient intakes.* Tape no. 6525, version 3 (Hyattsville, MD, September 1991).

TABLE 8.4 Mean Daily Frequency of Consumption of Food Groups by Hispanic Women (24-hour Recall)

Food Group	Age Group (years)			
	18–24 (N)	25–39 (N)	40–54 (N)	55–74 (N)
Mexican-American (N = 1782)	(407)	(669)	(433)	(273)
Milk	1.85	1.68	1.57	1.44
Meat	2.69	2.65	2.45	2.07
Bread	2.48	2.55	2.39	2.35
Vegetable	0.60	0.71	0.76	0.68
Fruit	0.88	0.94	0.84	1.02
Fat	1.26	1.42	1.37	1.23
Sugar	2.25	1.99	1.98	1.53
Cuban-American (N = 444)	(58)	(116)	(142)	(128)
Milk	1.65	1.49	1.67	2.03
Meat	2.50	1.97	1.80	1.47
Bread	1.85	1.76	1.84	1.77
Vegetable	0.64	0.65	0.72	0.62
Fruit	0.78	0.88	1.01	1.05
Fat	1.13	1.28	0.96	0.87
Sugar	2.47	2.34	2.89	2.03
Puerto Rican (N = 269)	(60)	(97)	(77)	(35)
Milk	2.15	2.11	2.14	1.82
Meat	2.38	2.34	1.98	1.62
Bread	1.62	1.63	1.51	1.56
Vegetable	0.46	0.59	0.69	0.74
Fruit	0.57	0.93	0.94	0.95
Fat	1.10	1.19	1.15	1.04
Sugar	3.45	2.64	2.38	1.40

SOURCE: National Center for Health Statistics, *Hispanic Health and Nutrition Examination Survey (HHANES). Dietary practices, food frequency, and total nutrient intakes.* Tape no. 6525, version 3 (Hyattsville, MD, September 1991).

TABLE 8.5 Patterns of Micronutrient Intake among the U.S. Hispanic Population, as Percentage of the 1989 Recommended Dietary Allowances

Micronutrients	Men (18–54)	Women (18–54)
Mexican-Americans		
Vitamin A	95.7	99.7
Vitamin C	174.6	142.3
Thiamine	117.1	99
Riboflavin	130.1	110.2
Niacin	141.9	105.7
B_6	107.7	80.9
B_{12}	397.8	260.8
Folacin	168.5	118.9
Calcium	102.6	70.8
Iron	169	73.6
Zinc	112.1	85.9
Cuban-Americans		
Vitamin A	80.7	75.1
Vitamin C	166.5	105.7
Thiamine	117.1	98.6
Riboflavin	119.5	103.5
Niacin	135.8	100.5
B_6	101.7	77.2
B_{12}	401.2	229.1
Folacin	125.6	89.4
Calcium	97.4	70.3
Iron	166.0	76.1
Zinc	115.7	80.9
Puerto Ricans		
Vitamin A	82.4	78.6
Vitamin C	182.4	116.6
Thiamine	124.7	108.1
Riboflavin	123.6	106.7
Niacin	137.9	108.4
B_6	99.3	78.8
B_{12}	304.1	252.8
Folacin	143	98.7
Calcium	93.9	67.6
Iron	164.5	75.8
Zinc	96	77

source: National Center for Health Statistics, *Hispanic Health and Nutrition Examination Survey (HHANES). Dietary practices, food frequency, and total nutrient intakes.* Tape no. 6525, version 3 (Hyattsville, MD, September 1991).

TABLE 8.6   Micronutrient Intakes

A.   Percentages of Total Food Energy Among the U.S. Adult Population

Macronutrient	Men (18-54 yrs.)	Women (18-54 yrs.)
Fat	36	37
Protein	16	16
Carbohydrate	45	46

B.   Percentages of the 1980 (RDAs)

Micronutrients	Men (18-54 yrs.)	Women (18-54 yrs.)
Vitamin A	122	127
Vitamin C	182	133
Thiamine	124	110
Riboflavin	129	115
Niacin	146	130
B_6	85	61
B_{12}	245	156
Folacin	76	51
Calcium	115	78
Iron	159	61
Zinc	94	60

SOURCE: USDA Continuing Survey of Food Intake, 1985, from U.S. Department of Health and Human Services; *The Surgeon General's Report on Nutrition and Health* (Washington, DC, 1988).

TABLE 8.7 Typical Diets of Mexican Adults at Three Caloric Levels

	Menu 1		
	1500 cal	*2000 cal*	*2500 cal*
Breakfast 8–10 a.m.	1 scrambled egg 1 ½ cooking tsp. of fried beans 1 tortilla 1 cup of coffee with sugar	1 scrambled egg/tomato, onion, and green hot pepper 1½ cooking tsp. of fried beans 1–2 tortillas 1cup of coffee with sugar	2 scrambled eggs/tomato, onion, and green hot pepper 2 cooking tsp. of fried beans 1–2 tortillas 1 cup of coffee with sugar
Lunch 1–3 p.m.	1 medium grilled beefsteak/tomato, onion, and green hot pepper 2 cooking tsp. of fried beans 1–2 tortillas 1 large glass of lemonade 2¼ medium baked potatoes	1 medium grilled beefsteak/tomato, onion, and green hot pepper 2 cooking tsp. of fried beans 1–2 tortillas 1 large glass of lemonade 1 cooking tsp. of fried potatoes	1 medium grilled beefsteak/tomato, onion, and green hot pepper 2 cooking tsp. of fried beans 3–4 tortillas 1 large glass of lemonade 1 cooking tsp. of fried potatoes
Dinner 6–9 p.m.	1 cooking tsp. of fried beans 1 tortilla 1 cup of coffee with sugar	2 cooking tsp. of fried beans 1–2 Tortillas 1 cup of coffee with sugar	2 cooking tsp. of fried beans 1–2 tortillas 1 cup of coffee with sugar
Snack 5–6 a.m. 3–4 p.m.		½ tortilla	Coffee with sugar Coffee with sugar 1 tortilla

By substituting flour tortillas with corn tortillas, the caloric content will decrease by approximately 19%. One cooking teaspoon is equivalent to a serving spoon.

TABLE 8.7 Typical Diets of Mexican Adults at Three Caloric Levels (cont.)

	Menu 2		
	1500 cal	*2000 cal*	*2500 cal*
Breakfast 8–10 a.m.	1 scrambled egg 2 cooking tsp. of fried beans 2–4 tortillas 1 cup of coffee with sugar	1 scrambled egg/tomato, onion, and green hot pepper 1 cooking tsp. of fried beans 2–4 tortillas 1 cup of coffee with sugar	2 scrambled eggs/tomato, onion, and green hot pepper 2 cooking tsp. of fried beans 3–4 tortillas 1 cup of coffee with sugar
Lunch 1–3 p.m.	2 tacos of grilled beef/tomato, onion, and salsa (tomato, onion, and green hot pepper) Water	2 tacos of grilled beef/tomato, onion, and salsa (tomato, onion, and green hot pepper) Water	2 tacos of grilled beef/tomato, onion, and salsa (tomato, onion, and green hot pepper) 1 beer
Dinner 6–9 p.m.	1 cooking tsp. of fried potatoes with pork chorizo 1 cooking tsp. of fried beans 1–2 tortillas 1 cup of coffee with sugar	1½ cooking tsp. of fried potatoes with pork chorizo 1 cooking tsp. of fried beans 2–3 tortillas 1 cup of coffee with sugar	1½ cooking tsp. of fried potatoes with pork chorizo 2 cooking tsp. of fried beans 2–3 tortillas 1 cup of coffee with sugar
Snack 5–6 a.m.	Coffee with 1 tsp. of sugar	Coffee with 2 tsp. of sugar	Coffee with 2 tsp. of sugar
3–4 p.m.		½ tortilla	Coffee with 2 tsp. of sugar

By substituting flour tortillas with corn tortillas, the caloric content will decrease by approximately 19%. One cooking teaspoon is equivalent to a serving spoon.

SOURCE: I. Ortega and A Castañeda, personal communication, Center for Food Research and Development, Hermosillo, Sonora, Mexico, October 1992

TABLE 8.8 Typical Diets of Puerto Rican Adults at Three Caloric Levels

	Menu 1		
	1500 cal	2000 cal	2500 cal
Breakfast	Orange juice	Orange juice	Orange juice
	Oatmeal with	Oatmeal with	Oatmeal with
	milk ½ cup	milk ½ cup	milk 1 cup
	Ham 1 slice	Ham 1 slice	Ham 1 slice
	Bread (toast) 1 slice	Bread (toast) 1 slice	Cheese 1 slice
	Margarine 1 tsp.	Margarine 1 tsp.	Bread (toast) 1 slice
	Milk, low-fat ½ cup	Milk, low-fat ½ cup	Margarine 1 tsp.
	Black coffee ½ cup	Black coffee ½ cup	Milk ½ cup
	Artificial sweetener	Artificial sweetener	Black coffee ½ cup
			Artificial sweetener
Lunch	Ham 1 slice	Ham 1 slice	Ham 1 slice
	Cheese 1 slice	Cheese 1 slice	Cheese 1 slice
	Lettuce and	Lettuce and	Lettuce and
	tomatoes 1/2 cup	tomatoes 1/2 cup	tomatoes 1/2 cup
	Bread (toast) 2 slice	Bread (toast) 2 slice	Bread (toast) 2 slice
	Margarine 1 tsp.	Margarine 1 tsp.	Margarine 1 tsp.
	Pear 1 med.	Fruit cake 1 piece 3"	Plain cake 1 piece 3"
	Milk, low-fat ½ cup	Milk, low-fat ½ cup	Milk, low-fat ½ cup
Dinner	Steak with onions	Steak with onions	Steak with onions
	(P.R. style) 2 ounces	(P.R. style) 2 ounces	(P.R. style) 3 ounces
	Rice ½ cup	Rice 1 cup	Rice 1 ½ cup
	Stewed *rosita*	Stewed *rosita*	Stewed *rosita*
	beans ½ cup	beans ½ cup	beans ½ cup
	Peas and carrots ½ cup	Peas and carrots ½ cup	Peas and carrots ½ cup
	Oil/vinegar 2 tsp.	Oil/vinegar 2 tsp.	Oil/vinegar 2 tsp.
	Apple 1 med.	Pineapple	Pineapple
		custard ½ cup	custard ½ cup
	Milk, low-fat ½ cup	Milk ½ cup	Milk ½ cup

TABLE 8.8 Typical Diets of Puerto Rican Adults at Three Caloric Levels (cont.)

	1500 cal		2000 cal (Menu 2)		2500 cal	
Breakfast	Pineapple juice	½ cup	Pineapple juice	1 cup	Pineapple juice	1 cup
	Scrambled egg	(1 egg)	Scrambled eggs	(2 eggs)	Scrambled eggs	(2 eggs)
	Toast	2 slices	Toast	2 slices	Toast	2 slices
	Milk, low-fat	½ cup	Margarine	1 tsp.	Margarine	2 tsp.
	Black coffee	½ cup	Milk, low-fat	½ cup	Milk	½ cup
	Artificial sweetener		Black coffee	½ cup	Black coffee	½ cup
Lunch	Baked chicken	3 oz.	Baked chicken	3 oz.	Baked chicken	3 oz.
	Mashed potatoes	1 cup	Mashed potatoes	1 cup	Mashed potatoes	1 cup
	Peas	½ cup	Peas	½ cup	Peas	½ cup
	Margarine	1 tsp.	Margarine	1 tsp.	Margarine	2 tsp.
	Fruit salad	½ cup.	Fruit salad	½ cup	Cheese cake	2½"
	Milk, low-fat	1 cup	Milk, low-fat	1 cup	Milk, low-fat	1 cup
Dinner	Stewed pork chop with vegetables	2 ounces	Stewed pork chop with vegetables	2 ounces	Stewed pork chop with vegetables	3 ounces
	Stewed rice with pigeon peas	1 cup	Stewed rice with pigeon peas	1 cup	Stewed rice with pigeon peas	1½ cup
	Oil	1 tsp.	Bread	2 slices	Bread	2 slices
	Pear	1 med.	Margarine	1 tsp.	Margarine	1 tsp.
	Milk, low-fat	½ cup	Guava paste	1 piece 2"	Guava paste	1 piece 2"
			Cheese	½ slice	Cheese	½ slice
			Milk	½ cup	Milk	½ cup

SOURCE: Sara Alicea, personal communication, Bayamón Regional Hospital, Puerto Rico, October 1992.

and Zayas[17] for an excellent source of information on diet counseling of Puerto Rican clients.)

Tables 8.9 and 8.10 (see pp. 272, 273) show menus for Mexican-Americans and Mexicans and Puerto Ricans, respectively that meet the U.S. Dietary Guidelines. In Table 8.10, it can be seen that different weekday (menu 1) and weekend (menu 2) consumption patterns emerged for Puerto Ricans, as opposed to patterns reflecting urban/rural differences. Consumption of elaborate-to-prepare traditional dishes was negligible during the week. Increased consumption of vegetables and decreased frying of foods were healthy trends apparent in these menus. For more in-depth background about food consumption patterns among these two major Hispanic groups, see Chapters 3 and 5.

SUMMARY

This chapter discussed the most recent U.S. Dietary Guidelines for consumption of a nutritionally adequate diet by the American population.[18] Discussion of the guidelines was followed by a presentation of dietary data gathered through the 24-hour recall method by HHANES for three major Hispanic subgroups: Mexican-Americans, Cuban-Americans, and Puerto Ricans. The data were compared with similar data for the total U.S. population.

Because the Dietary Guidelines are general recommendations for all Americans, sample menus that translate these recommendations into culturally acceptable diets for both Mexican-Americans and Puerto Ricans were provided. Complementing the sample menus are the following glossaries of common Mexican-American and Puerto Rican foods and mixed dishes, with descriptions of ingredients, weights, and energy values.

Dr. Malden C. Nesheim, chairman of the 1990 Committee on the U.S. Dietary Guidelines, has made invaluable contributions in this chapter. His knowledge and understanding of the nutritional rationale behind the guidelines and his expert discussion of these issues is hereby gratefully acknowledged.

TABLE 8.9 Mexican and Mexican-American Menus Based on U.S. Dietary Guidelines

	Mexican-Americans	Central/South Mexico	North Mexico
Breakfast	Hard white rolls Vegetable oil, margarine Guava jelly Orange juice *Atole de arroz* (with low-fat milk and artificial sweetener) Cafe con leche (with evaporated skim milk)	*Licuado* (with low-fat milk and banana) Fried beans (small amount of vegetable oil) White bread *Salsa* (tomato, *chile*, onion, garlic, coriander)	Potatoes (cooked with tomato, onion, and green hot pepper) Fried beans (small amount of vegetable oil) Corn or flour tortillas (small quantity of shortening) *Licuado* (with low-fat milk and banana)
Lunch	Fish (broiled) Spanish rice Refried beans (fried in small amount of vegetable oil) *Picante salsa* Tortillas Lettuce and tomato salad topped with shredded goat cheese (vinegar/oil dressing) Sugar-free beverage	Cooked rice, with tomato, onion, garlic, and carrots Cooked egg Corn tortillas *Salsa* (tomato, *chile*, onion, garlic, coriander) Lemonade	Tacos of grilled beef with corn tortilla, lettuce, tomato, onion and salsa (tomato, *chile*, onion, garlic, coriander) Pasta, watery soup with vermicelli, tomato, onion, carrots, and squash Orange juice
Dinner	Chicken (baked) *Calabazita* (Mexican squash and *fidello* (vermicelli)) *Picante salsa* Tortillas Vegetable oil, margarine *Flan* (made with skim or low-fat milk) Fresh cold prickly pears Sugar-free breverage	Fried beans with cheese Corn tortillas *Salsa* (tomato, *chile*, onion, garlic, coriander) Tomato *Atole de harina* (with low-fat milk) Bread (biscuit)	Fried beans with low-fat cottage cheese Corn or flour tortillas Coffee with low-fat milk Oatmeal (low-sugar) cookies
Snack		Apple	Grapes

SOURCES: For Mexican-Americans—J. Perkin and S. F. McCann, Food for ethnic Americans: Is the government trying to turn the melting pot into a one-dish dinner? In L. Keller-Brown and K. Mussell (eds.), *Ethnic and regional foodways in the United States* (Knoxville: University of Tennessee Press, 1984). For Mexicans—I. Ortega and A Castaneda, personal communication, Center for Food Research and Development, Hermosillo, Sonora, Mexico, October 1992.

TABLE 8.10 Puerto Rican Menus Based on U.S. Dietary Guidelines

	Menu 1	Menu 2
Breakfast	Orange juice Oatmeal with milk Bread with margarine Coffee with milk	Cornflakes with ripe bananas Coffee with milk
Lunch	Hamburger Lettuce and tomatoes Bread Fruit salad Milk	Spaghetti with meatballs Baked ripe plantain String beans with oil, vinegar dressing Bread with margarine Apples Milk
Dinner	Beef stew with vegetables Seasoned rice with corn Bread with margarine Banana	Rice with chicken Stewed red kidney beans Cabbage and tomatoes Bread with margarine Vanilla custard Milk
Snack	Milk Milk	1/2 Grapefruit

SOURCE: Sara Alicea, personal communication, Bayamón Regional Hospital, Puerto Rico, October 1992.

GLOSSARY OF COMMON MEXICAN-AMERICAN FOODS AND MIXED DISHES

Mixed Dishes	Serving Portion	Weight (g)	Total Caloric Value (cal)
Main Dishes			
Avena con leche	½ cup	120	121.1
Barbacoa	Filling for 1 taco	60	131.4
Bisteck	1 med.	141.7	237.3
Bolillo o birote	1 piece	80	248
Burrito	1 piece	44	137.85
Calabacitas con queso	½ cup	120	114.6
Caldo de albóndigas	1 med. plate with 8 meatballs	214	257
Caldo de papa/queso	1 med. plate	300	159.9
Carne adobada	4 oz.	113.3	415.4
Carne de puerco y chile	4 oz.	113.3	219.9
Carnitas de puerco	Filling for 1 taco	25	67.5
Chicharrones	3 oz.	85	506.6
Chiles rellenos/queso	1 piece	113.3	246.6
Chilaquiles	1 tortilla	75.2	211.1
Chivichangas or chimichangas	1 piece	142	383.9
Chorizo con papas	½ cup	180	664.2
Cocido o puchero	1 cup	235	209
Ejotes/chile colorado	½ cup	300	277.4
Enchilada	1 piece	43	94.4
Ensalada de pollo	1 cup	87.3	80
Guisado de lengua	5 oz.	141.7	217.9
Huevos rancheros	1 egg	72.8	134.3
Menudo	1 med. plate	280	378.6
Nopales	½ cup	78	17.9
Picadillo	Filling for 1 taco	41	69.3
Pollo en mole	3 oz.	114	201
Pozole	1 med. plate	180	517.4
Quesadillas	1 piece	75	179.3
Salpicón	3 oz.	85	87.5
Sopes	1 piece	69.5	196
Taco with beef and fried	1 piece	68	100.9
Tamal salado	1 piece	84.1	213.9
Torta	1 piece	208.8	386.8

Side Dishes

Frijoles de la olla	½ med. plate	166	195.9
Frijoles machacados	½ cup	160	227.2
Frijoles refritos	½ cup	150	495
Guacamole	1 teaspoon	18	26
Papas fritas	21 pieces	85	232.9
Salsa	1 teaspoon	13.3	11.6
Sopa de arroz	½ cup	120	130.8
Sopa de fideo	1 cup	226	123.5
Sopa de Macarrón	½ cup	120	130.8
Tortilla de harina	1 piece	31	123.7
Tortilla de maíz	1 piece	40	91.6
Tripas de leche	3 oz.	85	187

Desserts

Ate	1 small piece	25	110.2
Bollo	1 piece	50	192
Buñuelo	1 piece	46	123.1
Cajeta	1 package	45	179.5
Churros	1 med.	39	152.5
Concha	1 piece	57	205.8
Empanada	1 piece	100	278.8
Tamal dulce	1 piece	187	493.4

Beverages

Atole	3/4 cup	188	206.8
Champurrado	3/4 cup	188	158.6
Chocolate	3/4 cup	188	188
Licuado/plátano	1 med. glass	240	174.9

GLOSSARY OF PUERTO RICAN FOOD WITH PORTION SIZE, WEIGHT IN GRAMS, AND CALORIC VALUE

Mixed Dishes	Serving Portion	Weight (g)	Total Caloric Value (cal)
Bread and raisin pudding	1 3"x2"	95	260
Breadfruit fritter	2	29	64
Breaded beef	3 oz.	145	339
Carbonated beverages	1 cup	240	100
Cassava with creole sauce	1 piece	230	311
Chicken fricasseé	1 piece with potatoes	195	410

Codfish salad	1 cup toast	170	372
Codfish with starchy vegetables	2 tablespoons plus veg.	573	1091
Codfish fritters	1 3½" diam.	34	173
French fried potatoes	10	65	113
Green banana, pickled	½ cup	75	286
Green plantain fritter	2	80	113
Ham and cheese sandwich	1	113	338
Ham and fried egg sandwich	1	131	360
Ice cream	½ cup	74	168
Malt beer	1 cup	250	222
Mango	1 med.	200	113
Mashed green plantain with pork cracklings	1 ball	64	223
Meatballs	3 med.	150	387
Meat turnover	1 piece 4"x2x¾"	55	281
P.R. meat and vegetable stew	1 cup	450	497
Pork blood sausage	1 piece 1½"	28	111
Pork chop, fried	3 oz.	85	355
Pork cracklings	1 oz.	28	103
Pork, roasted	2½oz.	100	230
Ripe plantain meat pie	1 piece 4"x2"	190	596
Ripe plantain meat rolls	1 piece 2x"2"	58	296
Roast chicken	¼ chicken	147	120
Scrambled eggs	¾ cup	64	94
Seasoned ground beef for stuffing	1/2 cup	86	372
Seasoned rice with chicken	1 cup	205	468
Seasoned rice with pigeon peas	1 cup	178	385
Seasoned rice with squid	1 cup	160	440
Seasoned rice with Vienna sausages	1 cup	180	477
Soda crackers	2	10	44
Sofrito (P.R. seasoning)	1 tablespoon	15	46
Soupy rice with chicken	1 cup	366	415

Spanish coffee cake	17" diam.	86	325
Spanish omelet	1 piece 3"x⅜" diam.	175	629
Steak with onion P.R. style	1 piece 5"x2"	125	397
Stewed chicken gizzards	½ cup	130	257
Stewed corned beef	½ cup	140	293
Stewed liver, kidney, heart, lungs (*gandinga*)	1 cup	165	195
Stewed pig's feet	1 cup	290	341
Stuffed potato fritter	1 piece 4"x2 ¼"	95	219
Sweet orange	1 med.	163	61
Tannier fritter	1	60	230
Tripe stew	1 cup	300	359
Vanilla custard	½ cup	120	259
Vienna sausage	1 cup	175	298

NOTES

1. J. Perkin and S. F. McCann, Food for ethnic Americans: Is the government trying to turn the melting pot into a one-dish dinner? In L. Keller-Brown and K. Mussell (eds.), *Ethnic and regional foodways in the United States* (Knoxville, University of Tennessee Press, 1984).

2. E. N. Whitney and E. M. N. Hamilton, *Understanding nutrition,* 2nd ed. (St. Paul, MN: West, 1981).

3. Perkin and McCann, Food for ethnic Americans.

4. Whitney and Hamilton, *Understanding nutrition.*

5. U.S. Senate, Select Committee on Nutrition and Human Needs. *Dietary goals for the United States,* 2nd ed. (Washington, DC: U.S. Government Printing Office, 1977).

6. U.S. Department of Agriculture and U.S. Department of Health, Education, and Welfare, *Nutrition and your health: Dietary Guidelines for Americans* (Washington, DC, 1980).

7. U.S. Department of Agriculture and U.S. Department of Health and Human Services, *Nutrition and your health—Dietary Guidelines for Americans,* 3rd. ed., Home and Garden Bulletin no. 232 (Washington, DC: U.S. Government Printing Office, 1990).

8. U.S. Department of Health and Human Services, *The Surgeon General's Report on Nutrition and Health.* DHHS (PHS) Publication no. 88–50210 (Washington, DC, 1988).

9. National Research Council, *Diet and health: Implications for reducing chronic disease risk.* (Washington, DC: National Academy Press, 1989).

10. Health and Welfare Canada, *Nutrition recommendations,* Report of the Scientific Review Committee (Ottawa: Canadian Government Publication Centre, 1990).

11. Department of Health, *Report on health and social subjects—41 Dietary reference values for food energy and nutrients for the United Kingdom* (London: HMSO Publication Centre, 1991).

12. National Research Council, *1989 recommended dietary allowances,* 10th ed. (Washington, DC: National Academy Press, 1990).

13. M. Frezza, C. Di Padova, G. Pozzato, M. Terpin, E. Baraona, and C. Lieber, High blood alcohol levels in women: Role of decreased gastric alcohol dehydroge-

nase activity and first-pass metabolism. *New England Journal of Medicine, 322* (1990), 95–99.

14. National Center for Health Statistics, *Hispanic Health and Nutrition Examination Survey (HHANES). Dietary practices, food frequency, and total nutrient intakes.* Tape no. 6525, version 3 (Hyattsville, MD, September 1991).

15. U.S. Department of Health and Human Services, *Surgeon General's Report on Nutrition and Health.*

16. M. Fanelli-Kuczmarski and C. Woteki, Monitoring the nutritional status of the Hispanic population: Selected findings for Mexican-Americans, Cubans and Puerto Ricans. *Nutrition Today,* May/June 6–11, 1990.

17. M. Coll-Camalez, E. Sánchez, and E. S. de Zayas, *Siluetas que pueden cambiar,* 4th ed. (Isabela, Puerto Rico: Isabela Printing, Inc., 1991).

9

Reaching Hispanics Through Diet Counseling and Nutrition Education

THE PROCESS OF DIET COUNSELING

Understanding and Counseling Culturally Diverse Clients

Recent years have witnessed increasing interest in the role of multicultural awareness in counseling. Cultural diversity is a reality in the United States, and many health providers counsel people who are different from themselves.[1] There is disagreement, however, on how best to meet the needs of culturally diverse clients. Some believe that existing counseling strategies are effective for all people and that trying to categorize the traits of different cultural groups only perpetuates stereotypes.[2] Others believe that existing counseling models—based on middle-class—dominant cultural values, are ineffective with people from other cultures. The main thrust of this chapter, however, is to emphasize that learning, understanding, respecting, and accepting diverse cultural ways are imperative if one is to become an effective diet counselor or health or nutrition educator.

Table 9.1, adapted from Casas and Vásquez,[3] illustrates a framework for dietary counseling with Hispanic clients. A key issue, they argue, is for counselors to be aware of their own professional and personal beliefs and values. Similarly, it is important to understand clients' cultural beliefs and practices that could conflict with those of the counselor. In every culture it is common to assume that much of the world is "just like us." In the health care and nutrition field, there may be even more of a tendency to consider "our" medicine and foods as better than "theirs." However, what we describe as "good tasting food" or "good for you" food may not be considered so by a Hispanic client.

In short, effective diet counseling begins when a counselor develops respect and cultural empathy for the values, beliefs, and feelings of others. *Cultural empathy* refers to the capacity to understand many individuals who are vastly different from the counselor. An empathic counselor is one who has the ability to generate a maximum number of thoughts, words, and behaviors to communicate with a variety of diverse groups inside and outside the counselor's culture.[4] The ability and willingness to understand both one's own world view and that of others is the key to effective counseling.

Even though Hispanics are a major segment of the American population that influences Anglo culture, Hispanics are little understood by most other Americans. Axelson cites a Harris poll that found that 62% of non-Hispanics nationwide have had no real contact with the Latino community.[5] In view of this lack of contact, this chapter discusses key issues involved in providing effective, sensitive dietary counseling for Hispanics.

A complex and challenging task for nutrition workers is to identify the factors that affect health- and food-related behavior. Many health and nutrition textbooks review theories for understanding and explaining how individuals decide to change their health behavior. The health belief model, health locus-of-control theory, social cognitive theory, person-centered approach, behavior modification, modeling, theory of reasoned action, and innovation dif-

TABLE 9.1   A framework for counseling Hispanic clients

Counselor Variables		Client Variables		
Professional	Personal	Sociocultural	Sociohistorical	Environmental
Assumptions	Assumptions	Values	Life Experiences	
Values	Values	Attitudes	Statistics	
Attitudes	Attitudes	Norms	Demographic Characteristics	
Biases	Biases	Behaviors	Racial/Ethnic Background	
Sterotypes	Stereotypes	Value Orientations	Socioeconomic Status	
Behaviors	Behaviors		Immigrant Status	
			Health Status	

SOURCE: Adapted from J.M. Casas and M.J.T. Vásquez, Counseling the Hispanic client: A theoretical and applied perspective. In P.B. Pedersen et al.; Counseling across cultures, 3rd ed. (Honolulu: University of Hawaii Press, 1989).

fusion theory are a few of the most common theories used to explain nutrition and health behavior.[6] Because effective diet counseling also leads to behavioral changes, it is important to consider the impact of changes on people. Terry notes that health behavior research during the last 20 years has emphasized that individuals have logical reasons for such behaviors as eating certain foods or feeding children in particular ways.[7] Health behaviors are consistent with attitudes, beliefs, and resources and are adapted to use in cultural and physical environments. To affect any nutrition or food behavior, the etiology of that behavioral pattern must be well understood and respected.

As described in Chapter 1, *Hispanic* is a generic term that connotes a culture shared by several ethnic subgroups. Common features of these different subgroups include the use of the Spanish language, influence of Catholic traditions, respect for the traditional family, and warm, interpersonal relationships. But beyond these similarities, there is also much intracultural diversity among Hispanic subcultural groups.

Diet counseling has been defined as "providing individualized professional guidance to assist a person in adjusting his/her daily food consumption to meet his/her needs."[8] Listening is an important component of interviewing and counseling, and the very first step in establishing good communication with the client. Other counselor qualities that contribute to a successful interview are an ability to establish rapport, attentiveness, openness, and an understanding of the client's situation.[9]

Understanding Why People Eat the Way They Do

A fundamental principle of diet counseling is that nutrition information must be introduced so that an individual discovers *personal meaning* in it. A health provider who takes time to collect nutrition information through interviews or informal conversation will be able to provide more meaningful counseling. Information about food preferences and consumption of traditional foods and patterns of eating away from home is helpful in mapping out strategies for effective diet counseling. Further information about household economics

(Who is the main breadwinner? Is the mother employed full or part time?), family size and composition, and the person responsible for food purchasing, preparation, and distribution within the household can also be invaluable. In short, effective diet counseling must be appropriate within an individual's particular context.

Respect, Not Tolerance, for Traditional Foods

As discussed in Chapter 2, traditional foods or staples that are deeply rooted in an indigenous culture have important symbolic and emotional meanings. People do not tire easily of staple foods, and it is difficult to find substitutes for such foods in their diet. Therefore it is useful for health practitioners to know whether particular traditional foods are an integral part of an individual's diet, for they will perhaps offer the greatest emotional resistance to dietary change.

Traditional food practices have a logic of their own, even if it is not immediately apparent to outsiders. Too many well-intentioned efforts have been founded on a paternalistic, almost condescending, attitude without respecting an individual's right to make food choices. If diet counseling is to establish a closer meaningful relationship between a health practitioner (teacher or change agent) and a Hispanic client (learner), then it should be based on respect for the learner's values and customs. To be an instrument of change, diet counselors must recognize the *moral burden* inherent in attempting to change people's diets.

Spicer notes that assuming responsibility for changing people's customs is greater than that of conducting surgery:

> When a surgeon takes his instruments, he assumes the responsibility for a human life, whereas a change agent carries a heavier responsibility. Whenever he seeks to alter a people's way of life, he is dealing not with one individual, but with the well-being and happiness of generations of men and women.[10]

Dealing with change, including dietary change, involves values. If they conflict, should the values of the educator or those of the learner take precedence? In recommending that a learner change a particular food practice, the change agent also assumes that his or her values are superior to those of the learner. The responsible and sensitive diet counselor must respect the personal and cultural values of others. Simple tolerance is not enough. A perceived threat or lack of respect often causes people to cling more tenaciously to their traditional dietary values and practices. The ethics of helping individuals change food behaviors begins with an understanding of their culture, recognizing the good in it and the assumptions that underlie it.

Diet Counseling in a Culturally Relevant Context

Diet counseling begins with an interview, to obtain specific diet history from the client while maintaining an interpersonal environment conducive to disclosure by the client. According to Lee and Nieman, conditions that increase

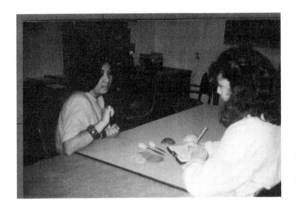

Diet counseling should begin with respect for the personal and cultural values of the Hispanic clients.

interviewing effectiveness include comfortable physical surroundings, freedom from interruption and interference, and privacy.[11] Interviewing about diet history may be perceived as threatening by a Hispanic client because it concerns personal control over food, especially if the interview is conducted in English. Again, it is imperative for health practitioners to establish initial trust and rapport by respecting the personal and cultural values of clients.

There is an old saying that if you want to know about water, never ask a fish. The point is that we take our own language, ideologies, and culture for granted. Most of us are not aware of the extent to which culture affects everything we see, or do, or think. Each of us is held hostage by our cultural heritage in thousands of subtle ways. Range notes that it is critical for health providers to know their own culture, values, assumptions, and expectations, including what they expect in a clinical or hospital setting, how they expect their clients to behave, and what the clients define as health, disease, and good nutrition.[12] Health providers bring all of their cultural orientations when sitting down with clients, who, in turn, bring another set of values, assumptions, and expectations.

Adult human behavior is directed more by cultural values than by basic biological needs, including the need for food. Thus biological needs are usually met within what the culture or subculture prescribes as suitable. Culture, paradoxically, also encourages *ethnocentrism*, the uncritical acceptance of one's own values and lifestyle as the most appropriate. Yet people can move across ethnic boundaries. Health practitioners must overcome natural ethnocentric perspectives and biases if they want to become better nurturing agents of change.

Beyond cultural considerations, diet counseling should also involve goal setting. Goals should be set and agreed to by both client and counselor, and these must be specific, reasonable, measurable, and most important, attainable. Dietary change must be approached with flexibility and anticipation of lapses. Clients and counselors must be aware that the resumption of unwanted habits or behaviors is possible; therefore corrective actions must also be discussed and planned as integral parts of the goal-setting process of dietary change.[13]

Intracultural Variation

As stated earlier, culture has a profound effect on the way health is defined and experienced. For example, some cultures may view health as being determined by fate, acts of God, or as an imbalance of supernatural forces, rather than by biological or environmental forces. A nonjudgmental understanding of these different beliefs and practices can enhance the effectiveness of dietary counseling. On the other hand, it is equally important to recognize that not all members of a cultural group have the same beliefs.

Like many other subcultural groups, Hispanics have different life experiences in the United States, according to their language skill, socioeconomic status, educational background, racial/ethnic background, and legal and citizenship status. The covariables of race and ethnicity illustrate diversity among Hispanics. Depending on geographic origin (Costa Rica, Dominican Republic, Guatemala, or Panama), Hispanics may be classified as Caucasian, Negroid, Indian, Oriental, or various combinations of these races. Economic status and educational background provide other examples of diversity. These differences in socioeconomic status among various Hispanic groups affect health and nutritional status (as discussed in previous chapters). Though Hispanics share a common history, ancestry, language, and traditions, each of the many ethnic subgroups follows its own unique social and cultural practices.

Another difference among Hispanic subpopulations is their use of medical care. In analyzing national data on medical care expenditures, Schur et al. found that persons of Puerto Rican origin used health care services very differently from persons of Cuban or Mexican origin.[14] Puerto Ricans were almost twice as likely as other Hispanics to use a hospital outpatient department or emergency room as a primary source of care. Puerto Ricans also were almost twice as likely as Mexicans and more than four times as likely as Cubans to be covered by Medicaid. Cubans, on the other hand, were most often privately insured. These data point to the importance of developing health strategies for particular Hispanic audiences. For example, in areas with a high concentration of Puerto Ricans, it might be most effective to focus on improving the public health care system and making it biculturally accessible. In areas with many Cubans or Mexicans who tend to visit doctor's offices, it might be more important to focus on educating private practice doctors about special health needs of these groups.

Casas and Vásquez also note that when health practitioners are familiar with particular Hispanic ethnic groups, the practitioners are less likely to make stereotypical assumptions about Hispanic clients.[15] The authors further suggest that differences in socioeconomic status among subgroups of Hispanics are related to immigration factors and degrees of acculturation and assimilation.

A person's cultural identity is dynamic, changing as a result of contact with different groups. This process of change, or *acculturation*, occurs naturally over time. Fieldhouse defines acculturation as the process by which groups and individuals adapt to the norms and values of an alien culture.[16] Acculturation also refers to the acquisition of a new cultural identity, but does not preclude retention of the old; a person may become bicultural, identifying with a new culture, without discarding any elements of the old culture.

As described previously, many Hispanic immigrants to the United States have maintained their original language, religion, and food customs, while also acquiring some of the values, practices, and language of the new culture needed to function in the new society. People have become bilingual and bicultural, identifying with and blending two cultures. As González et al. explain, the extreme of acculturation is *assimilation*, where an individual or group completely adopts a new culture.[17] Gradually the values, practices, or traditions of the original culture are replaced by those of the new.

Assimilation is sometimes a painful process for Hispanic migrants, who feel severe conflicts between the pressure to assimilate and of maintaining loyalty to their original culture. The decision to assimilate is one of many coping strategies that migrants use to survive or to avail themselves of opportunities in the newer society. Because cultural identity is dynamic, there is always intracultural variation regarding tendencies toward continuity and change within subcultural groups. In short, socioeconomic variables as well as cultural variables help account for the intracultural diversity found among different Hispanic groups.

Guidelines for Effective Cross-Cultural Counseling

As stated earlier, perhaps the key component of successful cross-cultural counseling is the ability to respect cultural differences in behaviors, feelings, and cognitions and to understand the socioeconomic and environmental issues relevant to particular ethnic groups. To understand the health and nutritional consequences of the diet prescription, a considerable knowledge of the patient is central to effective counseling. Following is a list of guidelines one can apply in a cross-cultural counseling interview.

1. Become familiar with your own beliefs and values and how these differ from your client's beliefs and values.

2. Become familiar with client's traditional foods and what role these play in social and religious activities.

3. Do not act on first impressions. Understand a client's nonverbal communication and cultural expressions of concern. Gestures and facial expressions are sometimes more indicative of a person's true feelings than are words.

4. Explain diet rationale and inquire about the client's own conception of the illness (cause, prevention, and treatment) and how he or she views the consequences of it.

5. Be aware of the extent of the use of traditional medicine or healers among your clients.

6. Be patient during the interview, and use common words while attempting to understand their ideas and feelings.

7. Explain health and nutritional behaviors that are beneficial, detrimental, and neutral. Try to modify only those behaviors that you deem harmful.

Individual Hispanics are often at different stages of the acculturation process, as illustrated by the apparently acculturated Hispanic in the workplace who returns to traditional values and attitudes at home. Ruiz points out that Hispanics can range from "completely Hispanic" to "completely Anglo," but most fall somewhere in between.[18]

Casas and Vásquez cite the following ways in which Hispanics often differ from Anglo-Americans:[19]

Hispanics often display a great concern for immediacy and the "here and now."

Hispanics frequently attribute control to an external locus, such as luck, supernatural powers, or acts of God.

Hispanics often take a concrete, tangible approach rather than an abstract approach to life.

Hispanics may show respect for authority by avoiding eye contact and remaining silent.

Hispanics may develop multilingual communication skills, using English, Spanish, and "Spanglish," a hybrid of the two.

It is helpful for diet counselors and other health providers to be aware of such general culturally dictated traits. However, it is also as important to be aware of individual intracultural variations.

THE PROCESS OF DIETARY COMPLIANCE

Diseases of Overconsumption

A paradox of today's world is that while most of it contends with problems of undernutrition, the industrialized segment is faced with problems of overnutrition or, as they have been called by an expert committee of the American Society of Clinical Nutrition (ASCN), "the diseases of overconsumption."[20] The ASCN report describes atherosclerotic disease, diabetes, hypertension, liver disease, dental caries, and obesity as diseases that may be influenced by dietary practices. These diseases are also called "diseases of affluence" because they are relatively rare in low-income segments of developing countries and become more common as economic conditions improve.

Development of atherosclerotic disease is associated with diets high in fat, especially saturated fat, and cholesterol. Diets that are high in animal products are also high in fat and cholesterol, and the use of animal products almost invariably increases as economic conditions improve. Liver disease, on the other hand, is associated with excessive alcohol consumption, hypertension with high salt intake in some individuals, and dental caries with consumption of certain forms of sugar.

Obesity, a common condition in industrialized countries, is of complex etiology. Although obesity can be controlled by reduced caloric intake, few obese people have had success at losing weight and maintaining the loss. The complex etiology of obesity involves variations in efficiency of energy utilization, control of caloric intake, physical activity, and social and psychological factors.

There is also some evidence that certain dietary patterns are associated with the development of certain cancers. High consumption of fat has been linked with increased incidence of breast cancer in women, and increased consumption of dietary fiber has been linked with lowered incidence of colon cancer.

However, most evidence associating dietary intakes with chronic diseases is not definitive. Most of these diseases are of complex etiology, and diet is only one of several environmental variables that may affect incidence. Because diet counseling and nutrition education may be of paramount importance in treating these diseases, becoming an effective counselor among urban multicultural clients will be useful for health practitioners working in these communities.

Factors Affecting Dietary Compliance

Dietary compliance refers to commitment and adherence to a medically prescribed dietary regime or treatment that requires fundamental change in present food behaviors. It is generally agreed that dietary compliance offers the best hope for control of some diseases, such as diabetes. As important as this is in clinical nutrition, there has been very limited research to assess factors that affect whether a person does or does not comply with a particular diet therapy. Psychologists seem to recognize, more than other health professionals, that medical outcomes depend on both behavioral and psychosocial factors. Following is a brief review of three conceptual models affecting diet compliance. Readers are also encouraged to review other excellent resources, including Terry's and Lee and Nieman's recent texts, which include sections on this topic.

Many factors affect an individual's ability to comply.[21] Rosenstock's health belief model, reviewed by Becker and Maiman,[22] identifies the following elements as predictors of preventive health care behavior:

The *individual's perceptions,* determined by his or her subjective notions of susceptibility and severity of the condition or disease state.

The *likelihood of action,* determined as a patient weighs the perceived benefits against the barriers involved in the treatment.

The *cues to action,* which must be present to trigger appropriate behavior. These can come from the family, media, or interaction with a health professional.

A central assumption of Rosentock's health belief model is that demographic, personal, situational, and social factors can affect an individual's ability to follow a course of treatment. This underlying assumption is well supported in the literature as a predictor of compliance behavior.

Another model, the Janis-Mann conflict theory model,[23] also assumes that people weigh the benefits of the recommendations against the costs or barriers, but it goes further by suggesting that compliance occurs only when the following three conditions are satisfied:

1. Conflict is aroused—the patient is aware of the risks of any alternative.

2. The person is optimistic about finding a satisfactory solution to the problem.

3. The person believes there is adequate time to search and deliberate before a final decision is required.

When these three conditions are satisfied, the patient is said to be coping in a "vigilant manner."

A common drawback of some of these conceptual frameworks is the underlying assumption that people's behavior is basically a function of reasoned action. However, extraneous mediating factors may delay or impede people from taking entirely rational, logical actions. Furthermore, it is estimated that an average of about 50% of patients comply with prescribed dietary or medical regimens.[24]

A compliance model has been developed by Jenny for diabetic instruction.[25] Three groups of elements or factors make up the model: *enabling* factors that have a positive effect on motivation, *modifying* factors that have a negative effect on motivation, and *facilitating* factors that operate to promote a positive adjustment between enabling and modifying factors. According to Jenny, because compliance results from a patient's decision, there is no direct connection to the facilitating factors.

A culturally adapted version of Jenny's model might be useful for facilitating diet compliance among Hispanics, given that high prevalence rates of diabetes have been reported among Hispanics, especially among Mexican-Americans.[26]

Selected Issues Associated with Noncompliance

Demographic Characteristics   Good health does not serve as a motivational force for healthy people to change eating patterns. Usually only when health is threatened will dietary action be taken voluntarily, and even then, a client's perception of health is affected by age, sex, income, and other biomedical and sociomedical factors.[27] In general, pessimism, alienation, skepticism, and fatalism—factors that contribute to noncompliance—appear to be associated with lower income and educational levels. Becker and Maiman note a relationship between extremes of age and noncompliance.[28] The very young are often resistant to making dietary changes and ingesting bad-tasting medicines; the very old may experience problems with memory and self-neglect. Howard and Herbold[29] give the example of the adolescent diabetic who is in poor control of his illness. Concerned with the here and now and with peer relations, this teenager will not be motivated by the threat of secondary diabetes complications. Social or academic incentives might be better avenues through which to motivate diet change.

The effective dietary counselor needs to be aware that for older Hispanics, for example, past history has great relevance to the present problem. With time constraints, a clinical nutritionist may be more interested in finding out how a client's "present food intake is related to weight loss" rather than in listening to the client describe what she "used to eat back home." The diet counselor may tune out the client's past history. However, the past and the present interrelate so complexly for most Hispanics that understanding and appreciating the past is essential to an understanding of the present situation.[30]

Individual Dispositions   Fear and anxiety are normal responses to serious diagnoses. Moderate levels of fear and anxiety are positively correlated with treatment compliance, whereas extremely high or low levels are associated with noncompliance. Locus of control (one's perception of control over the outcome of events) is also associated with compliance. Some Hispanics view fate or God's will (external locus of control) rather than personal behavior (internal locus of control) as responsible for their health condition. The stronger the client's commitment to external locus of control, the less likely is compliance.

Situational Demands   Dietary compliance often requires that a client make profound personal changes. The more rigid the recommendations for change in lifestyle and the longer the duration required, the less likely is compliance. Psychological costs exact a toll. For example, a Hispanic mother who cooks for family and friends will have difficulty complying with a diet that does not include core staple foods. Recommendations to change consumption of secondary core foods or complements to the main foods would be easier for the woman to comply with.

Other innovative approaches, such as establishing groups or "buddy" systems, where senior members of the group are assigned to newer members to help them on an individual basis, have been successful in the treatment of obesity and alcoholism. Educational activities could include supermarket tours, exploration of food labels, and/or short concrete demonstrations. Through these activity-oriented experiences Hispanic clients can learn, visualize, and practice, for example, how to reduce sodium, fat, or sugar in the diet. Activities can accomplish more in promoting dietary change than the distribution of written materials, even if they have been translated into Spanish. Connor et al. demonstrated that clients successfully reduced consumption of dietary fat by visualizing daily fat intake and practicing substitution of complex carbohydrates for fat.[31]

Networking and Developing Support Systems Family members, relatives, neighbors, and friends are the primary support system for Hispanics. Family, in particular, confers a sense of identity and self-worth and provides social support.[32] Perhaps more than a clinical counselor, the family can help a patient adhere to a particular dietary treatment; thus, the counselor might try to involve other family members in any plan for change. This might be particularly helpful for older patients, especially if they are limited in English or reading skills.

When restriction of salt, fat, sweets, or alcohol or an increase in daily exercise is recommended, family members might be able to provide encouragement for the client. Similarly, family members could remind patients of appointments and medication schedules and help remove any barriers to compliance. For example, the whole family might agree to stop salting food at the table.

Counselor-Client: Partners in Treatment Lewis notes that health professionals bear much of the responsibility for treatment,[33] but this may be by choice. There is a certain degree of ego involvement in the patient-clinician relationship. Having the authority to prescribe a treatment gives the health professional a sense of importance; sharing this responsibility also requires sharing recognition for successful treatment. Involving clients as active members in their own health care demands that they have knowledge, responsibility, and active participation. A culturally empathic counselor can begin by thoroughly describing any treatment, including the benefits and risks of compliance and noncompliance. What compliance really entails is a series of trade-offs, where the patient changes certain behaviors to obtain certain benefits.

Realistically speaking, it is difficult for most people to make radical changes all at once. In a real client-counselor partnership, with family support, it is possible to compromise in order to come as close to the ideal as possible. When clients finally take responsibility for their health, dietary compliance will be of minor concern to clinical nutritionists and health providers. The traditional medical model presents a clinician with a particular problem or illness, but not with a complex person who lives in an environment that shapes his or her behavior. Viewing the patient as a whole person, with multiple physical and emotional needs, may help health providers to develop successful strategies to improve the quality of life of their clients.

THE PROCESS OF NUTRITION EDUCATION

As an extension of Freire's message—"Literacy means reading not only the word, but also the world"—[34] nutritional literacy, and thus nutrition education, should mean more than knowing technical aspects of nutrition. It should also involve examination of the world and the issues that generate nutrition problems, so that any proposed solutions are culturally relevant and valid.

Views on Nutrition Education as a Process

The American Dietetic Association (ADA) takes the position that nutrition education should be available to all individuals and families. ADA views nutrition education as "the process by which beliefs, attitudes, environmental influences, and understandings about food lead to practices that are scientifically sound, practical, and consistent with individual needs and available food resources."[35] The underlying assumption is that nutrition education should focus on establishing and protecting nutritional health rather than on crisis intervention. Thus everyone, regardless of income, culture, social, or economic practices or level of education, should have access to nutrition education throughout the life cycle.

Two decades ago Berg recognized that an information gap could lead to poor nutrition.[36] Berg observed rampant malnutrition among youngsters in third world countries, even when adequate foodstuffs were available to their families. Based on his observations, Berg defined nutrition education as "the process of acquainting people with the value of resources already available to them, and persuading them to change existing practices."

From any viewpoint, nutrition education involves a conscious effort to alter food-related practices or attitudes when the need exists. It is also a multidisciplinary process that involves transfer of information, development of motivation, and modification of food habits. For nutrition education to take place, there must be a diagnosis of the nature and magnitude of the problem and a plan of action. For any plan to work, recommended foods must be available and acceptable, according to cultural customs and attitudes. Furthermore, the desired behavioral change must be doable, sensible, and practical for the client, and the learning experience should give the learner immediate or long-term satisfaction.

Nutrition education is like a bridge that carries science-based information to a client who will use it. During this transport, nutrition educators must adapt the information so that it can be applied in a variety of everyday situations by people with different cultures. Reaching a large number of people may require use of the mass media and involvement of governmental and private agencies, universities, and food industries.

The Concept of "Habit Strength"

How simple nutrition education would be if only it required teaching people what was "good" for them. People would immediately follow suggestions, and everyone would live happily and healthily ever after. Needless to say, modification of food habits is a much more involved process.[37] One task that has eluded many community nutritionists is identifying factors that affect food behavior and that can predict dietary change. Instead of asking how to change food habits, the nutrition worker may find it more productive to ask how food habits are formed.[38] Asking the question is simple; securing its answer is more complex. Other questions to consider are: How are new food habits learned? How strong is a habit being considered for change? What personal skills need learning/relearning in order to implement change? What situational factors are involved? Who should change food habits? What are the economical, nutritional, and ethical implications of particular diet modifications? Any search for answers must be systematic and holistic.

Habit strength, an important concept in achieving dietary change, refers to the degree to which a habit resists efforts to extinguish it. Empirical observations suggest that people may have more difficulty unlearning old food habits than accepting the validity of new dietary practices. There is a difference between knowing what to do and how to do it.

The importance of establishing a friendly, nurturing setting where learning can take place is essential. No matter what teaching strategy is chosen, the learner must have the chance to become actively involved in the process of diet change. Learning must occur within the learner.

Empowering Nutrition Education

Dietary modification, as one goal of nutrition education, requires a *change in human behavior.* Emphasis is often on how an individual should change, even though the environment may contribute to the problem. An enlightened nutrition educator tries to facilitate a client's *empowerment* in that environment. Casas and Vásquez[39] note that Hispanics in the United States experience in varying degrees feelings of second-class citizenship, oppression, and discrimination. Empowering nutrition education could focus on developing assertiveness skills, improving self-efficacy and self-growth, encouraging awareness of and participation in community food programs, and supporting clients' efforts to make their own decisions about what is best for them.

The effective nutrition educator opposes the unhealthy attitude of blaming the victim, helps community programs change any discriminatory rules, helps eliminate oppressive elements in a bureaucratic system, and creates a partnership with Hispanic clients that is based on mutual respect and trust.

If educators lack awareness, training, and information to deal with multicultural groups, they may rely on stereotypical misinformation and distortion. Direct personal and professional contacts with a variety of Hispanic clients may help nutrition educators counteract ethnic biases and distinguish between stereotypes and the truth.

The underlying assumption in "empowering nutrition" is that clients need to achieve equality in society and within the family. To be empowered, people must not only know (cognitive) but also act (behavior).

A question related to empowerment is whether nutrition education can stand alone, or whether it is more effective when complemented by services or food aid. Hornik notes that nutrition education complemented with additional resources such as food supplements is more persuasive, and education may ease the adoption of newly recommended practices.[40] He argues that conventional nutrition education within clinic settings has been somewhat ineffective. In fact, some critics question whether nutrition education can bring about improvement in nutrition. Perhaps it is more relevant to ask whether nutrition education is effective for specific populations. Different audiences have different needs. Furthermore, certain educational strategies may work better with one audience than another. Empirical observations in some Latin American villages have shown that nutrition education was more effective when it was coordinated with health services such as deworming programs for children. These health services attracted more mothers to nutrition education programs, with more enthusiastic participation.

The Use of the Mass Media in Health and Nutrition Education

There are a variety of different approaches to nutrition education, but the objectives, audience, timing, and message should be planned with a clear understanding and knowledge of the health and nutrition problems and the felt needs of the learners and their community.

Cerqueira et al., formerly with the National Institute of Nutrition in Mexico, in a control group study, tested the effectiveness of mass media techniques as compared to direct methods of education for transmitting basic concepts of hygiene, health, and an adequate diet in three Mexican villages.[41] It was found that nutrition concepts were learned equally well using the traditional classroom setting as with mass media.

The use of radio in particular as an effective educational tool for reaching Hispanic audiences has merited some attention recently, mainly due to the large number of Spanish radio stations in major cities in the United States, and also because of the widespread use of radio among Hispanics.[42] A study conducted by Ramírez at Baylor College of Medicine in Texas showed that education using the radio (five five-minute radio episodes) increased awareness of such chronic diseases as hypertension, obesity, and diabetes among Hispanics, and 39% of them took action to improve their health.[43] Romero-Gwynn and Marshall, in a study conducted among Mexican-American women in California, showed that radio is an accepted and successful medium for conveying nutrition education to low-income Hispanic mothers.[44] These authors suggest that "some of the new challenges facing Cooperative Extension in the United States today include the need to serve a culturally diverse population and the need to reach larger geographical areas with the same or reduced staffing."

Ethical Issues in Nutrition Education

Uneducated people may be misinformed about health and nutrition, but unless a nutrition educator is reasonably sure they are wrong on a particular point, it might be ethically questionable to try to "improve" them. A new way, because it is modern and scientific, is not necessarily better than a traditional way. Furthermore, not all traditional beliefs and practices are deleterious to health. Most cultural patterns are reasonably appropriate and functional; otherwise they would not have survived.

Thus the nutrition educator's job is not to tell people what food choices to make but rather to point out the interrelation among good health, food, performance, and the quality of human life, so that people can make their own decisions based on the best information available. If food practices are truly harmful, the nutrition educator is justified in guiding efforts to improve them. But change should be compatible with existing cultural traditions and should be introduced in a way least disruptive to traditional values and practices.

Many nutrition educators and health providers who have worked with needy families have asked themselves some of these questions:

What right do we have to change people's health attitudes and behavior?

What right do we have to change the food habits of an individual, group, or community?

Is it ethical to alter traditional ways or beliefs by demonstrating the advantages of the good and new?

If we want to move people in another direction, how can we best communicate with them so that the benefits are larger than the detriments?

What are the trade-offs in any proposed diet change?

Health professionals generally agree that clients must be informed, persuaded, and motivated to adopt health patterns for their personal benefit and the benefit of society. This places an enormous moral burden on those nutrition educators who accept the challenge.

Exercise and Activity Patterns

The current focus on health in American society includes quality of life as well as absence of disease.[45] The salience of the "wellness" concept is illustrated by the promotion of wellness programs by universities, private companies, and other groups. Many of these programs emphasize the benefits of physical activity for health, as inactivity has been identified as a risk factor in the development of stress-related disorders and coronary heart disease.[46] Although activity should be regular, it need not be unduly strenuous. People who engage in light to moderate exercise, equivalent to sustained walking for about 30 minutes a day, can achieve substantial health gains.[47]

Dishman outlines biological, psychological, and situational factors that can influence both willingness and ability to exercise.[48] The most consistent biological discriminator between people who exercise and those who do not is body composition. On the other hand, Dishman notes, lean individuals may have led more active lifestyles before enrolling in exercise programs, so that it is easier for them to continue to exercise.

Self-motivation also affects whether people continue to exercise. This behavioral trait is socially learned and depends on the capacity for self-reinforcement and the ability to delay gratification. Self-motivation is independent of other motivational concepts, such as approval motivation, achievement motivation, locus of control, ego strength, and exercise attitudes.

Exercise setting is a situational characteristic that can vary according to whether an exercise program is designed for an individual or a group, whether it is convenient or accessible, and whether it fosters interpersonal relationships between exercisers and leader. Such situational characteristics can influence whether or not a person starts and continues to exercise.

These findings about exercise and activity have relevance for Hispanics. The report issued by the U.S. Department of Health and Human Services, *Healthy People 2000,* notes that overweight affects about 26% of the population age 20 through 74 years, as follows:

OVERWEIGHT PREVALENCE (1976–80)

Low-income women age 20 and older	37%
Black women age 20 and older	44
Hispanic women age 20 and older:	
Mexican-American women	39
Cuban women	34
Puerto Rican women	37

The estimates of severely overweight or obese women range from 8% of the Cuban Americans to 16% of the Mexican Americans.[49] Overweight is multifactorial in origin, reflecting genetic, environmental, cultural, and socioeconomic factors. Socioeconomic status is especially linked to overweight. Between 1976 and 1980, 37% of all women below the poverty level were classified as overweight. Overweight was common among Hispanics, especially among Mexican-American women. However, this high prevalence of overweight may not be accounted for completely by socioeconomic differences. Mexican-Americans who participated in the San Antonio Heart Study had low levels of physical activity rates, lower than those for members of the gen-

TABLE 9.2 Percentage of New York State Adults with Sedentary, Irregular, or Regular Activity Patterns

	Sedentary	Irregular	Regular
White	27	39	34
African-American	32	42	27
Hispanic	38	32	30
Asian	38	32	31
New York	36	36	38
Non-New York	30	38	33
Total	30	38	32

SOURCE:Division of Nutritional Sciences, Cornell University, in cooperation with Nutrition Surveillance Program, New York State Department of Health, *New York State Nutrition: State of the State* (Ithaca, NY, 1992).

eral population, after differences in socioeconomic status, residential location, and gender were taken into account.[50] On the other hand, a recent report in New York State found only small differences in the percentages of Hispanics, as compared to other racial/ethnic groups, who had physical activity patterns classified as sedentary, irregular, or regular (Table 9.2).[51] Because regular physical activity is important in maintaining appropriate body weight and confers a number of additional health benefits, the large percentage of New York State adults who do not engage in regular physical activity is a public health concern.

A major health concern among Hispanics is that over the past several years the rates of diabetes among Latino groups in the United States have escalated dramatically.[52] Obesity is a clear risk factor for noninsulin-dependent diabetes mellitus (NIDDM), the most common form of diabetes. Stern et al. note that though Hispanics have higher prevalences of diabetes with advancing age than do members of the general population, prevalence in the Hispanic barrio is an astonishing 35% among people age 55 to 64 years.[53] Davidson notes that sedentary lifestyles contribute indirectly to NIDDM, in that calories consumed in excess of energy expenditures result in obesity. He adds that low physical activity leads to a deterioration of glucose tolerance and a reduction in insulin secretion, whereas exercise improves both.[54] Benefits of exercise, particularly during middle age and beyond, are not emphasized as much by some ethnic groups as it is by others. In general, Davidson argues that Latinos place very little, if any, emphasis on the beneficial effects of exercise.

Encouraging regular physical activity among Hispanics is a special challenge for nutrition counselors, who must consider economic barriers, cultural orientations, safety issues, time constraints, and other issues confronting the urban poor. It might be important for a nutrition counselor to take time to learn about the cultural attitudes of clients toward overweight and exercise. An emphatic counselor may be able to help Hispanic clients change or modify any negative attitudes. Not surprisingly, leisure-time physical activity may be a low priority for poor urban women who are struggling for physical and economic survival.

Cuidando el Corazón: A Successful Behavior Intervention Program for Mexican-American Women

Reeves reports on a successful behavioral intervention program for weight loss in obese Mexican-American women that highlighted the role of the family in the intervention.[55] Over a three-year period, 168 Mexican-American women between the ages of 18 and 45 years who were 20% or more over ideal body weight were recruited for the study. All subjects were married and had at least one preschool-age child. Most of the subjects lived in households with an annual income of less than $20,000 and on the average had completed the tenth grade.

Subjects meeting the criteria were assigned to one of the three treatment groups: the manual-only comparison group, the individual group, and the family group. In the third group, spouses were encouraged to attend class with the women. The children of these women also attended classes to learn simple concepts about heart-healthy foods and physical exercise. The women who were randomly assigned to the individual and family groups attended 24 weekly classes and a six-month follow-up class taught by bilingual registered dietitians.

According to Reeves, culturally relevant educational materials and behavior strategies contributed to the success of this program. These included:

1. *Weight-loss manual*—All participants received a bilingual weight-loss manual, divided into four sections.

   Section I: Nutrition. Each nutrition lesson reviewed the material from the previous week, presented the new topic, discussed the weekly behavioral strategy, and listed the assignment. Information on following a 1200-calorie, low-fat eating plan with calories consisting of 30% from fat, 50% from carbohydrate, and 20% from protein was provided. In the family group manuals, nutrition lessons contained sections on parenting and partner techniques to teach subjects how to gain support of their families and spouses in making changes in eating and exercise habits.

   Section II: Exercise. The exercise lessons emphasized the positive relationship between exercise and health and the beneficial effect on weight loss. Instructions for initiating a walking program were included in this section.

   Section III: Food lists. Foods commonly eaten by Mexican-Americans living in Texas were included. Foods were grouped into eight different food guides and classified as "green" for usual intake and "red" for occasional intake.

Section IV: Recipes. This section included traditional recipes modified in fat and sugar. Nontraditional recipes were also included after participants indicated a desire for "American-style" foods. All recipes were calculated for calories and food exchanges.

2. *Bilingual videotapes*—Five bilingual videotapes were developed to reinforced basic nutrition concepts presented during the classes. These tapes focused their nutrition messages on fats and cholesterol, meat, fish and poultry, seafood, obesity, and cardiovascular disease.

3. *Food records*—During the intervention, subjects were taught to record their daily food intake by placing a red (occasional) or green (usual) dot, which represented an average portion size, on the food record forms. This approach was adopted because of subjects' limited reading and writing skills. It was also a visual method for subjects to track their changes in eating behaviors.

4. *Cooking demonstrations*—Dietitians demonstrated how to prepare traditional dishes using less fat. They occasionally served low-fat foods not typically eaten by participants in order to increase their acceptance of these foods.

5. *Exercise*—Subjects were encouraged to adopt an exercise program, and the recommended form of exercise was walking. Time for exercising was included in each class session. Because of popular demand, aerobic dance classes led by certified instructors were later offered.

6. *Prizes*—Contests were organized to encourage participants to comply with their exercise programs. One point was earned for each 15-minute exercise session completed and recorded. Prizes were awarded based on the number of points earned. This proved a very successful incentive to encourage participants to maintain their exercise programs.

7. *Parties/fiestas*—Christmas parties and graduation dinners were held each year. At these occasions recognition certificates were handed out to participants for complying with different aspects of the intervention.

For the subjects who actively participated in the study by attending class and exercising regularly, the 12-month results were encouraging. The study demonstrated that the women were very receptive to information on improving their nutrition and health and were able to adopt many techniques that produced weight loss. Both the family and individual groups lost more weight than did the manual-only control comparison group at 12 months.

SUMMARY

This chapter has examined three issues that are critical if Hispanics are to achieve better health and quality of life by the year 2000 and beyond.

Diet counseling was discussed as a process, where behavioral change, that is, dietary change, is most likely to occur within a nurturing environment. Emphasis was placed on developing communication based on mutual knowledge and understanding about the counselor's and client's beliefs and values. Understanding intracultural differences as well as similarities among the Hispanic subgroups is important for effective dietary counseling.

Dietary compliance was discussed from a more theoretical basis, where models explaining compliance in other settings could conceivably guide a nutrititon counselor in helping Hispanic clients. Specific guidelines for cross-cultural counseling were also provided. Finally, the process of nutrition education, viewed from the perspective of fully understanding the habit strength, empowering nutrition, ethical issues, and exercise and activity patterns are all important components in packaging effective nutrition education, was discussed.

NOTES

1. R. B. Howard and N. H. Herbold, *Nutrition in clinical care* (New York: McGraw-Hill, 1978).
2. V. M. González, J. T. González, V. Freeman, and B. Howard-Pitney, *Health promotion in diverse cultural communities* (Palo Alto, CA: Health Promotion Resource Center, Stanford Center for Research in Disease Prevention, 1991).
3. J. M. Casas and M. J. T. Vásquez, Counseling the Hispanic client: A theoretical and applied perspective. In P. B. Pedersen et al., *Counseling across cultures*, 3 ed. (Honolulu: University of Hawaii Press, 1989).
4. González et al., *Health promotion.*
5. J. A. Axelson, *Counseling and development in a multicultural society* (Monterey, CA: Brooks/Cole, 1985).
6. R. D. Terry, *Introductory community nutrition* (Dubuque, IA: Wm. C. Brown, 1993); R. D. Lee and D. C. Nieman, Counseling theory and technique. In *Nutritional assessment* (Dubuque, IA: WCB Brown Communications, 1993).
7. Terry, *Introductory community nutrition.*
8. Howard and Herbold, *Nutrition.*
9. G. Corey, *Theory and practice of counseling and psychotherapy*, 4th ed. (Pacific Grove, CA: Brooks/Cole, 1991); K. E. Hoelzel, Counseling methods for dietitians. *Topics in Clinical Nutrition*, 1 (1986), 33–42; B. B. Holli and R. J. Calabrese, *Communication*
and education skills: The dietetian's guide, 2nd ed. (Philadelphia: Lea and Febiger, 1991).
10. E. Spicer, ed., *Human problems in technological change* (New York: Wiley, 1962).
11. Lee and Nieman, Counseling theory and technique.
12. M. Range, Knowing our own culture, Mimeo. (Washington, DC: WIC Conference on Cross-cultural Counseling, 1988).
13. Lee and Nieman, Counseling theory and techniques.
14. C. Schur, A. B. Berstein, and M. L. Berk, The importance of distinguishing Hispanic subpopulations in the use of medical care. *Medical Care, 25,* (July 1987), 7.
15. Casas and Vásquez, Counseling the Hispanic client.
16. P. Fieldhouse, *Food and Nutrition: Customs and Culture* (London: Croom Helm, 1986).
17. González et al., *Health promotion.*
18. R. A. Ruiz, Cultural and historical perspectives in counseling Hispanics. In D. W. Sue (ed.), *Counseling the culturally different: Theory and practice* (New York: Wiley, 1981), pp. 186–215.
19. Casas and Vásquez, Counseling the Hispanic client.
20. American Society for Clinical Nutrition, symposium report of the task force on "The evidence relating six dietary factors

to the nation's health." *American Journal of Clinical Nutrition* (suppl.), *32* (1979) 12.

21. C. Lewis, Dietary compliance, term paper for NS-631, Dietary Assessment, DNS, Cornell University, Ithaca, NY, 1987; M. H. Becker and L. A. Maiman, Sociobehavioral determinants of compliance with health and medical care recommendations. *Medical Care, 13* (1975), 10–24; R. K. Dishman, Compliance/adherence in health related exercise. *Health Psychology, 1* (1981), 237–267.
I.L. Janis, The role of social support in adherence to stressful decisions. *American Psychologist, 38* (1983), 143–160.
J. Jenny, A compliance model of diabetic instruction. *Rehabilitation Literature, 44* (1983), 258–263; A. Harwood, ed., *Ethnicity and medical care* (Cambridge, MA: Harvard University Press, 1981).

22. Becker and Maiman, Sociobehavioral determinants.

23. I. L. Janis, The role of social support in adherence to stressful decisions. *American Psychologist, 38* (1983), 143–160.

24. A. J. Stunkard, Adherence to medical treatment: Overview and lessons from behavioral weight control. *Journal of Psychosomatic Research, 25* (1981), 187–197.

25. J. Jenny, A compliance model of diabetic instruction. *Rehabilitation Literature, 44* (1983), 258–263..

26. U.S. Department of Health and Human Services, *Healthy People 2000*, National Health Promotion and Disease Prevention Objectives, DHHS Pub. 91–50213, 1991.

27. Stunkard, Adherence to medical treatment.

28. Becker and Maiman, Sociobehavioral determinants.

29. Howard and Herbold, *Nutrition*.

30. Casas and Vásquez, Counseling the Hispanic client.

31. S. L. Connor, J. M. Gustafson, and S. R. Vaughan, Promoting dietary change: Demonstrating reduction of dietary fat. *Journal of the American Dietetic Association, 85* (March 1984), 3.

32. N. S. Salgado and A. M. Padilla, Social support networks: Their availability and effectiveness. In *Health and behavior: Research agenda for Hispanics*. Simón Bolívar Research Monograph Series no. 1, University of Illinois at Chicago, 1987.

33. Lewis, Dietary compliance.

34. P. Freire, *Pedagogy of the Oppressed* (New York: Herder and Herder, 1970).

35. Position paper on nutrition education for the public. *Journal of the American Dietetic Association, 62* (1973), 520.

36. A. Berg, Educating for better nutrition. In *The nutrition factor* (Washington, DC: Brookings Institution, 1973).

37. D. Sanjur. Ethnicity and food habits. In *Social and cultural perspectives in nutrition* (Englewood Cliffs, NJ: Prentice Hall, 1982).

38. Diva Sanjur, Nutrition education materials: A sociocultural approach. *Human Ecology Forum* (Ithaca, NY: New York State College of Human Ecology, Cornell University, 1970).

39. Casas and Vásquez, Counseling the Hispanic client.

40. R. C. Hornik, The roles of information in nutrition. In *Development communication: Information, agriculture, and nutrition in third world countries* (New York: Longman, 1988).

41. M. C. Cerqueira, et al., A comparison of mass media techniques and a direct method for nutrition education in rural Mexico. *Journal of Nutrition Education, 9* (1979), 2.

42. E. Romero-Gwynn and M. K. Marshall, Radio: Untapped teaching tool—Effective nutrition education for Hispanics. *Journal of Extension.* (Spring 1990), 9–11.

43. A. G. Ramírez, Vivir o morir? The effects of radio on health education for Hispanics. Paper presented at the Annual Meeting of the American Public Health Association, November 13–17, 1983.

44. Romero-Gwynn and Marshall, Radio.

45. Dishman, Compliance/adherence.

46. H. Blackburn, Physical activity and cardiovascular health: The epidemiological evidence. In F. Landry and W. Orban (eds.), *Physical activity and human well-being*, Vol. 1 (Miami: Symposia Specialists, 1978).

47. U.S. Department of Health and Human Services, *Healthy people 2000*.

48. Dishman, Compliance/adherence.

49. L. M. Lopez and B. Masse, Comparison of body mass indexes and cutoff points for estimating the prevalence of overweight in Hispanic women. *Journal of the American Dietetic Association, 11* (November 1992), 1343–1347.

50. National Coalition of Hispanic Health and Human Services Organizations, *Delivering preventive health care to Hispanics: A manual for providers* (Washington, DC, 1988).

51. Division of Nutritional Sciences, Cornell University, in cooperation with Nutrition Surveillance Program, New York State Department of Health, *New York State Nutrition: State of the State* (Ithaca, NY, 1992).

52. Jaime A. Davidson, Diabetes in Hispanics—Diabetes in ethnic and minority groups: A growing challenge. *Diabetes Care and Education: On the Cutting Edge, 12*(6) (December 1991).

53. M. P. Stern et al., Sex difference in the effects of sociocultural status on diabetes and cardiovascular risk factors in Mexican-Americans. *American Journal of Epidemiology, 120* (1984), 834.

54. Davidson, Diabetes in Hispanics.

55. Rebecca Reeves, Successful behavioral interventions for Mexican American population—Diabetes in ethnic and minority groups: A growing challenge. *Diabetes Care and Education: On the Cutting Edge, 12*(6) (December 1991).

10

Assessing Food Intake Among Hispanics

The Process of Collecting Dietary Data
Choosing the Appropriate Methods
Minimizing Methodological Errors
Selecting and Training Interviewers
Bilingual Interviewers and Use of Interpreters
Local Interviewers or Outsiders?
Unfamiliarity with Ethnic Foods
Kinds of Training
Assessing Portion Sizes and Mixed Dishes

The Need for a National Data Bank on Ethnic Foods
Need for a National Nutrient Data Bank on Ethnic Foods
Need for Using Nutrient Data from Existing Food Composition
Tables and from Cross-Sectional Studies to Create a Nutrient
Data Bank for Hispanic Foods

THE PROCESS OF COLLECTING DIETARY DATA

In a multicultural society such as urban America, nutrition fieldworkers may collect information about food habits and other dietary information from people with different cultural and ethnic backgrounds and socioeconomic milieus. Foster[1] and Spicer[2] have provided invaluable anthropological insights into conducting this type of fieldwork. Both advise conducting a limited number of in-depth interviews with principal informants from the community at the beginning of any major investigation. Several of these somewhat lengthy sessions are usually required to gain an understanding of cultural ways and cues. These interviews also serve as points of entry into the community from which to continue observing food behaviors, and they are of utmost value in training interviewers who will collect dietary information.

When conducting dietary surveys among ethnic groups three questions arise:

1. How well were dietary intakes assessed?

2. How well were diets and nutrient intakes estimated, given that nutrient data bases for indigenous, ethnic foods are often lacking?

3. Did dietary intakes reflect ethnicity, or given that many ethnic groups have low incomes, did intakes more likely reflect a low socioeconomic status?

Undertaking dietary surveys as part of community nutrition research helps nutrition practitioners learn more about the diets of clients and about the community at large. Combining nutrition research and nutrition education is a productive strategy, with tangible benefits for participants, as it enhances their cooperation and improves rapport.[3] This is particularly true when subjects are treated with respect and researchers provide feedback on the data collected.

Cassidy notes that culturally sensitive dietary research recognizes differing values and the primacy of the respondent, while acknowledging that data accuracy is a function both of how well researchers know the people they want to understand and of how much respondents trust researchers.[4] On this issue, she suggests two important questions:

1. How do the ways people perceive food affect their reporting of intake?

2. How do the ways people relate to the interviewer, the setting , or the assessment instrument affect their reporting of intake?

This chapter addresses these and other issues relative to assessing food intake among Hispanic families, with particular emphasis on how to collect good-quality dietary data. No matter how sophisticated the subsequent statistical analysis, it cannot make up for poor diet assessments.

Choosing the Appropriate Methods

There is no one ideal method for assessing what people eat. Rather, the objectives of an investigation determine the best methodology for collecting, processing, and interpreting dietary data.

Needless to say, all nutritionists would like to find a method that is valid, reliable, and objective, as well as simple and inexpensive. To be *valid,* a method must truly measure what the investigator wishes to measure. To be *reliable,* a method must give the same results on repeated trials or the same results as another widely accepted method. And to be *objective,* a method must be standardized, or systematically applied, so that results can be compared with results of other investigators.

Clearly defined objectives are crucial in choosing an appropriate method. Different methods are most appropriate under certain circumstances. For example, to estimate the quantity of food consumed, food records or food weighing methods are possible choices; to obtain qualitative dietary profiles from large groups, 24-hour recall methods are valid. Information about present or past food intakes can be collected by using repeated food recalls, food frequencies, or diet histories.

Other factors that influence the choice of dietary method include sample size, cost, interviewers' training, education of respondents, languages spoken in homes and research sites, and age and maturity of respondents. Some methods work better than others with certain people. Reese studied response/nonresponse rates to measures of individual food intake among low-income populations, by sex and age, over a two-year period.[5] Reese specifically examined problems encountered when collecting data from the poverty-income population. Results from the study indicated that low-income people had difficulty in recording three days of intakes quarterly over a year for all household members. Asking respondents to mail in their records was unsatisfactory because it placed too much burden on them. Also, people living in rural areas were more responsive than residents of central cities. In general, adult males had the lowest response rates, whereas women over 50 years of age had the highest response rates.

Minimizing Methodological Errors

No method of dietary assessment is free of technical errors or reflects for any length of time the true biological variation of dietary intakes of free living individuals. Because no method is consistently best, nutrition researchers have to make trade-offs and decide which method will best accomplish their objectives. Although errors or biases in dietary surveys cannot entirely be eliminated, they can be minimized by sampling a large number of subjects (the larger the sample size, the smaller the variation) or by repeating the diet measurements with the same subjects over time. (In the statistical sense, an *error* is any source of variance that serves to reduce the reliability of the individual data and the group mean. In a dietary study, standardization and other data control procedures are used to reduce such error to a minimum.[6])

Two other issues are critical when choosing dietary methods to collect data, especially among low-income families who may be unfamiliar with American culture or with the English language.

1. *Minimize respondent's burden:* Interviews that are too demanding can compromise the validity and reliability of the data. Thus beware of long questions and complicated diet instruments (scales for weighing leftover foods), prolonged interviews (over an hour), and particularly, obtrusive and invasive methods (using tape recorders to record information about income and expenses for food). Collecting data in a sensitive way can make the difference between uncooperative and friendly and eager participants. Minimizing respondents' burden maximizes the validity and reliability of the information.

2. *Minimize technical errors:* Two particular kinds of variation that may lead to biases or errors in dietary surveys are interpersonal variation and intrapersonal variation. Each of these inherent sources of variation has two components: variation owing to true or biological variation (true differences among individuals reporting the food intake) and variation owing to measurement technique (measurement errors).

To minimize these sources of errors in dietary surveys one can increase the number of subjects in the study to reduce interpersonal variation and increase the number of days of collecting information from each subject, thus reducing intrapersonal variation. Errors owing to the measurement techniques employed can result from the effect of the interviewer on the respondent, the effect of the respondent on the interviewer, and the interaction between the interviewer and respondent.

Measurement errors of an attitudinal nature can result from the way the question is asked, intentional omission of questions, or even worse, fabrication of responses. On the other hand, situational effects, such as the physical setting of the interview, the need for confidentiality and anonymity, or accidental distractions, can also contribute to measurement errors. Relational effects such as whether the interviewer likes the respondent, whether the respondent trusts the interviewer, or whether there is general rapport between them can also affect the validity of the data. Finally technical errors can result from background factors, such as degree of interviewers' familiarity with respondents, urban/rural orientations, or ethnicity.

It is helpful to anticipate and recognize these potential sources of bias that may be encountered in conducting dietary surveys in order to try to minimize them.

Selecting and Training Interviewers

Selecting and training interviewers to assess food consumption among Hispanic families is an important consideration. There are many decisions regarding selection of interviewers, such as whether to use bilingual, indigenous paraprofessionals from within or outside the community. Familiarity with Hispanic foods and their availability, cost, and composition, cultural variation in estimating portion sizes, use of recalled or written food records, time dimensions and different value orientations are also important considerations when selecting and training interviewers.

Bilingual Interviewers and Use of Interpreters

Lack of common language can be a major barrier for an interviewer, who must then rely on an interpreter. However, using an interpreter can cause additional problems. There are several reasons why it is preferable to avoid relying on interpreters to collect dietary data. When interpreters collect food consumption data, they filter the data through their own personality and status. Furthermore, if an interviewer who does not speak the language wishes to study other diet-related topics, such as food beliefs, taboos, breast-feeding attitudes, and practices or traditional methods of weaning, validating the information becomes a serious methodological problem.

Because of these difficulties, it is best for interviewers who will be working with Hispanics to be fluent in Spanish. However, speaking the language is not enough. Methodological issues go beyond the language barrier. As Foster notes, serious difficulties may exist between people who presumably speak the same language in a large and complex society such as the United States.[7] The total range of food names and brands and their associated meanings is so great that no one can master them all. When intracultural Hispanic diversity is considered, the difficulty in having an untrained person, unfamiliar with the language and the culture, collect dietary information becomes apparent. Exact translation from one language to another is virtually impossible, and translating out of context is also very difficult.

A nutrition supervisor who hires bilingual Spanish interviewers must make sure to build into the study cross-checking validation techniques in order to ensure quality control of the data. In other words, the field coordinator should spot-check the data to make sure interviewers are measuring what the investigator wishes to measure. In addition, learning and acquiring a minimal working knowledge of the culture-specific language and observing the Hispanic group to be studied are helpful. The amount of time devoted to studying the culture-specific ways varies, depending on the interviewer's ability to learn new foodways.

An additional pitfall for the novice interviewer working in another culture is the desire to appear "intelligent and understanding." The interviewer may nod and say, "Oh, yes, I understand," when in reality she or he does not. Learning to say, "No, I do not quite understand that" or asking for clarification of specific points is important.

Local Interviewers or Outsiders?

Another dilemma facing a nutrition researcher is whether to select dietary interviewers from the same community or from a similar neighboring community. Although the added cost of transportation may prohibit using interviewers from another community, empirical observations among Hispanic low-income women have found them more willing to discuss openly food intakes with interviewers who do not know them or their relatives.

The age and gender of the interviewers may also affect responses. Are mothers more willing to talk about food with younger or older interviewers? Do women make better dietary interviewers than men? Again, empirical observations suggest that there are trade-offs. Although younger interviewers may lack familiarity with traditional foods and experience in food preparation, they are likely to be flexible, willing to learn and be trained, and are good at keeping food records and estimating quantities. Conversely, older interviewers may have more credibility concerning food preparation and be more patient and better listeners. However, older women may be more difficult to train because, as one remarked, "What can you teach me about food, when I have cooked all my life."

In addition, with the advent of more men into the nutrition and dietetics profession, several field studies are employing more male interviewers for diet surveys. Their success as interviewers is also a function of cultural acceptance. A good mix of indigenous interviewers, young and mature, men and women, who are enthusiastic, experienced, and willing to learn about how to assess food intake (which is distinctly different from cooking), might make a terrific team of bicultural dietary interviewers.

One last point is that it is advisable to select two or three more trainees than actually needed to conduct the dietary surveys. During the investigation if interviewers get sick, have family emergencies, or face other extenuating circumstances such as a death in the family, extra investigators will be invaluable. Interviewers in training should be paid and also advised that some will serve as substitutes whenever needed.

Unfamiliarity with Ethnic Foods

This book provides detailed glossaries of the foods most commonly consumed by specific Hispanic subgroups. It also provides serving portions, weight in grams, and energy values for selected foods. The glossaries are included in the chapters rather than in a separate appendix because learning about clients through food is a good way to start communicating with them. The basic reason for these glossaries is to help people become familiar with various foods and methods of preparation. The symbolic meanings cannot be overemphasized in counseling, education, and nutrition research. The same foods sometimes have different names and associations for different groups of people.

For example, for an American nutritionist, starchy vegetables are just that; for a Puerto Rican mother they are *viandas;* for a Dominican they are *víveres;* and for a Panamanian they are *verduras.* Rice and beans are just that for the health practitioner. Yet for a Puerto Rican mother, they carry a strong symbolic meaning and are called *arroz mamposteado;* in the Dominican Republic they are called *moros y cristianos;* in Cuba they are called *congrí;* and in Costa Rica they are called *gallo pinto.* Bananas are called *guineos* in El Salvador; in Mexico they are called *plátanos.*

One does not expect American nutritionists or dietary interviewers to learn all the Spanish names at this level of specificity, but recognizing that they exist and acknowledging their diversity among different Hispanic subgroups may help create sympathetic, friendly, and cooperative Spanish-speaking audiences. In fact, the underlying theme of this book is that nutrition practitioners who understand that cultural food patterns have a *functional significance* will find it easier to comprehend and explain variations in food intake among different ethnic groups in any society.

A selected list of food items, with their English names and common Spanish names variations is shown in Table 10.1.

Kinds of Training

A good way to begin training interviewers is to visit *bodegas* and markets where indigenous traditional foods are sold and to observe women prepare common and well-liked mixed dishes. Discussing household dynamics relative to food purchasing and preparation is also helpful. For example, when training interviewers, ask them who buys and prepares the food in their households, or whether the food preferences of husband or children dictate what foods are eaten. Training that includes observations and questions will contribute valuable information about the cultural setting.

The amount of training needed will vary according to the methodological approach chosen and the financial resources available. In general, if data are to be collected through home visits, it takes extra time to train the interviewers how to take control of the interview, to avoid distractions, and to make sure that questions are answered by the designated respondent rather than by spouse, children, or other relatives. Home visits can also be expensive in terms of transportation and identifying study participants with corresponding addresses. However, they do provide opportunities to learn about the food dynamics within the household. The validity and reliability of the data can be potentially increased if home observations complement the reported intakes.

Training of the interviewers should cover such issues as use or misuse of tape recordings; how to handle "don't know" responses; how to deal with families that are too intense or talkative about food or who volunteer unrelated information; how to handle unresponsive families; how to use any diet scales; and to understand why particular questions are included in

TABLE 10.1 Glossary of Selected Foods and Common Spanish Name Variations*

annato	achiote, aciote, colorante, bija
apple banana	guineo niño, guineo de oro, guineo de dedo
avocado	aguacate, palta, zaboca
bacon	tocineta, tocino, panceta
banana	guineo, plátano
beefsteak	bistec, bife
beet	remolacha, betarraga
black beans	frijoles negros, habichuelas negras
blackberries	moras, zarzamoras
bread	pan, bolillo, panecillo, michita
breadfruit	pana, panepén, fruta de pan, agualpán
brown sugar	panela, raspadura, azúcar morena
butter beans	porotos de mantequilla, frijoles blancos, habas lima, piloy
cabbage	col, repollo de col
cassava	yuca, manioca
cereal gruel	atole, atol
cashew	pajuil, marañón, jocote marañón
chives	cebollina, cebollino, cebollana
clove	clavito de olor, clavo de especie
coconut	coco, agua de coco, pipa
coriander	recao, culantro, cilantro
corn	maíz, choclo, elote
custard apple	anona, corazón
dasheen	malanga blanca, taro
fried green plantains	tostones, patacones
genip	quenepa, mamón, mamoncillo
grapefruit	toronja, pomelo
green beans	habichuelas tiernas, vainitas, frijolitos verdes, judías
guacamole	guacamol, guacamole
guava	guayaba, guava, goyave
hot pepper	chile, ají picante, pimiento picante, ají chombito, chile congo
ice cream	helado, nieve, mantecado
june plum	jobo de la india, jobo, ciruela, mangostín
kidney beans	porotos, caraotas, frijoles de riñón
lemon	limón, limón agrio, limón pica
mango	mangó, mango, mangue
meatballs	albóndigas, bolas de carne
mushrooms	hongos, setas, callampas
navel orange	naranjas naval, naranjas injertadas
okra	ñajú, quimbombó, molondrón
omelette	tortilla de huevo, revoltillo de huevo, torta de huevo
orange	china, naranja
papaya	papaya, lechoza, fruta bomba
parsley	perejil, perejil colocho
passion fruit	parcha, maracuyá, granadilla
peach	durazno, melocotón

peanut	maní, cacahuate
peas	arvejas secas, petit-pois, chícharos, alverjas
pigeon peas	gandules, gandures, frijol de palo, guandú
pineapple	piña, anana
potato	papa, patata
prickly pear	tuna, fruta del cactus
pumpkin	ayote, guicoy, pepitoria
red banana	guineo morado, plátano morado
red snapper	pargo, chillo
rice and beans	arroz con habichuelas, arroz con frijoles, arroz masposteado, moros y cristianos, gallo pinto, congrí
ripe plantain	plátano maduro, amarillo
root celery	apio, apio nabo, papa de apio, arracacha
sausages	longaniza, salchichón, chorizo, salchicha, butifarra, morcilla
sea grape	icaco, uva de playa
shrimp	camarones, gambas
soft drinks	bebidas gaseosas, sodas, refrescos
soup (thick)	salcocho, sancocho, sopón, sopa
spanish plum	ciruela española, jocote
squash	zapallo, auyama, calabaza
star apple	caimito, zapote, caimite
starchy vegetables	viandas, verduras, víveres
stringed beef	ropa vieja, carne vieja
sweet potato	batata, camote, boniato, patate
swiss chard	acelga, mostaza
tamarind	tamarindo, tamarín
tannier	yautía, otoe, papa de pobre
turnips	nabo, colinabo
white pear	chayote, tayota, calabacita china
yam	ñame, yampie, ñampí

SOURCES: B. Cabanillas, C. Ginorio, and C. Q. Mercado. *Cocine a gusto*, Department of Home Economics, University of Puerto Rico, San Juan, I968; M. Coll-Camalez, E. Sánchez F., and E. S. de Zayas, *Siluetas que pueden Cambiar*, 4th ed., San Juan, P.R., I991; Women's Auxiliary of the Union Church of Guatemala, *Kitchen fiesta*, Guatemala, I960; V. R. Mann, Food practices of the Mexican-Americans in Los Angeles County, mimeo. Los Angeles County Health Department, I966; Ministerio de Educación, Comida Tradicional Salvadoreña, El Salvador, I991.

tionnaires. Role playing can be helpful for practicing different approaches. Training usually takes from seven to ten days to cover all of these issues.

A final important issue related to training interviewers is the cultural value accorded to time. In general, Americans and Latin Americans view and handle time differently. In the American culture, time is used as an organizing system and a way of communication; words carry most of the messages, which must be written and communicated on time. Activities are organized on a time basis, which is linear and stresses a "one-at-a-time" system. In contrast, in the Latin American culture, activities are more group oriented, and less emphasis is placed on written and more on verbal communication. The nutrition practitioner who trains Spanish interviewers must spell out the expectations at the beginning of the training period. The practitioner should explain to interviewers when they are expected at the office, how long they should wait for anyone before going to the field, how the group's work is affected if someone is consistently late, and the consequences of persistent tardiness.

Laying out the rules and expectations at the very beginning of the training shows both respect for the trainees and the seriousness of their tasks. Being aware of potential cultural conflicts over time can help prevent serious problems.

Assessing Portion Sizes and Mixed Dishes

Very little data exist on whether standard portion sizes vary among different ethnic groups or according to age or gender within particular groups. Investigations into this possible effect could improve the accuracy of dietary data. Using average servings (Table 10.2) for American foods, community nutritionists could conceivably adapt them to develop "average servings" of foods eaten by various ethnic groups. Accurate estimates of portion sizes are important because the nutrient composition of diets depends on the portions of foods consumed.

For example, although Table 10.1 shows that one-half cup of rice is an average American portion, for many Hispanics one cup of rice is an average portion. Furthermore, when rice is eaten at more than one meal, knowing common portions is even more important. As another example, the number of tortillas usually consumed at one meal varies significantly among different Hispanic groups. Furthermore, tortillas commonly vary in thickness, which also affects portion size. The macronutrient composition of beans and tortillas also varies, depending on preparation. Table 10.3 illustrates how water and fat content varies based on the way Mexican beans and tortillas are prepared.

Murphy, from the Department of Nutritional Sciences at the University of California at Berkeley, worked with the Stanford Center for Chicano Studies in California, to evaluate food group intakes by Mexican-American children.[8] The researchers raised several critical issues relative to defining and quantifying daily servings, food group servings, portion sizes, and other important dietary assessment topics. For example, Murphy et al. found that the wording of food frequency questionnaires can substantially affect the responses. In the case of the Hispanic Health and Nutrition Examination Survey (HHANES), participants were instructed to indicate "how often they usually ate the food items in a food group." Because no information on portion size was given, people might assume that the responses reflected the number of eating occasions during which the items were consumed rather than the amount consumed at each occasion. In other words, consumption of two glasses of milk at the same meal could be reported as a single serving, or

TABLE 10.2 Average American Serving or Portion of Food

Product	Weights or Amounts	Product	Weights or Amounts
Dairy Products		Fruits	
Cheese		Fresh	By the piece
Cheddar	2 oz.	Fresh, cut up;	1/2 cup
Cottage	1/4–1/2 cup	canned	
Milk		Fruit juices	1/2 cup
To drink	1 cup (8 fl. oz.)		
For cooked cereal	2 oz.	Meat	
For dry cereal	4 oz.	Fresh, frozen,	
Ice cream	1/2–1 cup	canned	1/2 cup
		Liver	2 oz.
Eggs		Bacon	2 slices
Fried, poached,		Frankfurters	2 pieces
hard, or	1	Luncheon meat	2 slices
soft cooked	1 1/2	Legumes, beans	1 cup cooked
Scrambled		Peanut butter	2 tbl.
Fats and Oils		Poultry	
Butter or		Chicken, turkey,	
margarine	2 tsp. or 1 pat.	boned	3 oz.
Salad dressing	2 tbl.	Chicken, broiler	1/2 bird
Mayonnaise	1 tbl.	Chicken, fryer	1/4 bird
Fish and Shellfish			
Fresh, frozen, and		Vegetables	
canned	3 oz.	Cooked, canned	1/2 cup
		Lettuce	1/4 head
Bread and Cereals		Asparagus	3-6 spears
Bread, rolls,		Brussels sprouts	4-6
muffins	1 slice	Corn, ears	1 piece
Cereals, cooked	1/2 cup	Potatoes, whole	1 medium
Cereal, dry	3/4–1 cup	Potatoes, french	
Macaroni, rice,		fries	8-10 pieces
cooked	1/2 cup		
Saltines	4 pieces		
Graham crackers	4 pieces		
Pancakes or	2 or 3		
waffles			

NOTE: These servings may not be the amounts personally consumed. Knowledge of the average quantity per serving is useful in estimating cost and nutritive value

SOURCE: V. A. Vaclavick, M. H. Pimental, and M. M. Devine, *Dimensions of food*, 3rd ed. (New York: Van Nostrand Reinhold, 1992).

consumption of several different vegetables at the same meal might be considered as one single serving of dark green and yellow vegetables.

In addition, commonly eaten mixed dishes such as Dominican *arroz con pollo* (chicken with rice) or *carne adobada* (beef stew) contain ingredients from several different food groups. However, people may neglect to count serv-

TABLE 10.3 Water and Macronutrient Composition of Various Preparations of Beans and Tortillas in Sonora, Mexico

Food		Composition (per 100 g of edible portion)				
Spanish Name	Description	Water (%)	Energy (cal)	Protein (g)	Fat (g)	Carbohydrate (g)
Frijol de la olla	Whole beans boiled; watery	69	128	5	8	10
Frijol guisado seco	Fried beans mashed and dried	61	173	6	12	10
Frijol refrito	Mashed beans dried and fried with an excess of fat	59	221	10	14	11
Tortillas de maíz	Corn tortillas	46	183	5	0.4	41
Tortillas de harina mediana	Flour tortillas, medium size, commercial or homemade	27	298	7	10	28
Tortillas de harina (manteca)	Flour tortillas, small size but proportionally more fat (lard)	18	351	8	16	69
Tortillas de harina (agua)	Flour tortillas large size but less fat	27	275	8	4	53

SOURCE: M. Valencia, unpublished data, Center for Nutrition Research, Hermosillo, Sonora, Mexico, 1992.

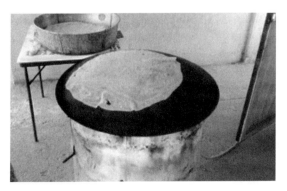

Tortillas de manteca *(flour tortillas with added fat)* vary in thickness, portion size, and composition.

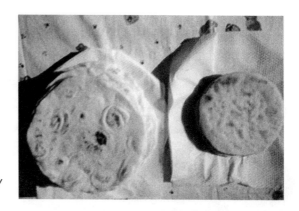

Tortillas de agua *(flour tortillas without added fat) are commonly thinner and of larger size.*

ings of individual ingredients when they are part of mixed dishes. Unless specifically instructed on how to count the number of servings, respondents are likely to vary in their interpretation of the questions and thus in their responses.

In assessing food intake, it is wise to assume that consumption of some foods, such as vegetables or fruits, may be underestimated because the range of possibilities within that particular group is very wide. In addition, overestimation of servings is also possible. For example, when Hispanic families are asked to estimate quantities consumed, they usually answer in terms of "serving spoons" (large spoons used to cook, stir, and serve the food) rather than of tablespoons or cups, which are more familiar to the nutritionist.

In assessing fruits, one could also argue that estimation could be favored by the fact that laypeople usually view them as units. For example, it is somewhat easier for people to report, "I had a medium banana or a small apple" than reporting what was in a cup of mixed fruits.

THE NEED FOR A NATIONAL NUTRIENT DATA BANK ON ETHNIC FOODS

Analysis and interpretation are central steps in the research process. The goal of analysis is to summarize the collected data in order to answer the questions that initiated the research. Interpretation refers to the search for the significance and implications of these answers within the framework of existing knowledge. In many parts of the third world, analysis of dietary data is still done by a handful of community nutritionists who are able to examine a limited number of diet records. In contrast, in technologically developed countries, dietary analysis occurs in many governmental, industrial, and academic institutions with computer centers to process dietary information.

Computers allow fast, efficient, accurate, and uniform handling of dietary data through the use of nutrient data banks. However, nutrient data banks (computerized nutrient data bases) are only as complete and as accurate as the nutrient composition data entered into them. Certainly, it is possible for people to make mistakes when presetting and precoding the information to enter in the data bank.

Tables of food composition, useful for large-scale or epidemiological studies, are available for various Latin American and Caribbean countries.[9] Such tables could certainly be employed to create a nutrient data bank of Hispanic foods for use in the United States. The ethnic or traditional Hispanic foods available to many individuals in urban America are already included in these tables. However, in general, food composition tables have certain limitations because they provide only approximate nutrient values. Furthermore, the effect of home cooking on nutrients is ignored in the calculations, and many convenience and processed foods are not included in some of the Latin American food composition tables. Also ignored is the loss of nutrients at home through plate waste, spoilage, and amounts given to domestic animals. Yet, although all food composition tables have these recognized limitations, they still provide important indirect estimates of a group's food intake.

Nutrient intakes can also be assessed by analyzing the chemical or caloric content of representative meals, single foods, or prepared "composites" of foods. This method is useful for individual dietary surveys or metabolic studies when a precise assessment of nutrient intake is needed. However, chemical analysis also presents certain limitations. Samples can be contaminated during storage or transport. Furthermore, chemical analysis is much more expensive than using food composition tables for dietary evaluation. However, community nutritionists can sometimes make use of existing industry labs, academic labs, or food and nutrition research institute labs to analyze the composition of specific ethnic foods.

On a more practical level, many academic institutions or nutrition research institutes are conducting dietary surveys of specific population groups, and these are another source of nutrient data. One useful strategy to compensate for limited data on Hispanic foods is to substitute data on similar foods for which food compositions are available. Respondents are asked to name ingredients used in any mixed dishes. Then researchers can obtain nutrient data for these known components, even though nutrient data for a mixed dish are unavailable. Although the appropriateness of this strategy could be questioned, there are also problems associated with relying on USDA databases for Hispanic foods.

Loria et al. maintain that the nutrient data for Mexican foods in the USDA databases are based on analysis of commercially prepared, Americanized versions of these foods, rather than on foods as they are prepared by Mexican-Americans at home.[10] For example, Americanized tacos usually consist of a fried tortilla, filling, and shredded lettuce, whereas Mexican tacos most often consist of a tortilla cooked without fat, which is wrapped around a filling and eaten without lettuce. Tamales (filled dough steamed in cornhusks) may also have very different nutrient profiles, depending on whether traditional or Americanized versions are prepared. Mexican tamales are made with *masa ha-*

rina, a flour made from lime-treated corn, commercially prepared tamales, such as those in the USDA databases, are prepared with degermed cornmeal. A tamale made with *masa harina* contains 47 mg of calcium per 100 g,[11] whereas one made with degermed cornmeal contains only 11 mg of calcium per 100 g.[12]

The need to develop nutrient databases for Hispanic foods through cross-sectional studies or other means, again, cannot be overemphasized. This is not a job for a community nutritionist but for governmental institutions charged with monitoring our food supply and its nutrients. Questions about the true dietary intake of Hispanic groups is of legitimate concern, given the limited nutrient data available for foods they commonly consume. Celebrating cultural diversity is fine, but more information is needed to unravel the nutritional adequacy or inadequacy of these ethnic diets.

SUMMARY

This chapter has raised some important concerns relative to assessing food intake among Hispanics. Undertaking dietary studies in a multicultural society is an important part of nutrition work. However, such issues as choosing the appropriate dietary method, selecting and training indigenous interviewers, becoming familiar with ethnic foods, and assessing portion sizes and composition of mixed dishes do merit special consideration, particularly if field staff is working in an unfamiliar frame of reference.

The need for a national nutrient data bank on ethnic foods has been discussed, and practical suggestions on using existing data from food composition tables for Latin America and the Caribbean and from cross-sectional studies were offered. A nutrient value dictionary for commonly used Hispanic foods provided in the Appendix was developed from various existing sources. This could prove useful for nutrition students and others doing research on food intake among Hispanic families.

NOTES

1. G. M. Foster, *Traditional societies and technological change*, 2nd ed. (New York: Harper & Row, 1973).

2. E. Spicer, ed., *Human problems in technological change* (New York: Wiley, 1962).

3. K. G. Dewey, E. S. Metallinos, M. A. Strode, E. M. All, Y. R. Fitch, M. Holguin, J. A. Kraus, and L. J. McNicholas, Combining nutrition research and nutrition education—Dietary change among Mexican-American families. *Journal of Nutrition Education, 16*(1) (1984), 5–7.

4. C. M. Cassidy, Walk a mile in my shoes: Culturally sensitive food-habit research, *American Journal of Clinical Nutrition, 59* (Suppl.)(1994), 1905–1975..

5. R. B. Reese, Pilot study of measures of individual food intakes of the low-income population. In *Research on survey methodology*, USDA, Human Nutrition Information Service, Adm. Report no. 382 (Washington, DC, May 1987).

6. G. H. Beaton et al., Sources of variance in 24-hour dietary recall data: Implications for nutrition study design and interpretation. *American Journal of Clinical Nutrition, 32* (December 1979), 2546.

7. Foster, Traditional societies.

8. S. P. Murphy, R. O. Castillo, R. Martorell, and F. S. Mendoza, An evaluation of food group intakes by Mexican-American chil-dren. *Journal of the American Dietetic Association, 90* (March 1990), 3.

9. L. C. Reguero and S. M. Rodríguez de Santiago, *Tabla de composición de alimentos de uso corriente en Puerto Rico*. Editorial Universidad de Puerto Rico, Rio Piedras, 1978; M. Hernández, A. Chávez, and H. Bourges, *Valor nutritivo de los alimentos Mexicanos: Tablas de Uso Práctico*, 8th ed. (Mexico: División de Nutrición del Instituto Nacional de la Nutrición, 1980); Centro de Investigación en Alimentación y Desarrollo, Aporte de nutrientes de platillos regionales de Sonora, unpublished data. Hermosillo, Sonora, Mexico, 1992; Instituto de Nutrición de Centro América y Panamá, *Tabla de composición de alimentos para uso en América Latina*. Guatemala, 1978.

10. C. M. Loria, M. A. McDowell, C. L. Johnson, and D. E. Woteki, Nutrient data for Mexican-American foods: Are current data adequate? *Journal of the American Dietetic Association, 91*(8)/(August 1991), 919-922.

11. U.S. Department of Agriculture, Nutrient data base for individual food intake surveys. Release 4.0, unpublished working version, 1990.

12. U.S. Department of Agriculture, *Nutrient data base for individual food intake surveys*. Release 2.1, 1986.

Appendix: Nutrient Value Dictionary for Hispanics Foods

Spanish	English	Kcal.	Protein (g)	Fat (g)	Carbohydrate (g)	Calcium (mg)	Iron (mg)	Vitamin A	Vitamin C (mg)
Aceituna	Olive	233	1.7	25	4.3	122	3	7 (re)	0
Acelga	Chard	27	2.9	0.3	4.8	62	3.9	404 (re)	6
Acerolas	West Indian cherry	28	0.4	0.3	6.8	12	0.2	—	1300
Aguacate	Avocado	149	1.8	13.9	4.2	53	1	300 U.I.	14
Ajo	Garlic	137	6.2	0.2	30.8	29	1.5	Tr	15
Ajonjolí	Sesame seeds	575	14.9	52.2	21.1	728	9.5	2 (re)	0
Albaricoque	Apricot	57	0.8	0.6	13.8	30	1.1	670 (mcg)	10
Alcachofas	Artichoke	65	2.2	0.1	16.5	32	0.6	95 (re)	6
Alfalfa	Alfalfa, tender	52	6	0.4	65.1	12	51	3410 (mcg)	162
Almendras	Almonds, dry	598	18.6	54.2	19.5	234	4.7	0 U.I.	tr.
Alubias	Beans	332	20.8	2.8	58.6	132	6.7	3 (re)	3
Anacardo o nuez de pajuil	Cashew nuts	561	17.2	45.7	29.3	38	3.8	100 ui	—
Apio, tallo	Celery	104	0.8	0.2	24.9	29	1.2	60 U.I.	28
Armadillo	Armadillo	173	29	5.4	0	30	10.9	0 U.I.	0
Arroz blanco enriquecido	Rice, polished, enriched	363	6.7	0.4	80.4	24	2.9	0 U.I.	0
Atún enlatado en aceite	Tuna in oil	228	24.2	20.5	0	7	1.2	20 (re)	0
Avena	Oats	370	11.6	3.1	73.8	64	4.9	0 U.I.	0

Food								
Bacalao seco / Cod, dehydrated, salted	375	81.8	2.8	0	—	3.6	0 U.I.	—
Banana / Banana	110	1.2	0.2	29	7	0.5	65 (mcg)	15
Batata amarilla / Sweet potato, pale yellow	122	0.53	0.28	29.4	22	0.8	200 U.I.	23
Batata blanca / Sweet potato, white	110	0.13	0.15	26.9	18	0.9	53 U.I.	11
Berenjena / Eggplant	25	1.2	0.2	5.6	12	0.7	10 U.I.	5
Berro / Watercress	26	3.6	0.8	2.9	155	2.6	312 (re)	51
Berza / Collard greens	45	4.8	0.8	7.5	250	1.5	9300 U.I.	152
Betabel / Yam (purple)	49	2.1	0.2	10.9	21	1.5	0 U.I.	20
Bizcocho sin azúcar / Plain cake without icing	364	4.5	13.9	55.9	64	0.4	170	tr.
Boquerón / Boquerón fish	95	17.7	2.2	0	566	1.2	0 U.I.	0
Cacao / Cocoa	552	15	47	26.1	134	1	0 U.I.	0
Calabaza / Squash	45	1	0.1	10	11	0.2	3300 U.I.	15
Calamar / Squid	78	16.4	0.9	0	12	0.5	0 U.I.	0
Camarones frescos / Shrimp fresh	91	18.1	0.8	1.5	63	1.6	—	—
Camote / Yam (orange)	103	1	0.4	24	41	2.4	81 (re)	23
Caña de azúcar / Sugarcane	64	0.5	0.5	17.2	18	0.7	0 U.I.	8
Cangrejo / Crab	93	17.3	1.9	0.5	43	0.8	650 (mcg)	2
Carne de liebre / Rabbit meat	135	21	5	0	12	3.2	0 U.I.	0
Carpa / Carpa fish	96	16	3.1	0	40	1.9	15 (re)	0
Cazón / Cazón fish	106	24.5	0.2	0	8	1.5	0 U.I.	0
Cebada / Barley	346	9	1.9	75.4	55	4.5	5 (re)	0
Cecina (salada y seca) / Hung beef	203	34.3	6.3	—	20	5.1	0 U.I.	0
Cerveza / Beer	37	0.3	0	5.1	0	0.1	0 U.I.	0
Chabacano / Apricot	52	1.3	1.7	9.4	33	4.4	0 U.I.	12
Chayote sin espinas / White pear	26	1	0.1	6.3	27	1	0 U.I.	8
Chícharo / Peas	140	9	0.3	25.5	37	2.8	52 (re)	60
Chilacayote / White pear (vegetable)	14	1.2	0.2	2.7	17	0.6	6 (re)	7

Spanish	English	Kcal.	Protein (g)	Fat (g)	Carbohydrate (g)	Calcium (mg)	Iron (mg)	Vitamin A (re)	Vitamin C (mg)
Chile pasilla	Red pepper long	327	12.7	9.6	60.5	154	6.3	9030 (re)	68
Chile serrano	Red pepper bush	35	2.3	0.4	7.2	35	1.6	56 (re)	65
China	Orange	49	1	0.2	12.2	41	0.4	200 U.I.	50
Chirimoya	Chirimoya	82	1.1	0.2	21.3	34	0.6	0 U.I.	17
Chorizo	Sausage	433	24	36.6	0	—	—	—	0
Chuleta	Pork chops	298	17.1	24.9	0	10	2.6	0 U.I.	—
Cilantro	Coriander	26	2.6	0.3	4.7	108	2.3	384 (re)	11
Ciruelas del país	Native plums	56	1.4	0.4	11.7	16	1.1	86 U.I.	50
Coco	Coconut	308	3.8	33.2	4.8	24	3.4	0 U.I.	2
Coliflor	Cauliflower	26	3.2	0.3	4.3	38	2.9	6 (re)	127
Colinabo	Kohlrabi	31	2	0.1	6.1	32	0.3	tr	60
Conejo (carne solamente)	Rabbit, flesh only	162	21	8	0	20	1.3	—	12.8
Costillas	Spare ribs	361	14.5	33.2	0	8	2.22	—	—
Crema de maíz	Corn gruel	373	18	6	62	513	18.5	250.4 U.I.	40
Crema de arroz	Rice gruel	364	7.2	0.6	79.7	9	1.3	0 U.I.	0
Crema de cebada	Barley gruel	355	9.1	0.9	76.4	18.2	—	—	—
Epasote	Goosefoot wormseed	42	3.8	0.7	7.6	304	5.2	1210 (mcg)	11
Esponjoso	Sponge cake	297	7.6	5.7	54.1	0	30	450 U.I.	tr.
Flor de calabaza	Squash, flower	16	1.4	0.4	2.7	47	1	77 (re)	15
Fresas del país	Puerto Rican raspberry	42	0.5	1	7.7	24	—	—	9
Frijol amarillo	Yellow beans	337	14.2	1.7	67.1	347	4.8	0 U.I.	0
Frijol negro	Black beans	322	21.8	2.5	55.4	183	4.7	1 (re)	1
Galletas marias	Marie cookies	20	0.5	0.5	3.3	1	0.1	0 U.I.	0
Galletas saladas	Crackers, salted	22	0.4	0.7	3.5	2	0	0 U.I.	0
Galletas de soda	Soda crackers	439	9.2	13.1	70.6	22	1.5	0 U.I.	0

Galletas de mantequilla	Butter cookies	457	6.1	16.9	70.9	126	0.5	650 U.I.	0
Galletas/emparedado	Cookies, sandwich type	495	4.8	22.5	69.3	26	0.7	0 U.I.	0
Gallina	Chicken	298	17.3	24.8	0	10	14	1080 U.I.	8.2
Gandules frescos	Pigeon peas, immature seeds	117	7.2	0.6	21.3	42	1.6	140 U.I.	39
Gandules secos	Pigeon peas, mature seeds	342	20.4	1.4	63.7	107	8	80 U.I.	—
Garbanzos secos	Chick-peas, dry	360	20.5	4.8	61	150	6.9	50 U.I.	—
Girasol, semillas	Sunflower seeds	573	25.4	51.3	13.6	105	8.1	5 (mcg)	0
Granada	Pomegranate	63	0.5	0.3	16.4	3	0.3	tr.	4
Grosellas	Gooseberry	34	1.1	0.7	5.9	12	4.1	—	8
Guanábana	Soursop	65	1	0.3	16.3	14	0.6	10 U.I.	20
Guayaba	Guavas	62	0.8	0.6	15	23	0.9	280 U.I.	242
Guineo gigante blanco	Banana, ripe white	85	1.1	0.2	22.2	8	0.07	190 U.I.	10
Guineo maduro	Banana, ripe	107	2	0.2	27.3	8	0.5	—	13
Guineo manzano maduro	Apple banana	92	1.1	0.1	21.6	3	1.4	50 U.I.	15
Guineo niño	Dwarf banana or banana lady	83	1	0.1	19.5	2.5	—	10 U.I.	—
Guingambó o Quimbombó	Okra	42	2.2	0.2	9.7	78	1.1	100 (mcg)	29
Guisantes verdes congelados	Green peas, frozen	73	5.4	0.3	12.82	20	2	680 U.I.	19
Guisantes verdes, enlatados	Green peas, canned, drained	88	4.7	0.4	16.8	26	1.9	690 U.I.	8
Guisantes, secos	Peas, dry mature seeds	340	24.1	1.3	0.364	5.1	120	—	—
Habas frescas	Lima beans immature	123	8.4	0.5	22.1	52	2.8	290 U.I.	29
Habichuelas blancas secas	Beans, navy, dry mature seeds	340	22.3	1.6	61.3	144	7.8	0 U.I.	—

Spanish	English	Kcal.	Protein (g)	Fat (g)	Carbohydrate (g)	Calcium (mg)	Iron (mg)	Vitamin A	Vitamin C (mg)
Habichuelas coloradas secas	Beans, red kidney dry	343	22.5	1.5	61.9	110	6.9	20 U.I.	—
Habichuelas soyas, secas	Soybeans, dry	403	34.1	17.7	33.5	226	8.4	80 U.I.	—
Harina de maíz	Cornmeal	368	7.8	1.6	76.8	6	1.8	340 U.I.	0
Hicaco	Cocoplum	47	0.4	0.1	12.4	38	0.6	tr.	0.9
Hígado	Liver	125	10.4	8.6	0.8	10	2.4	0 U.I.	18
Hígado de pollo	Chicken liver	131	20.6	3.7	2	10	19.2	12100 U.I.	23
Higo	Fig	54	1.6	0.4	12.7	52	0.4	9 (re)	4
Hongos	Mushrooms	27	3.2	0.4	4.4	19	4.3	0 U.I.	3
Horchata	Sesame seed/ pumpkin drink	37	0.8	0.1	7.9	1	0.1	0 U.I.	0
Iguana	Iguana meat	112	24.4	0.9	0	25	3.4	225 (re)	0
Jalea	Jelly	312	0.1	0.1	80.3	15	2.9	0 U.I.	4
Jamon ahumado	Ham, cured, smoked	389	16.9	35	0.3	10	2.5	0 U.I.	0
Jamon hervido	Ham cooked	374	23.2	30.5	0	10	3	0 U.I.	—
Jamonilla o carne	Luncheon meat	294	15	24.9	1.3	9	2.2	0 U.I.	—
Jobo de la India	Golden apple	53	0.8	0.2	12	20	—	—	50
Judías	Beans, snap or wax	36	2	0.2	6.6	55	1.7	100 (mcg)	18
Jueyes, enlatados	Crabs, canned	101	17.4	2.5	1.1	45	0.8	—	—
Langosta, fresca	Lobster, raw	91	16.9	1.9	0.5	29	0.6	—	—
Lengua	Tongue	207	16.4	15	0.4	8	2.1	—	—
Lentejas	Lentils	331	22.7	1.6	58.7	74	5.8	4 (re)	0
Lerenes	Sweet corn root	64	0.5	0.1	15.2	17	5.4	—	7
Lima dulce o limón dulce	Sweet lime	29	0.4	0.04	6.7	12	0.2	0 U.I.	44
Longanizas	Pork links	498	9.4	50.8	tr	7	1.4	0 U.I.	—
Maicena	Cornstarch	362	0.3	tr.	87.6	0	0	0 U.I.	0
Maíz amarillo	Yellow corn	350	8.3	4.8	69.6	158	2.3	17 U.I.	0
Malanga	Taro	88	2	0.2	20	25	1	40 U.I.	tr.

Mamey	Mammee apple or mamey	31	0.4	0.1	7.6	14	0.2	2855 U.I.	15
Mamoncillo	Mamoncillo	59	1.1	0.2	19.9	12	0.6	25 (mcg)	5
Mandarina	Tangerine	43	0.5	0.2	10.1	18	0.2	420 U.I.	31
Mango	Mango	70	0.3	0.2	16.7	6	0.3	1950 U.I.	28
Manzana	Apple	65	0.3	0.5	16.5	7	0.8	3 (re)	11
Marañon	Cashew fruit	46	0.8	0.2	11.6	4	1	40.1 U.I.	219
Melado	Cane syrup	263	0	0	68	60	3.6	0 U.I.	0
Melon	Cantaloupe	26	0.6	0.1	6.3	17	2.2	114 (re)	36
Membrillo	Quince, common	49	0.4	0.5	12.1	50	0	7 (re)	15
Miel de abeja	Honey	302	0.2	0	78	20	0.8	0 U.I.	4
Mojarras	Mojarras fish	106	19.2	2.7	0	15	3.7	5 (re)	0
Mollejas cocidas de pollo	Chicken gizzards	149	23.7	4.9	2.6	56.8	7.8	1.3 U.I.	0
Ñame	Yam, white	116	2.9	0.2	25.7	11	1.2	tr.	8
Nanche o nance	Byrsonima (fruit)	56	1.1	1.3	11.4	30	1.4	4 (re)	86
Naranja agria	Sour orange	50	0.7	0.1	13	43	0.6	60 U.I.	42
Nopal	Nopal cactus	29	1.3	0.1	6.9	—	2.7	220 (mcg)	16
Nueces de nogal	Walnuts, Persian or English	651	14.8	65	15.8	99	3.1	30 U.I.	2
Oregano	Spanish thyme	17	0.9	0.4	3.1	232	3.9	490 (mcg)	12
Pajuil	Cashew nut fruit	39	0.3	0.4	8.7	2	0.4	1052 U.I.	229
Palmito	Euterpe palm	26	2.2	0.2	5.2	86	0.8	tr.	17
Pan dulce	Sweet bread	288	6.8	8.7	45.6	26	0.9	0 U.I.	0
Pan francés	French or Vienna bread	290	9.1	3	55.4	43	2.2	tr.	tr.
Pan moreno de trigo integro	Whole wheat bread	243	10.5	3	47.7	99	2.3	tr.	tr.
Pana de pepita	Bread nut	144	3.7	1.8	28.2	78	0.6	—	15
Panapén	Breadfruit	122	1.7	0.4	28	15	1.2	50 U.I.	2
Papaya madura	Papaya, ripe	30	0.5	0.1	6.8	17	0.5	1750 U.I.	60
Papaya verde	Papaya, green	30	0.8	0.2	6.3	26	0.3	18 U.I.	29
Pargo rojo fresco	Red snapper	93	19.8	0.9	0	16	0.8	—	—

Spanish	English	Kcal.	Protein (g)	Fat (g)	Carbohydrate (g)	Calcium (mg)	Iron (mg)	Vitamin A	Vitamin C (mg)
Pasas	Raisins	315	3	3.3	77	79	3.2	3 (re)	0
Pasta de guayaba	Guava paste	364	0.3	1.4	87.5	25	—	713 U.I.	26
Patas saladas con hueso	Feet, bones included	102	7.1	8	0	4	1	0 U.I.	0
Patitas de cerdo	Pig's feet	285	20.21	22.09	—	12.5	2.92	0 U.I.	0
Pato	Duck	326	16	28.6	0	15	1.8	162 (re)	0
Pavo	Turkey	162	24	6.6	0	8	1.5	—	—
Pepino	Cucumber	15	0.9	0.1	3.4	25	1.1	250 U.I.	11
Pera	Pear	56	0.3	0.2	14.8	6	0.5	5 U.I.	5
Perejil	Parsley	43	3.2	0.6	8.5	5	3.1	1820 (mcg)	146
Pernil	Fresh ham	308	15.9	26.6	0	9	2.4	0 U.I.	—
Pescado seco	Dried fish	231	42.9	3	4.2	90	13.8	9 U.I.	0
Piloncillo	Molasses	356	0.4	0.5	90.6	51	4.2	3 (re)	2
Pimiento morron enlatado	Red Pimiento, canned	27	0.9	0.5	5.8	7	1.5	2300 U.I.	95
Pimiento verde	Pepper, green	22	1.2	0.2	4.8	9	0.7	420 U.I.	128
Piña fresca	Pineapple, fresh	52	0.4	0.2	13.7	17	0.5	70 U.I.	17
Piñon	Pine nut	634	15.3	61.3	16.8	14	4.4	10 (re)	1
Pitahaya	Fruit cactus	48	1.6	0.6	10.4	11	1.9	0 U.I.	16
Plátano maduro	Ripe, plantain	125	1	0.1	30.1	3	0.5	1080 U.I.	20
Plátanos en tentaciones	Ripe fried plantain in syrup	262	0.572	7.072	49.22	8	0.8	57.82 U.I.	15
Plátano verde	Green, plantain	165	1.1	0.2	39.2	3	0.5	1400 (re)	20
Platanutres	Plantain chips	425	0.72	35.72	25	45.56	2.4	0 U.I.	35
Pollo	Chicken	124	18.6	4.9	0	12	1.9	730 U.I.	—
Pomela		34	0.6	0.2	8.5	26	0.5	0 U.I.	35
Pulque	Pulque	43	—	1.1	12	0.7	0	6 U.I.	—
Quelite	Goosefoot, lamb's-quarters	39	3.2	1	6.4	230	6.2	401 (re)	42
Quenepa o mamoncillo	Genip	59	1.1	0.2	19.9	12	0.6	83 U.I.	5
Queso blanco del país	Cheese, native	398	34.4	—	—	930	1.3	2000 U.I.—	

Spanish	English							
Queso Chihuahua	Cheese, Chihuahua	458	28.8	37	1.9	795	5.8	184 (re)	0
Queso fresco	Cheese, fresh	127	15.3	7	5	684	0.3	70 U.I.	0
Queso Oaxaca	Cheese, Oaxaca	317	25.7	22	3	469	3.3	271 (re)	0
Rábanos	Radishes	17	1	0.1	3.6	30	1	10 U.I.	26
Remolacha, hojas	Beet greens	24	2.2	0.3	4.6	119	3.3	6100 U.I.	30
Repollo	Cabbage	24	1.3	0.2	5.4	49	0.4	130 U.I.	47
Riñon	Kidney	122	16.8	5	1.8	13	5.7	300 (re)	10
Romeritos	Herb seasoning	28	3.6	0.2	4.9	41	2.5	307 (re)	4
Salchichas de Frankfurt	Hot dog	296	13.1	25.5	2.5	—	—	—	—
Salmón, enlatado	Salmon, chunk canned	139	21.5	5.2	0	249	0.7	60 U.I.	—
Sandía	Watermelon	16	0.4	0.2	3.6	5	0.3	37 U.I.	10
Sangre (morcilla)	Blood sausage	159	18.2	8.6	0.9	12	44.9	20 (mcg)	1
Sardinas enlatadas en aceite	Sardines, canned in oil	311	20.6	24.4	0.6	354	3.5	180 U.I.	—
Sesos	Brains	125	10.4	8.6	0.8	10	2.4	0 U.I.	18
Sirop de maíz	Corn syrup	290	0	0	75	46	4.1	0 U.I.	0
Sorgo	Sorghum whole grain	342	8.8	3.2	76.3	19	3.7	10 (mcg)	0
Soya (Harina)	Soybean	331	37.3	3.9	40.2	187	8.3	0 U.I.	0
Tajadas maduros	Ripe fried plantains	271	1.2	14	35.2	6.9 +	0.7 +	49.8 U.I.	17.2
Tamarindo	Tamarind	239	2.8	0.6	62.5	74	2.8	30 U.I.	2
Tejocote	Yellow fruit	87	0.8	0.6	22	94	1.6	424 U.I.	46
Tomate del país	Tomato, native	19	0.9	0.1	3.7	8	0.2	320 U.I.	17
Toronja	Grapefruit	41	0.5	0.1	10.6	16	0.4	80 U.I.	38
Tortilla de maíz	Corn tortilla	224	5.9	1.5	47.2	108	2.5	2 (re)	0
Trigo	Wheat	337	10.6	2.6	73.4	58	0.9	1 (re)	0
Tripas de res	Beef tripe	220	11.3	19.1	0	12	1.8	177 (re)	0
Tuna	Fruit cactus	38	0.3	0.1	10.1	63	0.8	4 (re)	31
Ubre	Cow's udder	234	15.4	18.7	0	70	2.6	0 U.I.	0
Uchepo	Sweet tamal	97	2.8	0.3	21	29	2.1	0 U.I.	0

Spanish	English	Kcal.	Protein (g)	Fat (g)	Carbohydrate (g)	Calcium (mg)	Iron (mg)	Vitamin A	Vitamin C (mg)
Uvas	Grapes	69	1.3	0.1	15.7	16	0.4	100 U.I.	4
Uvas de playa	Sea grape	74	0.6	0.6	16.5	90	—	—	4
Verdolaga	Purslane (portulaca)	21	1.7	0.4	3.8	103	3.5	2500 U.I.	25
Yautía amarilla	Tanier, yellow	155	2.8	1.4	312.9	13	0.7	350 U.I.	18
Yautía blanca	Tanier, white	126	1.7	0.3	29	9	0.5	25 U.I.	10
Yuca	Cassava	165	2	0.1	38.9	27	0.9	tr.	29
Zanahoria	Carrots	44	0.4	0.3	10.5	26	1.5	664 (re)	19
Zapote amarillo	Sapodillo	79	1.2	0.4	20	34	2.1	19 (re)	59
Zarzamora	Berry	57	1.2	0.6	13.2	34	2	10 U.I.	18

SOURCES: L. C. Reguero and S.M. Rodríquez de Santiago, *Tabla de composición de alimentos de uso corriente en Puerto Rico*. Editorial Universidad de Puerto Rico, Rio Piedras, 1978; Centro de Investigación en Alimentación y Desarrollo, Aporte de nutrientes de platillos regionales de Sonora, unpublished data, (Hermosillo, Sonora, Mexico: 1992; Instituto de Nutrición de Centro América y Panamá, Guatemala, 1978; *Tabla de composición de alimentos para uso en América Latina*, *Guatemala*, 1978; M. Hernández, A. Chávez, and H. Bourges, *Valor nutritivo de los alimentos Mexicanos: Tablas de Uso Práctico, 8th ed. (Mexico: División de Nutrición del Instituto Nacional de la Nutrición, 1980).*

0 = zero value
— = data unavailable

Index